THE DIALOGUE OF TOUCH

Developmental Play Therapy

Viola A. Brody

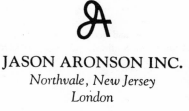

JASON ARONSON INC.
Northvale, New Jersey
London

THE MASTER WORK SERIES

1997 softcover edition

Library of Congress Cataloging-in-Publication Data

Brody, Viola A.
  The dialogue of touch : developmental play therapy / Viola A.
Brody.
      p.   cm. — (Master work series)
    Originally published: Treasure Island, Fla. : Developmental Play
Training Associates, c1993.
    Includes bibliographical references and index.
    ISBN 0–7657–0088–3 (alk. paper)
    1. Touch—Therapeutic use.   2. Play therapy.   3. Developmental
therapy for children.   I. Title.   II. Series.
[RJ505.T69B76   1997]
618.92'89165—dc21   97–9432

Printed in the United States of America on acid-free paper. For information and catalog write to Jason Aronson Inc., 230 Livingston Street, Northvale, New Jersey 07647-1731. Or visit our web-site: http://www.aronson.com

To Austin M. Des Lauriers,
a man ahead of his time.

To Austin M. DesLauriers,
a man ahead of his time.

ACKNOWLEDGMENTS

I would like to acknowledge the contributions of those who have worked with me to develop the Developmental Play approach to its present form. Mary Lenholt, who co-leads training workshops, has been involved in Developmental Play with me for over fifteen years. Her work as a Leader of the children's Circle Time is presented in Chapter 5. Developmental Play, as it stands today, is as much a product of her work as it is of mine. The effectiveness of our training workshops in Developmental Play is due, in large part, to the quality of the relationship between the two leaders. That quality of presence in the two leaders is felt by the participants. I appreciate having someone like Mary with whom I can both work and grow.

Others who have worked with me in my Florida period are Diana Ross, Susan Stephenson, and Anthony Quaglieri, each of whom has contributed an important part.

I would like to thank those who have helped me in the writing of this book: Carolyn Pinkard, Ph.D., who worked with me on the first part of this book and in its beginning stages; Naomi Lucks, who helped me organize the chapter headings and the focus of the book; Linda Ober, who handled the typesetting, editing, and printing of the book and who was very encouraging and fun to work with; Lynn Gordon, who helped out with typing the manuscript; and Mildred Reeves, who gave me the idea for the title.

And forever, I will be grateful to my mentor, Austin Des Lauriers. He and I were destined to meet when we both came to Michael Reese Hospital in Chicago at the same time, 1960: he as the new Head of the Department of Psychology and I as the recipient of an APA postdoctoral training award. We were meant for each other—he as the teacher and I as the student.

CONTENTS

PREFACE TO THE 1997 EDITION

Since the publication of *The Dialogue of Touch: Developmental Play Therapy* in 1993, I have received many letters from readers. They have come from Europe, the Far East, Africa, the United States, Canada, and Great Britain. From wherever they live the writers stated, often touchingly, eloquently, with excitement, that they have learned from the book how to touch children in ways that profoundly help them. They write that learning how, when, and why to physically touch a child—and the experience of doing so—made them more effective parents, teachers, and therapists. Very important to them, the readers of the book said, is that they have experienced for themselves, after reading the book, how touching enables a child, even a child stuck in emotional disturbance or violent response to earlier and terrible violations of his or her self, to heal and grow again.

For example, from London, a respondent who works in a psychiatric facility wrote:

I've opened myself to touch and it has had a remarkable effect on the children I work with both in class and in a therapeutic situation. A boy of 12 in twelve weeks has undergone an incredible transformation from being a violent, untouchable bully to showing a sensitive, more relaxed presence.

And there was this from a therapist in South Africa:

I asked a child care worker to use Developmental Play Therapy with a

3-year-old girl who had been sexually abused as an infant. The results have been amazing. In a period of four weeks we have a total change in this child. She smiles and laughs now. It was like magic. Thank you for all you've done for me and the children of South Africa.

In addition, many responses to the book have come from psychotherapists whose clients are children. Most of them employ play therapy in their work with children. But, they write, they did not touch a child client during play therapy except casually. Deliberate touching of a child had not been used as a therapeutic method in play therapy, reflecting that no rationale for the use of touching as a therapeutic tool had been put forward in any of the theories of play therapy. This book offers such a rationale, demonstrates that touching the child client is a potent therapeutic tool, and gives examples of its use based on theories of child development and the results of research on the effect of touch on humans.

An interest in touch as a therapeutic approach has arisen since publication of *The Dialogue of Touch*. Recently, for instance, I gave an invited keynote speech on the role of touch in play therapy at an international conference on play therapy. I believe that interest in the topic and recognition of its importance was stimulated by the first edition of this book and I welcome the broader readership this second edition makes possible. In this book I present three cases in which I used touch as the central therapeutic approach. The sessions of these Developmental Play therapies (with a 6-year-old autistic boy, a 6-year-old psychotic boy, and a 4-year-old hyperactive girl) are given verbatim with description of the touches I gave and my comments on why a particular touch or touching game was needed and the response of the child to the touching. Thus, the reader can follow the progress of these three children to greater self-appreciation, and can see in concrete detail the development in a child of the ability to relate to a caring adult. Readers have reported that they are amazed at the rapidity of desirable changes in these children once they have been provided with the needed touch by an adult who knows how to touch.

The first edition of this book offered my thinking on three issues affecting our society and current therapy for children. I feel that these are of continuing or of even greater importance today.

First, I wrote of child abuse and its consequences for the abused child, the abuser, and society. Statistics inform us that abuse darkens the lives of millions of children worldwide. We have evidence too that individuals abused as children can suffer strongly adverse effects of this treatment in their adult lives and may perpetuate the cycle of violence by abusing their own children. That our society is damaged by child abuse and that no adequate remedy for this horror has been found are beyond question. This book offers the hypothesis, and some demonstration through cases presented, that the effect on a child of violent handling may be counteracted by loving touches from adults cognizant of how touch can meet the emotional needs of an abused child. I hope that readers of this second edition of *The Dialogue of Touch*, so many of them undoubtedly already working with children so that they see how greatly the epidemic of child abuse harms children, will think about and test out how Developmental Play Therapy can help the abused child.

Second, I considered the taboo in American society and other world societies against touching children. Partly stemming from a perceived but probably exaggerated need to keep children from being sexually exploited, this taboo has been given the sanction of law in many places. A consequence is that those who work with children are afraid to touch them. I have noticed this fear spreading and increasing in intensity among teachers, case workers, even child therapists. Many who work with children have told me they would not dare to touch any child in their care, however much they believed that touching would help that child. I urge, even more strongly now than when this book was first published, that absolute prohibition against touching children be abolished. I contend that the advantages of touching children for their good should not be foregone because some touch children promiscuously for selfish ends. The latter should be, and in most countries already is, prohibited by law but the price of preventing it by forbidding touch altogether robs caring adults of one of the most useful and promising ways of helping children. I hope that the readers of this book will initiate and support efforts to remove barriers to the use of touch in education and therapy.

And third, the issue of what is therapeutic has engaged researchers and practitioners in the field of therapy for a long time. The facts now in tell us that the *person* of the therapist makes a more significant contribution to the outcome of therapy than do the particular therapeutic techniques he or she uses. In this context *person* refers not just to distinct personality characteristics but to the unique individual therapist who is infinitely more than the sum of his or her parts. Developmental Play Therapy recognizes that touching is not a therapeutic technique easily learned and applied. It is, instead, an expression of love and care by a truly loving and caring adult. Therapeutic touching is given in the spirit not the letter of a manual, cataloging ways of touching. To provide caring adults and therapists, to provide *persons* who can touch a child, not technicians who have learned some rules about touching, this book includes a training program for those who wish to learn about Developmental Play Therapy. Much of the program specifies touch experiences adults themselves need in order to be able to touch children in helpful ways. It is a unique program that explores and affects the person of the participant and so supports the view that the person who does the therapy makes the largest impact on the outcome of that therapy.

> *i know that touching was and still is and always will be*
> *the true revolution.**

Viola A. Brody
March 1997

---

* From "When I Die" by Nikki Giovanni (1992) in *The House*. New York: William Morrow. Copyright © 1996 by William Morrow & Co. and used by permission.

PREFACE

*"Pick me up and carry me like a baby.
Pretend I'm your tiny baby."*
— Request from a four-year-old
girl to her Developmental
Play therapist

Deep within each of us is the longing to be touched by someone willing and capable of caring touching. Within each of us is also the potential to become a toucher for another. This book is about the means of capable touching and the effects of touching.

In my first position as a psychotherapist in 1953—a second career begun after 20 years of teaching school—I worked in a hospital unit for the treatment of children with psychosomatic illnesses. I was asked to treat several children who had not been doing well under child analysis. I used touch as the main avenue for reaching these children. By *touch* I mean I carried them, held them, bathed them, sang to them and allowed them to touch me. My supervisors, who were internationally known child analysts, supported me in doing this—and these children got better (Brody, 1963).

The touching, however, was never mentioned either by them or by me as being a factor in these children's shift toward health. I didn't talk about touch because there was no place to talk about it. I had no frame of reference in which to put it. I had no name for it.

In 1970, I offered training in my approach to child therapy and named my approach Developmental Play therapy. Under the name of Developmental Play therapy, touch was considered an important contributor to a child's movement toward health. At that time I was encouraged by Des Lauriers, then chief psychologist of Michael Reese Psychosomatic and Psychiatric Institute in Chicago, to develop my use of touch with children. He also gave me a framework within which I could talk about touch.

Touch is essential for life. Various kinds of behavior in children who are deprived of touch are unconscious attempts by the child to cause adults to touch them: They get sick in order to be touched by doctors, nurses, parents; adolescents engage in sex to get touched; boys play contact sports to get touched. Much behavior in growing up, whether understood in this way or not, is in the service of trying to get the needed touch from a parent or other adult important to them. To be touched, however, requires someone who knows how to be present with a child, who knows what it takes to touch another.

The core of Developmental Play therapy is touching. Capable touching, when experienced by the child, builds the child's self and appreciation of the other's self (the one doing the touching) and establishes the possibility of dialogue between the two. This touching dialogue serves as an organizing force for everything the child does—moving, feeling, thinking and, above all, relating. The basic principle of Developmental Play therapy is that a child who experiences touch from a capable toucher will grow toward healthy maturity and will heal from earlier trauma and neglect.

In teaching adults the Developmental Play therapy approach, I ask my students to abandon the idea that their aim is to change the child and tell them their responsibility is to change themselves so that they are able to touch the child and lead the child to feel touched. Therefore, I built two emphases into training adults to use the Developmental Play therapy approach: 1) providing adults with the experiences needed for them to feel touched, so that they, in turn, can touch children; and 2) providing adults with experiences in taking part in Developmental Play therapy interactions in which adults play both roles—the one who touches and the one who is touched.

The focus of touch as the therapeutic tool in child therapy and adult training makes this book very different from other child therapy books. Most child therapists do not touch. The few who do tend to use touch in an aversive and punitive way to control the child. The use of touch in adult training is even more unusual. The ideas this book presents are not new at all, but the implementation of these ideas in the form of Developmental Play therapy is unique.

The ever-increasing number of abused and destructively acting-out children in our society is telling us that the basic needs of children are not being met. One of the unmet needs is to be touched in a loving way. We need to find some capable touchers for these children. Developmental Play training is designed to provide adults with the experience they need to become capable touchers of children—adults who know what it takes to be a capable toucher.

I feel privileged to have discovered touch as an effective therapeutic tool for helping children grow a core self. In this book, I have shared my experiences and learning to encourage you to explore the use of touch and to create your own new way of being with a child.

This book is specifically designed for four groups:

1. **College students and young clinicians in training to work with children.** In this book, students can experience themselves in the therapist's role because it includes verbatim case material as well as the theoretical foundation. With all of the recent research on the importance of touch, this book is a much needed text and supplemental reading for college courses in child therapy, play therapy, and child development.
2. **Play therapists.** Developmental Play therapy differs from other play therapy models in that it is a presymbolic form of play. It is the earliest form of play. It is basic to and precedes the symbolic play described in other play therapies. Developmental Play has been found to be especially effective for children with attachment and relationship problems. This includes the severely acting-out child, the psychotic and autistic child, the Attention-Deficit Disorder child, and the sexually and physically abused child.
3. **Experienced therapists.** Developmental Play presents a very basic and effective way to work with very disturbed children without medication (see Chapters 3 and 4). This book is for those interested in exploring an alternative approach—Developmental Play.
4. **Training therapists.** Developmental Play differs from most other training programs. Developmental Play training not only includes what to do with the child (the client) but also, and even more so, how to help the trainee experience what she needs to experience in order to do Developmental Play (see Chapter 6). The training goal is to help the trainee learn to be present.

In addition to the above, others involved with children (teachers, parents, daycare staff, administrators, judges) could gain new insights on ways to be with children. Developmental Play is for normal children, too. They love it!

Part I: What Is Caring Touch?

The Introduction describes the evolution of Developmental Play therapy, defines its principles, and describes the range of children who benefit from Developmental Play therapy. It includes a case-study example.

Chapter 1 sets the stage for the remainder of the book by illustrating the nature and intent of touch, how Developmental Play therapy works with "normal" children, describing the role and experience of the toucher and the role and experience of the one touched.

Chapter 2 looks at some Developmental Play sessions which demonstrate the effect of the structure of Developmental Play therapy—touching and being touched—on the behavior of different children. This chapter presents the different touching approaches, the use of the singing voice and, finally, limit setting—all illustrated in examples.

Chapter 3 presents a case study of Developmental Play therapy with a six-year-old autistic boy, Jason. The transcribed sessions over a three-year period show the effect of touch on this boy's behavior.

Chapter 4 is a case study of a six-year-old psychotic boy demonstrating the way touch organizes behavior.

Part II: Putting Developmental Play Therapy Into Practice

Chapter 5 presents the Developmental Play group therapy approach for small groups of children—for "ordinary" children in school and daycare settings, Headstart, and for disturbed children in residential settings. This program involves weekly meetings with six children, six adults, and a Leader. It includes a child-adult one-to-one time and a group time (Circle Time). This chapter shows how touch is used in a group program and its effect on the behavioral of the children.

Chapter 6 describes the training approach used with the adults learning to play with their child in the group program described in Chapter 5. This training takes place in a one-hour pre-session meeting and a one-hour post-session meeting. This chapter includes material from transcribed sessions in which the participants share their experiences with the Leader and with each other in their work of getting to know themselves and in their work with the children.

The Appendix contains Developmental Play games for adults to play with children.

Note to the reader: I use the feminine pronoun for the children, the child-care giver, and the child therapist.

PART I: WHAT IS CARING TOUCH?

INTRODUCTION: THE HISTORY AND METHOD OF DEVELOPMENTAL PLAY THERAPY

We shall not cease from exploration
And the end of all our exploring
Will be to arrive where we started
And know the place for the first time.
　　　　　　　　　　　　　—T.S. Eliot

In this century, various approaches to psychotherapy have appeared. These differ in methods, although there is also much overlapping of helping techniques. By and large, modern schools of psychotherapy are known, and often named, for their singular methodology. The helping approach that is unique to a school of psychotherapy is usually a codification of discoveries made by a single psychotherapist—a practicing psychotherapist discovers and becomes convinced of the worth of innovative ways to do psychotherapy; the new ways are tested in practice; and, if they prove effective, a new approach to psychotherapy can come into being.

THE EVOLUTION OF DEVELOPMENTAL PLAY THERAPY

The history of Developmental Play therapy followed this pattern. In my work as a psychotherapist, I devised innovative methods for promoting the healthy psychological growth of children. I came to base what I did in psychotherapy sessions on my conviction that children must feel touched in order to mature in a healthy way. I came to understand that the task of the therapist of children is to provide the structure that allows the child to feel touched.

Any theory of psychotherapy is born of two parents: experience and thought. Like good parents, they work together.

In my formulation of Developmental Play therapy, both were of crucial importance. Before I began to work as a psychotherapist for children, I had years of experience as a teacher, and I was the oldest child in a large family of children.

Thus, I had much experience in knowing children, helping children in practical ways, and teaching them. My goal in helping children changed when I began to do psychotherapy with them. My aim then was to help them psychologically, but I soon came to define the specific goal of psychotherapy with a child as assisting the child to develop her *self*. The definition arose as I thought hard about severely disturbed children who were my first psychotherapy clients. As I came to know these children, I realized their self-development was arrested. They lacked or had only a vestige of what we call various names—identity, ego, I, or self.

I came to know, personally or through their writings, others who had ideas about the development of self in children. I considered their ideas in relation to my experience.

Three people in particular gave me a great deal to think about: psychologist Austin Des Lauriers, philosopher and theologian Martin Buber, and movement therapist Janet Adler. What they taught me about self-development and psychotherapy with children has guided me on my path to discovering the theory of a therapy I came to call Developmental Play.

Austin Des Lauriers: In 1960, Des Lauriers was chief psychologist at the Michael Reese Psychiatric and Psychosomatic Institute in Chicago, where I was working under his supervision as a psychotherapist for children. The situation offered me the opportunity to observe Des Lauriers in therapy sessions with children diagnosed as autistic or schizophrenic—all, of course, severely disturbed.

What I saw was physical contact. In therapy sessions Des Lauriers repeatedly touched the child. Some of his touches were quick, others lingering, some forceful, some gentle, soft. To make contact he used his fingers, hands, other parts of his body, and even most of his body. Many times I saw him position himself in front of a child who, in order to move, would have to touch him—either to invite contact or to push him away. With this variety of contacts, he touched a small area of a child's body or larger areas—sometimes almost the child's whole body (Des Lauriers, 1962).

As I observed Des Lauriers' sessions, it quickly became clear to me that, sooner or later, the child had to acknowledge or deal with his physical presence in one way or another. Clearly, Des Lauriers believed physical contact to be curative. I asked him why.

Des Lauriers' reply began with his theory about the development of self in the child. He reminded me that the self of the infant and very young child is, as her mind and body are, vastly different from what it will become in adulthood. One of these differences is in awareness of the self. The adult is aware that *she* wills, feels, wants, evaluates. The newborn baby has no such sense of a subjective center that chooses and acts. Yet the sense of a self emerging begins at birth.

The earliest self-experience is recognition of the body. This body awareness comes about through the physical contact and playful and loving attitudes the mother provides. The infant recognizes as hers those parts of her body the mother touches, kisses, and holds. The infant comes first to perceive parts of her body as distinct entities, and then that her body has distinct boundaries which enclose her and separate her from the world about her. At this stage, the child can distinguish herself from what is not her.

Des Lauriers maintained that the development of the self began with the appreciation of the body. He called this early consciousness of body "the bodily self." Des Lauriers believed the bodily self had to emerge before there could be the further development of the self. The schizophrenic child, he said, does not experience herself as separated and differentiated, and hence is lacking the structures or the bodily self needed to be able to relate to others. The aim of psychotherapy with the schizophrenic child, then, had to be to do whatever encourages awareness of the bodily self.

To accomplish this therapeutic aim, Des Lauriers provided carefully chosen and carefully executed touches. He called these touches *sensory stimulating contact* and defined such contact as any concrete touch that makes the child who is touched aware of her body, aware that she is being touched, and aware of who is touching her. In other words, this sensory stimulating contact creates a relationship between the toucher and the one touched. Thus, not every touch is a sensory stimulating contact. To make sensory stimulating contact, the therapist must use the particular touches that encourage emergence of the bodily self in a particular child.

An excerpt from a Des Lauriers therapy session with a 13-year-old catatonic girl illustrates his use of sensory stimulating contact. (The girl, Sue, was mute and immobile most of the time.) The session is recorded in Des Lauriers' book, *The Experience of Reality in Childhood Schizophrenia* (1962, pp. 72-73):

Therapist: It's time to go, Sue. I'm here again.
    Sue: (Silence)
      T: (Shakes her shoulder, a pained expression appears on her face) You felt that! I'm glad you know I'm here.
      S: (Slowly, she turns her head around toward him, and her eyes take on what seemed to be a languorous and pathetic look)
      T: Let's go. We're going outside.

The therapist gets Sue to go outside by pulling her up and pushing her out the door. She begins to enjoy being pushed. The session ends like this:

3

T: (Places hand in front of her face, forcing her to look at it)
S: (Grabs his finger and pinches hard, gritting her teeth, but still half smiling)
T: Ouch, that hurts, Sue! You hurt me! (As he said this, he slapped her hand. She looked at him, looked at her hand, then looked at him again)
S: Go away. Leave me alone. I hate you!
T: Sue, honey, you can talk! You talked to me!
S: What did you think, you stupid! Go away. I hate you!

In this meeting with Sue, Des Lauriers' persistent, intrusive, hard touches enabled Sue to experience *his* body (when he pushed her, when he slapped her hand) and *her* body (when she grabbed his finger and pinched it). Experiencing her own presence and at the same time experiencing his presence provided the conditions for relating—two people being present to each other (Sue: "I hate you!" Des Lauriers: "You can talk!").

Des Lauriers had set in motion a process of recognition by Sue of her bodily self and that self as a separate entity. With this recognition, Sue could choose what to do and do it. She could act as a separate person in relation to another, also a distinct person. When she yelled at Des Lauriers, she showed herself capable of encounter with another. For Sue, it was a tremendous step toward selfhood, and Des Lauriers showed her how much that pleased him and emphatically described to her what she had done as a meeting ("*You* hurt *me*; *You* talked to *me!*").

According to Des Lauriers, the bodily self is the foundation for the subsequent development of the psychological self (the sense of I-ness, the center within that chooses and acts). This development goes on through childhood and adolescence and, at a much slower pace with much less alteration, into adulthood. In essence, this development is the constantly evolving and progressively more complex awareness of who I am, of my self.

Des Lauriers said the growth of this psychological self depended on relating to other selves and, particularly for the young child, on relating to a mother who was invested in nurturing the self of her child. The mother, he said, could act to support and encourage the growth of her child's autonomous psychological self. But he believed her attitudes and feelings toward her child were of even greater influence. These were, he believed, the most potent shapers of the psychological self of the child. Des Lauriers had in mind the influence of the mother's attitudes and feelings on the child's self when he said the therapist working with children must *be* a mother. I thought he meant play the *role* of a mother.

"No," he said, "*Be* a mother."

With time, experience with children, and a lot of thought, I came to know what the *be* meant. The adult who assists the healthy growth of a child's psychological self cannot don attitudes and feelings like clothing. Nor, like clothing, can these be the only trappings. They must be integral and central in the self of the adult who relates to the child. In other words, the adult must be present when working with a child.

Martin Buber: In talking about the psychotherapist as mother, Des Lauriers used a metaphor that helped me form my own views about therapeutic relationship. I was able to expand and clarify these views further when I read the celebrated book, *I and Thou* (1958), by theologian Martin Buber. Buber writes that the only way an individual develops a sense of what he calls *I* is by meetings with another person, *Thou*. The *I*, Buber says, is never the product of the person acting alone—"We can't become an *I* by our own agency." On the contrary, for the *I* to be born and to grow requires that *I* and *Thou* meet.

The bulk of Buber's book describes the *I-Thou* meeting. Its heart, he says, is that the presence of *Thou* impacts on *I* and changes *I's* very self. The *I-Thou* meeting is not the words that are spoken or the actions that are taken while the two are together. It cannot adequately be described in words, but it can be categorized as dedicated relating. In the *I-Thou* relationship, self meets self and there is nothing but this meeting. *Thou* is wholly present with *I* and is wholly *for I*.

Buber's thought-provoking writing on the *I-Thou* meeting has helped me to understand the power inherent in being truly and simply and completely present with a child.

Janet Adler (1981): Some time after reading Buber's book, I attended workshops titled "Authentic Movement," with Janet Adler as workshop leader. In her workshop, Adler directed the interplay between two participants. First, naming one the Witness and the other the Mover, she instructed the Mover, with eyes closed, to attend to her body and to express with her body the feelings and impulses that arise within her body.

The Witness was instructed to observe the Mover and to note her own reactions to the Mover's expressions. Adler explained that this exercise modeled the therapeutic relationship (the Mover being the client, the Witness the therapist). Entering fully into this exercise, she said, taught how to allow oneself to be seen, how to see another, and how to see oneself. For me, understanding what Adler called seeing and being seen came from the sharing after each movement exercise. Being the Mover gave me an appreciation of the validating effect of being truly seen by another. Listening to my Witness tell me what she saw me doing and the effect it had on her was an unbelievable experience. She saw qualities in

5

me I didn't know I had. For me, being seen was a very heightened physical, bodily experience. There were no words. The experience of being seen provided me with what I needed to be a Witness. Adler said that one has to learn to be the one seen before one can become a Seer or Witness. Above all, participating in the workshops made clear to me the causal relationship between being seen, seeing another, and seeing oneself. I could also relate to a child's wonderful feeling of being truly seen.

More than 35 years has gone into creating Developmental Play therapy. My own experiences with many children guided me in its development and gave me a laboratory for trying and testing my ideas about effective psychotherapy. But these ideas were also strongly influenced by exposure to the thinking of Des Lauriers, Buber, and Adler. Des Lauriers' belief that the development of the self in the schizophrenic child begins with the bodily experience and awareness of being touched by someone who knows how to touch was confirmed in the therapy I did with children. I discovered that not only the schizophrenic child, but the child with fewer major mental health problems and the so-called normal child all lacked clear awareness of the bodily self, awareness every child needs as a beginning and foundation for further development. I found, as Des Lauriers had, that providing what is needed to foster awareness of the bodily self requires a therapist who chooses and directs the activities of a psychotherapy session.

Des Lauriers required that the psychotherapist be a mother, an adult with a loving, unstinting commitment to the child. He once demonstrated, by touching my hand, what he meant by the touch of a mother. These many years later, I can still feel that touch. The demonstration brought home to me, as words about touch could not, the impact of a touch by someone who knows how to touch. The experience of being touched by Des Lauriers provided a rationale for the emphasis I place on teaching how to touch in DP training. It also began my thinking on the need of adults to be touched and especially the need for those training to be DP therapists to be touched by someone who knows how before they can capably touch children.

As Des Lauriers' mother-to-child image describes his concept of the necessary features of therapeutic relationship, so does Buber's concept of the I-Thou meeting. Buber's view of a relationship as a dialogue has given me a way of looking at adult-child interaction in DP sessions. I look to see if the therapist is present with the child, is fully there for the child, responding to the child's cues in a way that enables the child to become aware of her own existence. The Developmental Play term of Buber's I-Thou meeting came to be the dialogue of Seeing and Being Seen.

Adler's workshops had suggested that Seeing and Feeling Seen were apt names for the essential therapeutic processes of Developmental Play therapy. As I thought about Seeing and Feeling Seen, I came to realize that we are first seen through touch. I then came to realize that touch *is* the method of Developmental Play therapy, touching and being touched.

Thus, I ended up with *touch* where I began and understood it for the first time—what it means to touch and what it means to be touched. I have come full circle, returning to where I started and knowing it for the first time. Experience and thought, the parents of the theory of Developmental Play, have come together.

PRINCIPLES OF DEVELOPMENTAL PLAY THERAPY

Although I have incorporated some of the ideas of my teachers, especially Des Lauriers, Developmental Play therapy and training are the product of my own experiences with children and adults over a 35-year period. The insights from training became the principles of Developmental Play.

Six guiding principles lie behind the interactions between an adult and child in DP sessions (Brazelton, 1990).

1. *A child who experiences herself as touched develops a sense of self.*
   In the context of Developmental Play therapy, the child's experience of being touched causes her to relate to the adult who touches her. The child who is touched is enabled to recognize herself as an *I* and to recognize the Toucher as an *Other* toward whom she has feelings and toward whom she can take action.

   Broadly speaking, the child who feels touched can either *accept* the Toucher (often shown by moving toward the Toucher) or *reject* the Toucher (often shown by turning away from the Toucher). The child who repeatedly experiences being touched cannot, however, fail to relate in some way to the adult who touches her. And relating, of course, means the interaction of separate selves. Being touched not only authors the sense of self in the touched child, it opens the child to the myriad formative influences of relationship. Through relationship the child grows.

2. *In order for a child to experience herself touched, a capable adult must touch her.*
   A capable adult is one who has had the experience of feeling touched. Because she knows what it feels like to be touched and she knows what the Toucher did to create that being-touched feeling, she is able to be the one who touches. She knows how to provide the relationship needed for a child to feel touched, too.

7

3. *In order to be a Toucher, the adult must first be willing to learn to be the One Touched.*

Allowing yourself to feel touched is not easy, especially if you are a therapist, a teacher, or a parent. It is often difficult because the experience of feeling touched opens you to childhood memories (some good, some not so good). Yet it is these being-touched experiences that make you capable of touching children.

4. *In order to feel touched, a child has to allow herself to be touched.*

Children who have been abused in one way or another may not allow themselves to be touched. For them, relating to an adult has been painful. Instead of responding by moving toward the adult who touches her, the abused child either turns away or remains unresponsive. Yet if the therapist is sensitive and remains quietly present without withdrawing, these children begin to experience their bodily selves. Little by little, they allow the adult to see them and eventually touch them.

5. *A child feels seen first through touch.*

We first experience being seen at birth. The experience comes when a parent touches us for the first time. For us humans, touch precedes more formal, more complex ways of relating. But other ways of relating do not supersede touch as we age. Throughout life, touch arouses emotions and embodies the quality of interactions between persons.

Both children and adults have reported that they felt seen and acknowledged when they were touched.

Touch as a way of being seen continues throughout the course of therapy embodied in a variety of physical contacts—those chosen by the adult as right for a particular child at each phase of the relationship that develops between them.

In Developmental Play therapy, the right touch is the one that helps a child feel touched, to acknowledge her own body signals, to experience her relationship to the adult touching her in the moment of their live meetings.

6. *To provide the relationship the child needs to feel touched, the adult controls the activities that take place in a Developmental Play therapy session.*

During a Developmental Play session, the adult creates the experiences in which a child feels touched. To this end, the adult initiates the action in Developmental Play sessions.

The adult takes charge because it is up to the adult, not the child, to act so that a therapeutic relationship between adult and child becomes possible and then grows.

8

The initiatives of the adult in a Developmental Play session fall into four broad, but not exclusive categories:

» Noticing the child
» Touching the child
» Responding to the child's cues
» Bringing to the attention of the child, in undeniable fashion, the presence of an adult who meets her needs

CHILDREN WHO BENEFIT FROM DEVELOPMENTAL PLAY THERAPY

Developmental Play therapy is effective for a wide range of disturbed children. Developmental Play therapy provides the basic relationship needed to develop a core self for all children, of all ages in varying stages of development. For severely developmentally delayed children (autistic, Chapter 3; psychotic, Chapter 4), DP therapy provides the beginning conditions needed for growth through touch. For more advanced disturbed children, DP therapy provides the opportunity of returning to an earlier stage to pick up what they need and bring it forward to the present—some touching experience they need to feel complete.

Three categories of disturbed children are currently receiving much attention: 1) The sexually abused child; 2) The ADD (Attention Deficit Disorder) child; and 3) The destructively acting-out child—the child who kills other children and adults. These children do not experience themselves having a core.

The Sexually Abused Child. Sexually abused children have a tremendous longing to be touched in a caring way. They don't know how to ask for it because they have rarely or never received it. Therapists tend to shy away from providing caring touch because they assume that it will be too painful or that it will not be acceptable to the child. Cradling the child with caring touching is very healing and helps the child to deal with the abuse when she is ready to do so.

The ADD (Attention Deficit Disorder) Child. Developmental Play therapy offers a very effective treatment for these hyperactive, distractible, and sometimes aggressive children. The touching, holding, and cradling relaxes them and helps them to experience their bodies. The cradling also creates a feeling of closeness between child and parent. DP therapy gives the parent permission to take charge—to hold and cradle her child. As a result, the parent feels less helpless and angry. DP therapy is more effective than drugs because it helps the parent become a capable toucher for her child—to feel connected to her child.

The Destructively Acting-out Child—the Child Who Kills Other Children and Adults. The rising number of children who kill is frightening and troubling. These children are shifting their acting out from property to people. These children are calling for help! They have no inner core. To feel alive for the moment, they act impulsively and destructively without feelings, and then the moment is gone. They don't remember. They don't learn.

The behavior of these children shows that they have been deprived of their most basic need—caring touch. Without the core self created by touch, they get attention through impulsive acts of destroying others.

DP therapy is extremely effective with this population. I have had considerable experience with these children, most of them boys. They respond very well to being physically contained in caring ways. They like it. They begin to feel and to relate. For the DP therapist, however, it is physically and emotionally hard work. Talking is not effective at all. (See Donald, pp. 31-33).

JANE: A CASE STUDY

The active role of the Developmental Play therapist is illustrated in my work with Jane, a nine-year-old who was talented in art but doing poorly in school.

When I first met Jane, she looked like a neglected orphan. She wore a dress that did not fit; it was too long, and the hem was coming out. Her nails were bitten and cracked. In our therapy sessions, I led Jane in front of a mirror. I had her look as I arranged her long hair in different ways. I asked her to choose the way she liked her hair best. I put lotion on her chewed-up nails. I helped her mend her dress. She showed she loved to have me comb her hair. She also liked me doing her nails.

I helped her celebrate her birthday because no one else did. I got some cake from the hospital cafeteria, put a candle on it and sang Happy Birthday to her.

In this therapeutic work I noticed Jane, touched her in a variety of ways, and was for her what Des Lauriers calls "a forceful, insistent presence" (Des Lauriers, p. 63).

None of the actions I took with Jane were exclusively one therapeutic activity or another—for example, in combing her hair I noticed her and touched her, and I did it in such a way that she knew *I* did it. *I wanted her to experience me touching her.* I wanted her to experience the sensations and energy changes in her body as I touched her—how her body got warmer all over and came alive. My main goal was to help her *feel* her body—*to help her get interested in herself.*

That the active Developmental Play approach did help Jane know and expand herself can be seen in her "Draw-A-Girl" sketches: No. 1 is a pre-therapy sketch; No. 2 was drawn at the end of six months of therapy. She was seen once weekly.

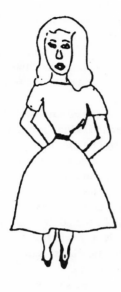

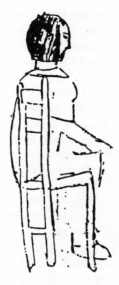

1. Pre-therapy   2. Six Months Later

No. 1—Pre-therapy: This sketch expresses Jane's experience of herself before therapy. She sees herself as an adult, but she doesn't feel real because she's not an adult. She has no inner life, hence no tools for relating to others. Psychologically, she is dead. The figure looks like a paper doll cut-out.

No. 2—Six months later: Jane's post-therapy sketch now reflects the effect of her Developmental Play experiences on the way she experiences herself. Now she's real. She's the child she is. She feels very alive and has an inner life; that is, she now has a self. The emphasis on her hair in the sketch may be a reflection on how much she enjoyed the hair combing. One can identify with this girl sitting in a chair with her back partly turned away from the viewer, as if trying to decide if she should turn around and make contact. Jane's talent as an artist shows in this drawing. She can show it because now she has something to express.

11

The Developmental Play therapist controls any DP therapy session by selecting what activities take place and the exact character of her own participation in them. At the beginning of a DP session, the therapist takes charge by initiating contact with the child. This means that the child experiences the therapist's presence right from the start. The child need not figure out what to do today, although many times a child comes knowing what she wants to do. The DP therapist goes along with the child's request just so long as what the child wants to do will create a closer relationship and is not a way for the child to control the therapist.

The central paradox in raising a child is that exercising control over the child is the means of developing independence in the child. What brings this off is the *kind* of control exercised. Neither arbitrary control by the adult—forcing a child to do things chosen by the adult—nor allowing the child to control the adult are effective in assisting the child to make choices that acknowledge her own existence and the life-enhancing possibilities of relating to others.

The DP therapist, therefore, does control the therapy but does not control the child by forcing the child to conform to rules made by the adult. The only exceptions to these rules are that the child must physically stay with the therapist (usually within touching distance) during a Developmental Play session, and the child may not physically hurt the adult or herself.

The active role of the Developmental Play therapist does not interfere with the child being in charge of herself because the child determines what response she makes to the therapist's initiatives. (The success of DP therapy is measured by the child's growth in her ability to express, either verbally or non-verbally, where she is at any one moment.) Following the child's freely chosen responses, the therapist chooses her own response, a response always guided by the intention to support the particular child's move toward an autonomous self.

1 TOUCHING THE SELF: THE DEVELOPMENTAL PLAY THERAPY DIALOGUE

The name for what a Developmental Play therapist does is *touch*. Touching the child is the central and crucial method of Developmental Play therapy.

The intent of touching the child is to bring about a fruitful dialogue between an adult therapist and the child she touches. The adult initiates and sustains the dialogue, acting not as a person who presents herself as stronger and wiser than the child, but one who, roles and pretenses aside, is truly herself. The true self is being, spirit, and essence.

DP is meetings between an adult's true self and a child. Over time, these meetings between an adult who touches and a child who is touched access the true self of the child.

The DP therapist is a skilled midwife birthing the child's self. In this, her essential tool is touching. Touching brings about the growth and expansion of the child's unique self. This outcome is both the intent and the fruit of Developmental Play (Brazelton, 1990).

Developmental Play therapy takes the form of a dialogue between true selves. In Developmental Play therapy, the worth of the touch is that it conveys the character of the true self. It brings the self of the one who touches to bear on the self of the one who is touched, and that is the way of a dialogue between selves.

How the self of the one who touches affects the self of the one who is touched is illustrated in the dialogues I had with three "ordinary" children—Lisa, Charles, and Mira.

The use of *I* in this chapter and throughout the book came about naturally as I wrote. I developed the methods of therapy that I describe, and I am the therapist in the examples that illustrate the methods. The use of *I*, then, tells it like it is. Besides, I did not want to put the reader through many repetitions of "the developmental play therapist" when "I" is so much less consuming of time and effort—and paper and ink. The same regard for ease and economy has also led me to use the abbreviation DP for Developmental Play therapy.

13

SOME EXAMPLES OF TOUCHING

LISA

Scene: I (the author) am standing next to Lisa, a 2 1/2-year-old girl, in the shallow end of a swimming pool. Her mother, who knows me, is nearby talking to friends. Lisa has seen me before at the pool, but, up to now, we have not interacted.

> Vi: (Touching Lisa's bare knee lightly with the index finger of her right hand) There's a knee.
> Lisa: (Smiles, moves closer and lifts her other knee towards Vi)
> Vi: Oh, here's another knee. (Gently touching it)
> Lisa: (Smiles, brings a foot out of the water, looks at Vi)
> Vi: And, here's a foot. (Gently touching it)
> Lisa: (Moves closer and brings up her other foot)
> Vi: (Touching her foot) Oh, this foot doesn't want to be left out. It wants me to say *Hello* to it, too. Shall I kiss it?
> Lisa: (Nods yes)
> Vi: (Kisses her foot) Did your foot like it?
> Lisa: (Nods yes)

At this point, Lisa's mother is ready to leave. I look at Lisa, smile and bend the fingers of my right hand in a little *good-bye*. Lisa smiles back at me and waves. Her mother, too, smiles at me, then takes Lisa's hand. The two walk away.

I began by just looking at Lisa. I found she was already looking at me and as soon as our eyes met, she moved, just a little, toward me. Her movement told me that Lisa was inviting contact with me. I decided to accept her invitation. That committed me to a meeting with her—and to nothing else but our dialogue—for the time we would be together.

I initiated our meeting by lightly touching Lisa's knee, a way of seeing her through touch. I chose her knee because knees are less personal parts of the body than would be the face, for example, when touching a child the first time. The quality of my touch and of my accompanying words as I spoke to her ("There's a knee.") told Lisa something of me. She learned a little about who I *am*. As a very young child, she could not put this understanding into words. She didn't have to. Lisa learned about me by experiencing my touch and my voice. Her responses (smiling at me; moving still closer; lifting her other knee) confirmed she knew we had met. They also showed she liked the meeting and

14

wanted it to continue. Lisa's responses told me that she felt me touching her and that she liked it.

Actually, I knew Lisa's responses to me even before she lifted her other knee. When I touched Lisa I felt, through my fingers, Lisa's skin and muscles accept my touch, receiving it gladly as if to say, "This feels so good. I need this."

Lisa's response to my initial touch and words determined what I did next. This was to touch her other knee. This second touch let her know more of me—that I was a person who understood her non-verbal language and that I wanted to meet the need she had expressed for more contact with me. Her responses to my second touch (smiling, lifting up her other foot) again guided me so that I could do what she wanted (touch her foot). And, her response to that touch led me to continue our dialogue by touching her other foot. My decision to kiss her foot also depended on looking at Lisa's responses and sensing her eagerness to have our meeting bring us into more intimate contact.

During our meeting, I spoke to Lisa several times. My words did not attempt to tell Lisa what she felt, and I did not directly ask how she felt. Instead, my words spoke to the part of her body reaching out to be touched (her foot). I was responding to her on *her* level, which was physical, direct, and very personal. My words also helped her become aware of her pleasure and delight in being touched when she responded affirmatively to my asking, "Shall I kiss it?" and "Did your foot like it?"

Lisa experienced me touching her. As a result, she experienced her bodily self. She knew then that she had a body because she could feel it. It could move and communicate. She and I had a dialogue without her saying a word. Her body said it for her.

Identifying wants and feelings and recognizing that *I* have them begins and then expands a child's sense that she is a separate and unique self. As with this brief game with Lisa, much of Developmental Play is intended to foster the realization of possessing a self. At this stage, it is a *body self*.

CHARLES

Scene: A large kitchen in a home in the country. At one end of the room the mother is cooking; her four-year-old son, Charles, is trying to get her attention; from the other end of the room I am observing Charles. I decide to contact Charles, who knows me because I have been in his home a couple of days and because I interacted with him a year ago. Up to now, I have not moved toward him except to say "Hello," to which he responded by averting his head.

Charles: (Walks by Vi)
    Vi: (Reaches over, picks him up, puts him on her lap and lightly touches his hand) There's a hand.
Charles: (Looks at his hand and closes it)
    Vi: My goodness, those fingers are all folded up. (Looking at them closely) Are they hiding? Is one going to move?
Charles: (Leaves his hand closed)
    Vi: Well, I wonder if I can find the magic button that would make one of those fingers move? (Touching one finger)
Charles: (Moves that finger, then moves his other fingers, then closes his hand again)
    Vi: Well, I guess I'll have to try the magic button again. (Touching his finger as before)
Charles: (His fingers remain still)
    Vi: (Reaching down and touching his foot) Maybe this is the magic button that makes them move this time.
Charles: (All at once, his fingers unfold; looks at Vi) This is what you have to do the next time. (He gently cradles Vi's face in his two hands, one on each side of her face)
    Vi: Oh, that's so nice! (Puts her two hands over his and holds them there on her face for a few moments; then puts his hands in his lap; takes her own hands and does to him what he just did to her; cradles his face in her two hands holding them there for a few moments before removing them) Your face feels so soft and nice.
Charles: (Holds both hands open)

At this point, father entered the kitchen and the game ended with his greeting everyone.

At first, Charles was not really experiencing me touching him because he was wanting a longer, closer kind of touch (when he held my face to show me). He was responding, playing my game, but his heart wasn't in it. When I responded to his request, we began to have a dialogue. When he requested a more intimate touching, I realized then why I had not reached him in the beginning. A year earlier, I had interacted with Charles, and at the beginning of these meetings he regularly turned away from me. Therefore, I expected he would turn away this time right after I put him in my lap. But he did not turn away, something I could have noticed if expectation had not biased my perception. Fortunately, Charles showed me the kind of touch he needed—a bold move on his part and one that also revealed how much he needed to be touched and accepted for

16

who he *was* at that moment in his life. I was surprised and touched by what he did, and I was able to experience his touching as approaching—not turning away—from me. With that, I was able to give him (by cradling his face) the kind of touch he needed.

MIRA

Scene: Mira, a four-year-old girl, and I are sitting on the floor facing each other. This is the 12th session of a Developmental Play group program. It follows a three-week break over the Christmas holidays. In this same room are four other child-adult pairs sitting on the floor playing.

Mira: (Whiny voice) I didn't get to bed until midnight.
   Vi: Let's rock then. (Putting Mira in her lap and cradling her [In cradling, child lies in adult's lap, head on adult's left arm. In this position there is close eye contact between them], singing a lullaby)
Mira: (Lies quietly in Vi's arms with eyes open. Seems to be thinking about something. At the end of Vi's singing, still cradled, she looks up at Vi) You know what? The other foot is the stuck one today. (Points to her foot which she holds up)
   Vi: (Ignoring Mira's foot, but looking at her face) Did you bring any kissable places today?
Mira: (Still cradled, looks up at Vi's face) No, I didn't. (Pauses, thinks, still looking up at Vi) Do *you* see one?
   Vi: (Laughing) Do I see one? Yes. I see one right here. (Kissing her on the cheek)
Mira: (Looking at Vi) That's not it.
   Vi: Is it here? (Kissing her on the other cheek)
Mira: No. (Holds up her foot, looks at Vi, smiles)
   Vi: (Taking her foot in her hand) Is it this foot?
Mira: Try. (Looks at Vi. She is smiling and has an impish look)
   Vi: (Kisses the held foot)
Mira: No. (Smiling. She is enjoying herself immensely)
   Vi: Is it this foot? (Touching her other foot)
Mira: Try. (Smiles. She is being playful)
   Vi: (Kisses her other foot)
Mira: Ouch! (Sits up and examines her foot) A sore toe.
   Vi: (Holding her, joins Mira in looking at her toe)

Looking told me Mira wasn't really tired. Her tone of voice, her posture, her looking at me said she wanted to feel herself with me again after a long break in our dialogue. So I cradled her and sang to her as a way to give her an immediate experience of renewed relationship with me.

When I cradled her, Mira first lay quiet. She was receptive to all she was feeling as I sang and held her. I sensed she was relaxed and content. She experienced me again (in the way that I held her and in the quality of my voice), and she showed me that she did by playing a part of a game ("Stuck Foot") that I had played with her in an earlier session.

At this point, I began a game that could be a vehicle for the relationship we could build that day. I did not want just to repeat "Stuck Foot" because I sensed that Mira was ready for an offer from me for action that would bring us closer than the action of that game does.

Then Mira delighted me so much that I laughed in my enjoyment of her. She playfully teased me; *she* played with *me*; she got her kisses where *she* wanted them. She enjoyed and shared her enjoyment of herself with me. In all of this, she was fully and openly herself.

As with Lisa and Charles, Mira expressed her reaction to touch in body language (holding up her foot, her smile and eye contact). She did use a few words, the meaning of which, however, was in her body movements. I, in turn, responded at her level by touching her other foot. I did not make any interpretations such as: "It feels so good you want to be touched all over." Mira used a body response to end this game ("Ouch! A sore toe"). I did not see any sore on her toe. Again, I responded at her level without giving her act any specific meaning. At this stage in her development, any verbalization on my part would not have been meaningful to her.

Yet, compared to her behavior in earlier sessions, Mira showed me she had matured. In our previous meetings, Mira had been more like a child younger than herself. She had been much more receptive than active as we related. For the first time, in this session Mira showed she experienced me, the adult, as not her, as separate from her when she asked, "Do *YOU* see one?" She has begun to know her true self, to be that self, to enjoy that self—through the pleasurable and playful touch she asked for. These will be the foundations for creative self-expression and self-esteem in her later life. It was exciting and moving for me to be present in that moment with her.

These three examples with Lisa, Charles, and Mira illustrate the Developmental Play dialogue. A model of DP dialogue would appear like this:

>Adult touches the child ⟶ Child reacts
>to being touched ⟶ Adult chooses a way
>of contacting the child based on the child's reac-
>tions ⟶ Adult contacts the child by touch-
>ing, hearing, or noticing.

This is a working model. The arrows stand for action and impact. The model depicts a dynamic relationship between the toucher and the one touched.

THE EXPERIENCE OF BEING TOUCHED

One of the parts of this dynamic relationship is a subjective experience— the feeling of being touched. If you recall a time when you experienced yourself touched by someone who understood you as you are, you will have a grasp of the experience of feeling touched.

One adult who recalled such an experience named its "ingredients" for her—she said she felt her body sensation heightened; she felt her tears; she could still feel the place on her hand where it had been touched; and she felt both joy and sadness. Your memory will probably include some of these feelings. In any case, feeling touched is a very significant experience remembered for years and years. The skin never forgets. When you really let yourself feel the touch from a person who is really present, you feel real. That's why you remember it.

A child does not usually try to describe the experience of being touched in words. An adult must look at a child's behavior to know if she feels touched. Or, an experienced therapist knows if the child is feeling the touch by the way her skin feels.

The behavior, the attitudes, the feelings of a child who feels the touch un-mistakably change. The touch is a bodily-felt experience that is reflected in the child becoming more relaxed and comfortable, yet also more energized and very much alive. The touched child is, simply, happy. She shows a heightened aware-ness of who she is, and she acts on this awareness by initiating new activities and relating in new ways to the adult. Finally, being touched is highly pleasurable for the child. Consequently, she wants to be touched again. The pleasure she feels is the pleasure of feeling alive and feeling her realness and her growing sense of self. She wants to keep that. She keeps it by asking the adult to repeat touching or do it a new way—"the other foot," for example. Such requests give the adult the opportunity to contact the child again and more fully and deeply, since the child is very open to being touched. These are some of the effects that being touched had on Lisa, Charles, and Mira (Des Lauriers, 1962).

19

THE EXPERIENCE OF THE TOUCHER

A second part of this dynamic Developmental Play relationship is the subjective experience of the one doing the touching. When I touch a child, I feel the energy and warmth of my hands. At the same time, I feel the quality of the child's skin. I experience the child's skin letting me in, or pushing me out, or ignoring me. The child's skin guides me and tells me how the child feels about me or about what we are doing.

When a child's body lets me in, I feel it relax and get heavier. I feel a flow of energy from her to me and from me to her. And there is nothing either of us have to do but be there in that quiet, wonderful space of presence—a feeling of unity and separateness at the same time.

When I feel a child's body shutting me out, I experience the blocked energy. In that case, I try other ways of contact—maybe just looking at the child or singing to her, noticing her so that she experiences my presence and learns that no matter what she does, I am not going away.

As the Developmental Play therapist who initiates the touching, I experience three main stages with a child. My subjective experience is different for each stage.

1. The beginning, the Hello, the "Getting to Know You" stage. The child and I do not have a dialogue yet. The child may be testing me. At this stage, I experience myself being very attentive to the child's cues and body to guide me. The energy between us feels uneven and sometimes rough.
2. The child allows and invites touch. She trusts the therapist. I experience this stage as "She is letting me love her." I experience love from the child. The energy feels smooth and quiet, but most of it seems to flow from me to her. We do have a dialogue, but I am providing most of the content of our dialogue. In Object Relations theory, this would be the attachment stage.
3. The child's behavior shows that she experiences the therapist as separate from her. The child has a self that speaks for her now. This is a very exciting stage for me. It is always a "peak" experience for me when a child moves into a more mature stage and does something she has never done before. It always feels like a miracle to me. It's always a surprise. I respond to this new behavior with heightened energy and a great deal of delight. I can identify with the child's immense joy at being able to do something on her own without the help of an adult.

At this stage, the therapist and child have a true dialogue because the child contributes some of the contents. The child treats the therapist more as an equal.

When this happens, I experience myself seen and touched by the child. The toucher becomes the one touched, and the one touched becomes the toucher (Levin, 1987). That is, both are being touched and touching at the same time—a very moving experience for me as a therapist. These are some of the effects of being the toucher.

The effect of Developmental Play therapy depends on touching the child and the child feeling touched. An objective description of touching is creating a relationship in which the true selves of the adult and child can meet and dialogue. An objective description of feeling touched is perceiving this relationship and the quality of its meeting. Developmental Play therapy is creating relationship through touching and creating new relationship as the child feels touched.

2 THE STRUCTURE OF DEVELOPMENTAL PLAY THERAPY: A LOOK AT SOME DEVELOPMENTAL PLAY THERAPY SESSIONS

The unrelated human being lacks wholeness, for he can achieve wholeness only through the soul, and the soul cannot exist without its other side, which is always found in a You.
—Carl Jung

In my work as a psychotherapist, begun in 1953, I devised innovative methods for promoting the healthy psychological growth of children. I came to base what I did in psychotherapy sessions on my conviction that children need to be touched in order to mature in a healthy way. The task of the Developmental Play therapist is to provide the structure that allows a child to feel touched.

In this chapter we will explore what is meant by structure through the ways the DP therapist uses touch. Sessions with different children illustrate how the Developmental Play therapist adjusts her touch to the child's ability to accept touch. How, for example, does she touch a child who is afraid of touch? An angry child? A child who pushes her away? Or a child who doesn't feel the touch?

This chapter also demonstrates how touch is an organizer of behavior. You will notice how the touching enables the child to utilize the therapist as a *You* so that she can find her *I* or core self. You will notice how the touching stimulates the child to move, feel, think, talk, and above all, to relate to the DP therapist.

THE SETTING

Sessions of DP are times for touching a child. I do DP in a room furnished with some or all of the following:

- » a rug (at least big enough for two to sit on)
- » a rocking chair
- » a table and chair

I usually have available

- » paper
- » crayons
- » a pencil
- » a bottle of skin lotion

The room needs also a door that shuts in order to make the meeting private. When I enter the room with a child for a DP session, I immediately shut the door. This act, recurring at each session, comes to mean to the child that she is in a special place where special things can happen. Very quickly the child comes to realize that in a DP session, she is free of an adult who judges her and demands obedience—the role which, in our culture, the adult adopts toward the child so much of the time. I have observed that shutting the door comes to symbolize the opportunity to be with an adult in a different way. Privacy creates and reproduces a paradoxical setting in which the child is both freer for self-expression and powerfully guided into a loving relationship with an adult, a relationship that is a partnership.

The props used in DP are both simple and limited. The rug and the rocking chair allow and promote close physical contact between the therapist and child. They also are aids to physical and mental relaxation. The table and chair, crayons, pencil and paper permit self-expression to the child through the medium of art, a natural medium of self-expression for a child and one most children readily can use. The bottle of lotion is used in DP games (see Appendix). The games are themselves ways of bringing about a meeting between the child and the therapist. Most DP games require only the physical presence of the child and the therapist.

Toys are notably *not* available in a room where a DP session is held. The helping force in DP is in the relationship developed between the child and the therapist. The helping force in DP is the experiencing of the therapist's physical presence directly. DP sessions can and do take place with nothing more in the room than a rug. This allows the child and therapist to be physically close. This means that DP can take place in schools or other institutions and in homes as well as in professional offices.

24

BETSY, AGE 5, A FEARFUL CHILD

This session took place in a room of a facility where Betsy was living while awaiting placement in a foster home. Staff members reported that Betsy had lived in four different foster homes over the past two years. She had become an insecure child with many fears. For the session, Betsy and I used a room in the facility which had two large beanbags in it. When I entered the room Betsy had hidden herself under one of the beanbags. I sat down in the other beanbag.

Vi: Hello, Betsy. I'm Vi, and I'm here to play with you. Is that you under that beanbag?

Betsy: (Makes a soft sound)

Vi: Oh, I hear something.

Betsy: (Makes another sound, a little louder)·

Vi: Is that a Betsy sound?

Betsy: (Peeks out from under her beanbag and then hides again)

Vi: Oh, it is Betsy. I saw you peek out. Here's my sound to go with yours. (Making a sound)

Betsy: (Makes her sound back)

Vi: (Goes over to Betsy's beanbag, makes her sound and then chants) Betsy come play with me. (Returns to her beanbag)

Betsy: (Comes out from her beanbag and comes over to Vi)

Vi: If I put my cheek next to yours, maybe we can make our sounds together. (Takes Betsy's face in her hands and puts her cheek next to hers. Makes a humming sound)

Betsy: (Hums a little, then pulls away and hides again under her beanbag)

Vi: Oh where is Betsy? She was here a minute ago.

Betsy: (Makes a squeaky sound)

Vi: I hear Betsy. Is she going to come over and play again?

Betsy: (Crawls out from under her beanbag and comes over to Vi)

Vi: (Takes her hand) Look at this wonderful hand. It has fingers.

Betsy: (Allows Vi to hold her hand; then holds up the other one for Vi to see and touch; then returns to her hiding place under the beanbag)

Betsy continued hiding and coming out to me for close to an hour. Each time Betsy came over to me, I held her a little longer. But when I felt her getting tense, I let go so that she could go back to her beanbag. Soon she began staying longer with me. Each time she hid under the beanbag I said, "Now where has that Betsy gone? She was here a minute ago." After I spoke Betsy would come out, then come over to my beanbag and invite more touching, which I supplied.

Once when she was hiding I kept still, not making my usual remark. Soon I heard a voice from under the beanbag: "You're supposed to say 'Where is Betsy?'" Toward the end of the session, Betsy stayed with me on my beanbag. She began telling me what she wanted: "Touch my face again. Do that game again." When it was time to leave the room, Betsy did not want to go. I said to her: "You had such a good time that you don't want to leave. What you can do when you're by yourself is to close your eyes and just pretend you're here with me and you can feel me touching your face." In the end, Betsy would not leave the room until I walked out with her.

This session with Betsy illustrates how the DP therapist takes the time to make a fearful child comfortable—how she recognizes and respects where the child is before touching her. In Betsy's case, I began by making my presence felt through my voice, to which she responded (making sounds back and peeking out). I noticed her (I see you peeking out) and moved close to her (still under the beanbag). She responded by playing the hide-and-seek come-find-me game, to which I responded. She, in turn, responded to me by coming over to me and allowing me to touch her. Even here, I allowed Betsy to withdraw when she felt tense in her body. Feeling in control of herself (and not forced to do anything by me), she returned to me on her own for more touching. From then on, she couldn't get enough.

Betsy's response to my opening contact started our dialogue—first carried out through sounds and movement, then through touch and verbalization ("Touch my face again"). This session shows the effect of touch on Betsy's ability to organize herself and relate to me. The pleasure of the touching moved her toward me to get more, to get the feel of who she is through touch.

Since this was a one-time meeting, I did not ask her about her foster home experiences. What I did was to offer her experiences in being touched and seen and enlivened in a relationship with a loving adult. She can carry the benefit from that DP experience wherever she goes.

My job as a therapist is to structure the situation so that the child will experience being touched. To do that, I must assess the child's response to my actions because the child's reactions to what I do determines what I do next to promote my therapeutic goals. Yet when I am with a child, I am not thinking about goals or anything else. I'm just being present, responding to and experiencing the child.

CRADLING

One kind of touch I use often is cradling. To do cradling, I sit in a rocking chair (or on a rug on the floor), holding the child in approximately nursing position. This makes eye contact easy, and it is possible to speak very softly if I wish.

During cradling I may rock, sing a lullaby, or sing a song I make up about the child. The song might be about what the child has done during the DP session, what she has shown she wants or feels, or what I have noticed about the child. Sometimes I chant the names of the parts of the child's body as I touch them. Quite often I cradle the child and do nothing else. In this instance we sit quietly, neither one of us doing anything but instead experiencing all that it means to be together.

What I do while cradling the child depends partly on what the child does. Many times the child asks, verbally or nonverbally, for specific touches. At all times during cradling I am keenly observant for clues that reveal the child's needs at the moment. I have found that a child may be particularly open to receiving these touches during cradling and may be profoundly moved by them while being cradled.

Moreover, cradling helps the child to feel safe and to feel her body calming and relaxing. Cradling eliminates distracting environmental stimuli and focuses the child's attention on her inner world of emotion and body sensation. She experiences the warmth and energy of the mother's body. She experiences what is her and what is not her. She experiences feelings and pleasure that come from inside her. They are hers.

By experiencing cradling, the child also learns how she can calm herself because I teach the child that she can, even though I am absent, imagine herself being cradled by me and so restore all the feelings she has had during cradling. Whether I teach it or not, children create their own ways of reliving their cradling experience. For example, at bedtime one child (age 4) would place a Polaroid picture of her and her DP therapist on her bedside table. Thus, cradling helps the child to accomplish two primary tasks of childhood: knowing who she is through recognizing and owning her feelings and needs; and becoming self-regulating.

All children—including "ordinary" children and especially Attention Deficit disorder children, acting-out children, and psychotic children—need the caring physical contact of cradling to help them experience their bodies so that they can become fully human. I do it in small doses with the child who is wary of cradling, who at first finds it strange or uncomfortable. When the child experiences cradling as pleasurable, even for a few moments, she almost always wants more cradling.

I fashion a DP session into three parts: (1) a beginning *Hello Time*, when I greet the child and begin to let her know that I am seeing her; (2) a *middle time* of play activities—sometimes initiated by me, sometimes initiated by the child; and (3) an *ending time* or *cradling*. After many deeply moving experiences for me and for the child, experiences that happened during cradling, I know that cradling is effective therapy, perhaps the most basic and effective therapy I do.

DP THERAPY CRADLING DIFFERS FROM "HOLDING" THERAPIES

The Developmental Play therapy cradling differs markedly from the forced "Holding" described by Welch (1988, *Holding Time*), Magid (1988, *Children at Risk*), and Jernberg (1979, *Theraplay*). I do not hold a child to force the child to feel, say, or do something. Developmental Play therapy provides cradling to enable the child to experience her bodily self, the pleasure of contact, and the joy of feeling alive. Through the cradling the child begins the process of discovering her core self.

If a child resists the cradling (as some children do in the beginning stages of therapy), I simply stop it and do the touching in a different way or make my presence felt without touch. In other words, I listen to the child, and the child feels heard. I can always find other ways to make my presence felt by the child. Thus, I get my way (doing what I think needs to be done), and the child gets her way (feels heard and that she counts). For example, Mira responded to the cradling in her third session by pushing me away, saying in a whiny voice, "You're hurting my neck." Stopping the cradling, I said, "Well where is your neck? (looking at it and touching it)." Children often use their bodies to describe their discomfort.

Later in the session, she accepted the cradling and was totally relaxed. Most children, however, welcome the cradling from the beginning.

In the DP approach, the cradling, sometimes accompanied with thumb sucking, comes about out of the desire for it from the child—very different from it being forced on her from the outside. When the children in a DP group are asked what they liked best of all the things we did, nearly all of them say, "The cradling." In other words, the children in DP have a voice. In the other three therapies, they clearly do not have a voice.

The Holding therapies have a specific agenda for each child for each session. The plan is made ahead of time. The child is required to say or do some specific thing—for example, nurse from a baby bottle. The therapist makes the decision, and the child has no say in it. It is a one-way communication process.

The DP therapist takes charge, not by forcing the child to do something, but by noticing and touching the child to enable her to feel touched. I am gentle but very persistent in making my presence felt by the child—if not by touch, by looking at her and saying what I see. No matter what the child does, she cannot get rid of me. I also listen to the child to encourage a dialogue which is often nonverbal in the beginning. DP therapy is a touching dialogue—a two-way communication that initiates the growth process.

Developmental Play therapy also has a well-defined underlying structure. This structure, however, does not take the form of a pre-planned agenda for each session. Each DP session creates its own dialogue of touch agenda as child and therapist dialogue.

The DP therapist *never tickles* a child. Tickling is the most invasive, intrusive, hostile thing to do to a child. The child has no defense at all.

Some therapists do not see the value of the cradling. They may see it as allowing the child to be passive, withdrawn, or in another world. They want the child to be active, working on something.

In DP cradling, the child is far from passive. She is actively focusing her attention on experiencing her body being touched and feeling what other places want to be touched. (See Mira, third example, p. 17.) Or the child may be simply enjoying the pleasure of being cradled. The child's attention is focused on experiencing this experience. She doesn't have to do anything, just be. The Developmental Play therapist has only one goal in offering the cradling—to provide the child with this wonderful life-giving experience of being touched and cradled by one whom she trusts. The DP therapist makes no demands that the child do anything or feel anything except to feel herself being touched and cradled by the therapist. I always end a session with cradling. This quiet time, besides being a good-bye ritual, helps to center the child in preparation for turning her attention to the outside world.

CRADLING MARIE, AN ANGRY CHILD

I had DP sessions for eight months with Marie, a talented child, age 6. The initial problem as described by her mother was Marie's aggressive behavior at school—she hit and bit other children, a behavior her mother could see no reason for, and Marie fought with her mother. This is how a DP session with Marie ended with cradling. (Throughout the session, Marie expressed anger toward her mother and toward me. Toward the end of the session—after Marie began to realize that she couldn't control me with her kicking, pushing, and yelling, she became quiet. I am helping Marie write a story about her feelings.)

     Vi: I'm going to write a story about you today with your help. (Prints as Marie watches) Marie was angry today because . . .

Marie: Mommy wouldn't give me the tablet.

     Vi: Very good. Were you mad at me too?

Marie: (Nods yes)

     Vi: (Writing) She was mad at Vi because she . . .

Marie: Wouldn't let me out (the door).

     Vi: What's nice is that you can say it. And now, I am . . .

Marie: Okay.

     Vi: (Writing) And Vi says she loves you.

Marie: (Reading it as Vi writes) What is the "s" for?

Vi: If I say "I love you," then we don't need the "s". (Reprints "I love you" and reads it aloud to her) Okay, let's have our quiet time—you know how we do before we say good-bye. (Sits in the rocking chair)

Marie: (Comes over and gets in Vi's lap)

Vi: It's nice to be together. I really love you. Do you have any kissable places?

Marie: (Turns her face up to Vi to be kissed)

Vi: (Sings a song sung before at the end of each session with her) Oats, peas, beans, and barley grow: oats, peas, beans and barley grow. Does anyone know? Does anyone know how oats, peas, beans, and barley grow?

Marie: (With smiles and looking at Vi, sings with Vi)

Vi: (After rocking her in silence, leaves the room with Marie)

Marie gave form to her feelings through the story I helped her write. In doing that, and in sharing her feelings with me, she took a big step toward self-understanding because she recognized herself as the source of her feelings. She could say both that she had been angry with me and that she was okay with me now. Once she was in touch with herself, she could relax and receive from me. She did not any longer have to try either to control or to take care of an adult, and so she could let herself be a child. She could allow herself to be loved by an adult in an uncomplicated way without a struggle for dominance. Cradling allowed Marie to experience my love deeply. She felt so happy and free during the cradling that she could join me in singing. This was a new experience for her. Later her mother reported that while driving home after this session, Marie said very firmly, "I love Vi." This statement shows that Marie has become aware of the shift in her from being outer-directed and controlling of others to experiencing and sharing her own inner self with another. Her ability to identify and express her feelings had carried over into her life outside DP.

TOUCHING AND CHANTING BODY PARTS

During a DP session, I very often touch parts of the child's body with my fingertips or hands. I touch the child's hands, arms, and face most often, and I may touch the child's feet and legs (we often have shoes and socks off during a DP session). I may name the body part as I touch it—either just saying or singing the name. Sometimes the touch is followed by holding the part so that the time of touching is lengthened. I may manipulate fingers or toes and comment on their movement.

These kinds of touches are basic DP methods. Tangible in themselves, they bring the crucial intangible of the therapist's total commitment to the child home to the child. The quality of the touches conveys the regard, the understanding, sometimes the playfulness of the therapist. These kinds of touches arouse immediate response from the child. They cannot help but do so given the nature of the human senses, mind, and brain. Put in broadly descriptive terms, the child responds by turning her attention on herself and on the therapist. She turns from attention to the outer to attention to the inner—her own self—and she responds to the therapist, thus beginning significant relating.

TOUCHING ANN, WHO DIDN'T FEEL THE TOUCH

Ann, age 4, and I are sitting on the floor, facing each other. It is early in our first DP session.

Vi: (Touching Ann's hand) Look at this hand.
Ann: (Points to a picture on the wall) What's that?
Vi: (Reaching up and taking the hand that is pointing) And this hand has fingers, and they move. (Moving one finger at a time)
Ann: (Starts to pull away)
Vi: (Continues to hold her hand) Let me see how soft your hand is. (Touching my cheek with her hand briefly, then placing her hand against her own cheek) Now you see how soft your hand is.
Ann: (Lets Vi hold her hand to her cheek)

When Ann pointed to the picture, I used her own body movement as an opportunity to begin touching to get her to experience my presence and feel me touching her. I touched her hand and the fingers on that hand. She experienced touches on her face and on my face. Even when she pulled away, she had to experience touch on her body and she experienced her hand and body doing the pulling. This feeling in the pulling came from inside her and belongs to her self. That self part of her let her know that she was enjoying her hand touching my cheek and then her cheek. She was surprised by these touches, as children almost invariably are.

Usually, the child never has been touched by an adult in this way. Ann did feel her own body, and she responded to me. By allowing my touching, even briefly, Ann took the beginning step in letting herself be touched.

DONALD

As a consultant to a residential facility for boys who had severe behavior problems, I was asked for help by a paraprofessional who was working without success with Donald, a boy living in the facility. Donald was a nine-year-old who

31

acted out a lot. He was a small, slightly built child with blond hair. When I walked into the home where the boys were being treated, Donald walked up to me. He showed me a trick with sexual content obviously intended to shock me.

The paraprofessional said he did not know how to help Donald. He had been unable even to keep Donald in a room, and the child was unwilling to do anything. First I observed the frustrated paraprofessional and Donald together. Then I said I would help by demonstrating how to work with Donald using the DP approach.

I asked the paraprofessional to physically hold Donald while I worked with him. (I knew I did not have the physical strength to contain this very strong, slippery child.) During the DP session, Donald (tight in the arms of the paraprofessional) and I are in a room of the residential facility.

> Vi: I know you, Donald, a little bit because you showed me your trick in the hall. (Touching Donald's hand)
> Donald: (Pulls hand away) Get your hands off me.
> Vi: Well, I can see you have hands! Did I hurt you?
> Donald: Just leave me alone.
> Vi: (Touching Donald's foot briefly) And you have a foot here.
> Donald: (Struggling to get free, trying to kick Vi) You're an old woman. You got gray hair and you got wrinkles on your face.
> Vi: You are absolutely right. You are so smart. (Moving closer and taking his face in her two hands, massages his face, gently but firmly) And *you* don't have any wrinkles at all. *Your* skin is so nice and smooth. (At this point I felt his whole body relax as I massaged his face) And your hair is blond.
> Donald: (Looking at Vi and holding out a hand to her) Give me five, old woman. (He smiles and relaxes even more)

This work with Donald is an illustration of persistence in providing the touches that cause a child to feel touched. Despite Donald's attempts to stop me and to get rid of me by taunting me, I continued to touch him. Because he was physically restrained, he could not discharge his feelings motorically, the usual behavior of an acting-out child. In the DP session, Donald had to stay with the situation. He could not leave me. He could not fail to recognize his feelings at being touched by me.

Donald discovered, as shown by his smile and the release of the tension in his body, that he liked my touches. He approached me (he held out his hand), signaling that he wanted more. The pleasure associated with being touched and being known is a strong, positive element in DP. When the child has experienced this pleasure, she is better able to tolerate any difficulty that arises in the relationship with the therapist. It is as though she has money in the bank and need not fear the adverse happenings of a rainy day.

HUGGING, KISSING, SPEAKING, SINGING

I often ask a child if she has any kissable places. This inquiry invites the child to share pleasure with me. Thus, a kiss can help a child recognize and place a high value on a part of her body, a first step toward knowing herself as valuable. From this experience, the child also learns to kiss—a very important developmental step. With a kiss, a child can learn to give and receive unconditional affection. Hugging offers these possibilities, too. It may be more acceptable to older children who shy from other expressions of affection with adults.

The spoken word also touches. The tone of voice of a speaker tells the listener how the speaker feels about what he is saying and often how he feels toward the person spoken to. One use I make of tone of voice in DP is to express delight.

I often describe how a child's skin feels. "Oh, your skin feels so soft," I say as I gently and slowly touch her face. I say this slowly and warmly, in tune with the rhythm of my hand doing the touching. Or, "You have a wonderful voice. Would you make that sound again?" My voice expresses my delight. This is not fake. I *am* delighted. Letting it show helps the child to experience this delight also. It helps the child experience herself as a delightful and fun person to be with. This translates into "People like to be with me." I let playfulness, affection, anger or whatever I am feeling come through in my voice. Such expression makes me real and comprehensible, both to myself and to the child. It also models for the child that expressing feelings is safe to do during a DP session.

A special use of voice for touching inheres in singing to the child. Without having to do anything, the child feels the adult's presence through the vibrations of her singing voice. If the child joins in, then she adds or matches her vibrations to those of the adult's—another way to touch—to be together that is fun and pleasurable. A frequent use I make of singing is to sing a lullaby while cradling. That combines rhythm, vibration of tone, the influence of words, the physical touch, and the impact of looking lovingly at the child into a powerful effect.

WILLIAM

William, age 7, rejected physical touch at first but could accept my voice reaching out to him.

William: Leave me alone. Don't touch me.

    Vi: Oh, Did I hurt you?

William: Just leave me alone.

    Vi: You said that with a higher voice that time. (Imitates his voice) You've got a good voice. Would you do it again? Would you sing it? (Her voice is enthused and playful as she makes this suggestion)

William: (Begins to smile. Playfully covers his eyes with his hands)

    Vi: (In a playful, singing rhythm) William's gone away but here are his hands. (Gently touches his hands)

William: (Peeks out at Vi between his fingers. He is willing to interact with her now and let her touch him)

The work with William is an example of how I use the child's own response to guide my subsequent response. I began by touching William in an effort to lead him to feeling and listening to his own body. I wanted him to know that I was the one touching him. He found my touch invasive or unacceptable, so I chose another touching method—use of voice. First I listened to William's voice and described it as "good." He felt noticed and seen when I did that and when I encouraged him to sing. As a result, he begins to experience his body, his existence, his aliveness and the wonderful pleasure in just being noticed—perhaps for the first time. He wants more of this feeling. To get it, he interacts with me. He forgets to be resistant and initiates his own "see-me" game. That he invites contact, is playful, allows the physical touching, and shows his shyness is evidence that he felt touched and seen by me.

The often recurring task of a Developmental Play therapist is to decide how to touch the child in a way that will help that particular child feel touched. The subsequent task is to observe and to comprehend the meaning of the child's response to touch.

The preceding examples of the touching methods of DP demonstrate that a child will feel touched by an adult who understands the power of touch and knows how to touch. The examples also demonstrate that learning to feel begins with touch. The responses to touch by the children in the examples show how touch starts a kind of chain reaction. A simple touch moves a child from experiencing the touch, to a feeling reaction to the touch, to experiencing self, to experiencing relationship to the toucher, to feeling good about the self, to taking charge of a self that becomes a loving, social, competent, thinking individual. *When you touch a child, you start something.*

SETTING LIMITS

A second major method of DP is the setting of limits. Limit setting involves both informing the child that certain behaviors are not permitted and making clear to the child that she cannot control the therapist.

In DP, the child's role is to respond to the structure which the therapist provides in whatever way she needs to. The child, therefore, must have great latitude of response so that her needs can become known, first to the therapist so that the therapist can meet them, and then, as the child matures, to the child herself so that she can learn to be self sufficient. There is no useful learning when a child is simply destructive, when a child goes out of control, on a rampage. When this behavior occurs, I forcibly hold the child. I prevent any child who is out of contact and out of control from hitting me or herself or from tearing up the room or the objects in it. While restraining the child, I do not attempt to help the child experience her blind fury; I do not ask her to say something specific. I do not try to force any change in her. What I do focuses the child's attention on herself. I say things like: "I will let go when you stop hitting me." "See how nice it is to let me hold you?" "Look at this hand I am holding."

What guides me in setting limits is my belief that a child needs to experience limits in order to mature. No human is omnipotent; the child must realize this natural state of affairs. The child must discover that she cannot control others or many of the physical aspects and events of her world. To know her capability, she must acknowledge what is impossibility. When a DP therapist sets realistic limits, the child is enabled, first, to recognize that limits exist. Then, with further experience of adequate response to limits, the child can experience a new capacity in herself, the competence to set limits for herself because she has experienced limit setting by another who knows how to do it.

I never allow the child to control what I do during a DP session. I constantly respond to the child, but the response is my own choice. Not being able to control me, the child turns inward to experience her feeling reactions to her inability to control. The energy that has gone to a futile effort to control me can then fuel a useful concentration on her inner feelings and wants. Turning within enables the child to experience herself as an individual separate from me. The touch methods of DP lead the child to connect with another and to experience her physical self and aliveness. Limit setting methods enable the child to separate from the adult and experience the dimensions and qualities of her own psychological self.

One effect of limit setting is to teach the child that she is not in charge of me and cannot control me. She learns, also, that she does not have to take care of me, since my actions make it clear that I can take care of myself. Because she cannot control me, the child cannot escape my presence or get rid of me. Limits hold the child to the desired role—responding to the structure I provide in whatever way she needs to.

A DP session with Marie, age 6, ended with cradling (pp. 29-30). Before cradling Marie, I had set limits on her controlling behavior toward her mother and me. Limit setting began even before the start of the session. The arrangement was that while Marie and I were in a DP session, her mother waited for Marie in an adjoining room. When I came for this session (I had been seeing Marie weekly for several months), I found Marie and her mother standing in the doorway fighting over a writing tablet which they both wanted.

Marie: (In a high-pitched, baby-talk sounding voice) I get the pad, Mommy. (Holding the tablet in her hands)

Mother: Well, let me use the pad. (Reaching for it)

Marie: (In whiny, crying-sounding voice) No . . . No.

Mother: Vi has other paper. That's what Mommy brought to do.

Marie: No. I get a sheet.

Mother: You can take two sheets.

Marie: I need a board.

Mother: I don't have a board.

Marie: I'll give mommy two pages.

Mother: (With resigned, angry tinge to her voice) Then I don't have anything to write on . . . and you have a table.

Marie: You have some paper.

Mother: It's not going to work. I don't have a table to write on.

Vi: (To mother) Be straight with her. Tell her to give you the tablet.

Mother: (With firm tone) I need this tablet.

Marie: (Whiny) No.

Mother: Yes.

Vi: Don't argue with her; tell her to give you the pad.

Mother: Give me the pad.

Marie: I want it.

Mother: You can have it when you're done, I'll give you the brown marker.

Marie: No. (Phony crying)

Vi: Don't bribe her.

Mother: (In firm tone) Give Mommy the tablet.

Vi: You don't need the tablet in here. (Taking the tablet from her and handing it to mother)

Marie: (Clings to mother)

Mother: (Stands there)

Vi: (Moves mother out the door and shuts the door; turns to Marie) You don't need the tablet in here. You and I have other things.

Marie: (Crying, close to screaming)

Vi: You haven't even said Hello to me.

Marie: (Screaming, getting louder)

Vi: Are you mad at your mother?

Marie: No. I wanted that tablet.

Vi: It wasn't your tablet.

Marie: mhm-mhm (meaning yes)

Vi: Mother's tablet.

Marie: My tablet.

Vi: I think you're mad at your mother, right?

Marie: (Crying subsides; she moves toward the door)

Vi: (Stopping her at the door) You're not going out to the other room.

Marie: (Starts crying again)

Vi: Tell me you're mad at mother.

Marie: (Crying sounds very angry now. Tries to get out the door)

Vi: (Stopping her by holding her) You're not going out to the other room.

Marie: (Pushing hard against Vi) I'm gonna. . .

Vi: I hear you say it. You're really mad.

Marie: (Lies on floor, kicks, and screams) Mommy, Mommy. (Gets up, tries to get out the door)

Vi: (Blocks the way) Look at that arm. (Picks her up and holds her in sitting position on a couch) We're going to sit right here.

Marie: I want my Mommy.

Vi: I hear you, and you can see your Mommy later.

Marie: (Screaming again) Let go of me!

Vi: You looked at me just then. (Lets go of her) (Several minutes of Marie trying to hit her. Grabs her arm, then she would kick, and Vi would grab her leg. She made sounds like an animal in a rage)

Marie: Let go of me.

Vi: I'll let go of you when you stop hitting and kicking.

Marie: (Stops screaming, goes to the door, speaking in a loud clear voice) I AM GOING OUT!

Vi: You looked at me just then.

Marie: I'm going out. (Said firmly, no screaming)

Vi: You looked at me just then. What did you see?

Marie: (Starts pushing against me, trying to get out)

Vi: *Stop pushing me!* (I'm angry) Pushing, hitting, kicking are no-no's. You don't do that!

Marie: You're hurting me.

Vi: Where am I hurting you?

Marie: Me go. (Baby-talk; said calmly)

Vi: You're staying right here. This is where we work. This is your time to be with me.

Marie: (For a moment she looks at me and almost smiles, but then she fights that and works up another screaming) Don't touch me!

Vi: I'm not even touching you. Look. (Holding my arms out) Is that new tooth in yet?

Marie: No. (Said quietly)

Vi: You looked at me just then.

Marie: Nope. (Starts for the door) I'll kick you. Don't touch me!

Vi: You're the one touching me. You're here to play with me.

Marie: Nope.

Vi: Would you stop pushing me. You're the one touching me now.

Marie: I'll bite you. (What she does to children at school)

Vi: You're really mad today. I'll get some paper and you can make a mad drawing. (She always liked to draw)

Marie: No.

Vi: Let's see what kind of a mad drawing you can do.

Marie: No. I'm getting out of here. (Pushing and scratching at Vi)

Vi: (Stopping her) *Don't you scratch me!* You're the one touching me now.

Marie: Mommy.

Vi: Your Mommy's okay.

Marie: (Screaming) No, she's not. (Looking straight at Vi, saying softly under her breath) *I hate you.*

Vi: I hear you. I think you're right. How about my getting some paper and you do your drawing, and then you can show it to your mother?

Marie: No. (Hits Vi and growls like an animal) I'm going out!

Vi: I'm the boss, and you can go when the time is up—just like we always do.

Marie: *(Starts to kick me but stops herself in the act)*

Vi: Thank you for not kicking me. Your eyes are still blue.

Marie: (Starts screaming again)

Vi: (Focuses her on her body. She doesn't respond but continues to scream— she doesn't want to be moved out of her anger; she has to be in control) When you get your picture done your mother can come in.

Marie: I want my Mommy now!

Vi: You are so mad.

Marie: I got to go to the bathroom. (She never has to go)

Vi: You can go when it's time to leave.

Marie: I'm thirsty. (Said calmly)

Vi: You can get a drink when the time is up.

Marie: (Starts to cough as if she's going to vomit; sits down in the center of the room and starts a hiccup-kind of crying. This is crying that comes from the inside—very different from the screaming kind of crying she's been doing) Mommy.

Vi: Your Mommy is fine.

Marie: (Angry tone) No, she's not.

Vi: You're mad at Mommy because she wouldn't give you the tablet, and you're mad at me because I wouldn't let you go out.

Marie: (Sits there very quietly, just feeling whatever she is feeling, feeling her own sobs) (Quiet moments: neither one of us saying anything)

Vi: (I feel for her when she sobs like this) Would you let me hold you?

Marie: No. (Quietly gets up, goes to the table where the drawing paper is, sits down, and starts to draw with the crayons. She draws a girl, the first full figure drawing she's made. She gives the girl a solid blue dress and blue eyes that have pupils)

Vi: Who is that? (Looking at her drawing)

Marie: (One last quiet sob) I don't know.

Vi: It's a nice drawing. Is it you?

Marie: (Nods yes)

Vi: (Turns the paper over, puts her hand on it, and draws around her hand and does the same with the other. This is something we have done before)

Marie: (Allows me to do it; then she draws a smiling face on one hand)

Vi: Oh, you've got a smiling face. Does that mean you had a good time at school today?

Marie: No. That was for nap-time, the only thing you get a happy face for. (She takes the crayons and fills in the two hand drawings with different colors)

Vi: (Looking at what Marie is doing) I've never seen anyone do hands like that. That's nice.

Marie: (Continues coloring in silence)
Vi: (Still looking at the coloring) That's very nice. I'm going to write a story about you today . . . (The balance of this meeting between Marie and me, the cradling segment where she let me hold her, is on pp. 29-30.)

I repeatedly set limits during this session with Marie because appropriate limit-setting was what she needed to feel touched. I knew, from earlier work with Marie, that she saw herself as ugly and unloved. In this session she showed her "ugly" side to me, forced it on me over and over. But I refused to confirm her as bad or ugly. I didn't go away, reject her, or punish her. I did ensure that she felt my physical strength when I stopped her from hitting and kicking, and my psychological strength when I accurately defined her extreme anger and showed her that her anger could not control me.

Although Marie tried hard, she could not manipulate me, destroy me, or make me go away. She learned that her anger was not that potent. She also learned that I could be angry with her and we could still be friends. She discovered that my anger did not destroy her or our relationship. By acting so that Marie would be sure to know how angry I was, I caused Marie to see me. She had to recognize my personhood. By setting limits, I helped Marie to see herself, to discover her own person separate from me. She came to know what she felt toward me and what she wanted from me. She had, as her behavior more than her words indicated, these insights: I am a child. I can let Vi see me and give to me. I don't have to control Vi or take care of her. I can feel. I am loved. I can love.

What Marie learned in this session changed her self-image. This is reflected in the drawing she made toward the end of the session. She had made another drawing during an earlier session. That one, Drawing A, shows my room with the outer door, with doorbell, doorknob, windows, roof, birds outside, and me sitting in a chair rocking her. The drawing she made months later during the limit setting session, Drawing B, is of Marie herself, complete with all her parts, in a blue dress, with blue eyes through which a person is looking out. Drawing A depicts Marie's experience of being seen through touch and Drawing B her experience of being seen through limit setting. Being seen through touch furnishes the relationship needed for her to experience herself seen through limit setting.

Touching methods usually precede or at least take up most of the time in the beginning phase of ongoing DP. They help to ready the child for later limit setting procedures. Of course, neither method is excluded at any time. Every session includes some of both as demonstrated in the examples in this chapter. What method I use is determined by what the child needs in the moment. Over a course of DP sessions, a child needs touching and limit setting to develop a healthy, diversified, and active self.

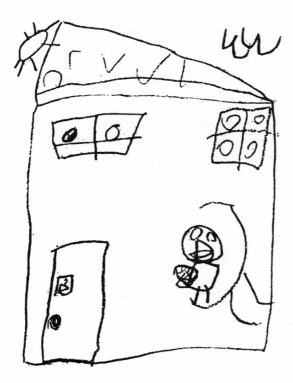

Drawing A

Drawing B

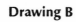

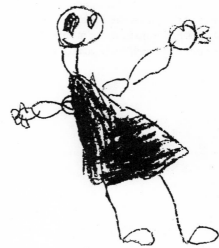

Parents who have not experienced appropriate limit setting from their parents or some adult will not know how to set limits for their children. Obviously, Marie's mother did not. Without understanding that they are doing it, these parents demand that their children take care of them. (Mother's fears of setting limits were reflected in her thinking that Marie would never want to come again.) When I work with a child in DP, I also work with her parents in separate, individual sessions. I teach a parent how to touch a child and how to set appropriate limits. I accomplish this by touching and setting limits within the context of the relationship that develops between us. In other words, I help them get in touch with their own childhood experiences with their parents. After they have these experiences with me, they become effective in touching the child and in setting appropriate growth-inducing limits.

DEVELOPMENTAL PLAY GAMES FOR CHILDREN

In my work with children—helping them feel touched by experiencing my presence through touch—I created a number of "games." Each DP game was originally created for one specific child. Yet, as I tried out these games on other children, including "ordinary" children, I discovered they loved these games. Teachers, parents, and child therapists have asked for these games. There is no set way to play them. Through these playful body-contact games, the adult and child experience an *I-Thou* relationship. You may have created games similar to these for a child. These games are presented throughout the text and in the Appendix.

Whether through "games" or simple touching, the child experiences her sense of self when she feels touched in those moments of "meeting." The adult touches her child in those moments of meeting. *To create these moments of "meeting" through touch is the goal of Developmental Play therapy.*

3   TOUCHING AUTISM: DEVELOPMENTAL PLAY THERAPY WITH JASON

Autism is a mental disorder best understood by recognizing its core: *Absence*. The very behavior and emotions that mark the human as a social being are absent in autism. In fact, diagnosis of autism depends largely on identifying the *lack* of appreciation that persons around one have feelings and wants that require response and that they offer an indispensable source of learning and love.

Thus, the autistic child is a withdrawn child. She deserts objective outer reality for a subjective, unpopulated inner world—and she zealously guards the gates to her sanctuary.

The autistic child shows the effects of withdrawal in inordinately disturbed perception and behavior. She does not, for example, feel pain. If she falls down and skins her knee, she makes no observable response. She does not cry (the earliest form of calling out to others and the earliest means of influencing others) either with or without tears. Typically, she seldom moves her body in an organized, goal-directed way. For example, she is not able to play ball or ride a bicycle. Conversely, she may make stereotyped, purposeless movements for hours at a time. Even more typically, the autistic child has no speech, instead making weird noises not intended to communicate. She does not initiate, and she refuses to touch. The autistic child has a need for sameness. For example, if one small thing in her environment is out of place, the child responds with bizarre behavior (making noises, flapping her hands, running around). Finally, the autistic child is apt to be beautiful. Even so, unanimated, she looks like a beautiful, lifeless doll. These behaviors describe Jason.

JASON

Jason, a six-year-old autistic boy, was brought to me by his parents for Developmental Play therapy. From his parents' account of Jason, their first and only child, I learned that by the time he was two they realized he was very different

43

from other children. He was very quiet; he didn't talk at all; he responded to them hardly at all. Thinking he might be deaf, they took him to the first of many examinations. The physician stated the results of this first examination negatively: Jason was not, he said, deaf or mentally retarded—or autistic.

At three, Jason, who had changed very little, was examined again. This time the examiner characterized Jason as "unrelated to people" and as "treating people like objects."

When Jason was five, a collaborative diagnosis by a pediatrician and psychologist labeled him mentally retarded and autistic. Ritalin was prescribed to control his hyperactivity and behavior modification to manage his daily life.

A year later, when I began therapy with Jason, neither drug nor behavior modification treatment had effected significant change in him.

Most autistic children I have known have a similar history of uncertain diagnosis and unsuccessful treatment. Their parents experience, as Jason's did, heartbreaking frustration, anger, and increasing alarm as their autistic child continues to live at a far psychological distance from them, a distance they are unable to bridge, however they try.

DEVELOPMENTAL PLAY THERAPY WITH JASON

I saw Jason in individual play therapy for 3 1/2 years. Sessions were held weekly in the first 24 months and less frequently in the last 18 months—102 sessions in all.

Many of the sessions (including most of those that follow) were videotaped, making the best possible record of therapy with a child who had almost no speech. I showed some of the videotapes to Jason's parents in order to demonstrate how an adult could help Jason and to discuss with them how Jason's behavior could be understood. I also required that one parent be present at each therapy hour. This was to support any helpful interaction between Jason and his parent and to give his parents "live" demonstrations of how to see him and the effects on Jason of being truly seen.

Before beginning psychotherapy with Jason, I asked that he be taken off Ritalin because his medicine was ineffective (according even to his pediatrician) and, more important, because I wanted his growth to depend on his own capacities and thus be solid and permanent. I felt Jason's problem was not a physical one that could be alleviated by medication. He had, rather, severe psychological problems.

The root cause of autism in the child is the lack of bonding with her parents, bonding that begins ordinarily almost immediately after birth. The bond forms as parents touch and feed the child and continues to be cemented by the quality of the interactions necessary between the very young and the parent. Such bonding is the essential soil for nourishing the growth of the child's self. Without it, the child is bereft of the center that chooses, directs, and evaluates her individual life.

My therapeutic goal, therefore, was to help Jason develop a sense of self. My method would be to see him (in the DP therapy meaning of touch) so that he could bond with me. Then I would promote transfer of bonding to his parents in part by teaching them how to touch him. Put in descriptive terms, I aimed for a journey for Jason from social isolation and a very limited existence to social participation and exercise of ability to understand, shape, and enjoy the world and himself. I thought it would be a long journey during which Jason had to grow up all over again.

The Setting

Jason's psychotherapy sessions were held in a room in my apartment that serves as my office. A fairly large, second-story room, it contains a couch next to which is a two-foot high metal filing cabinet. There is a rocking chair in the middle of the room and, opposite the couch, a desk with a swivel chair. The window, fronted by a very large sill, is next to the file cabinet. On the east wall is a closet with folding doors. This office adjoins my living room, which contains a piano. Off the living room is a porch. To get to my office, Jason and his parents have to climb a set of front stairs. I greet them at the top of the stairs and invite them into my office.

Session 1: First Month

Present: Jason, mother and therapist (Vi). Mother is sitting in the rocking chair. Vi is sitting on the floor in front of the couch.

Jason: (Running back and forth from one end of the room to the other, tearing at the curtains on the window as he goes by and making eerie high-pitched sounds. He doesn't look at mother or Vi)

Vi: (Watching him run as he goes by, grabs his hand)

Jason: (Tries to free his hand; not looking at Vi)

Vi: (Holds on to his hand for a few moments, then lets go of it)

Jason: (Returns to running back and forth, making sounds, not making eye contact. After a few moments of this, comes over to Vi and holds out his hand to her)

Vi: (Taking his hand in hers, looking at it and holding it) Look at this hand, Jason.

Jason: (Again tries to free his hand; no eye contact)
  Vi: (Still holding on to his hand) Pull, Jason, pull.
Jason: (Starts his high-pitched sounds; no eye contact)
  Vi: (Lets go of his hand) Oh, you pulled your hand away!

Comments

This excerpt from the first session illustrates how the Developmental Play therapist interferes with an autistic child's stereotypical behavior through touch, the only avenue open to her at this stage. I did this with Jason by grabbing his hand and holding it long enough for him to feel the muscles in his arm when he pulled away. I was surprised that Jason came back for more touching when the first one seemed to be so uncomfortable. Feeling discomfort, however, is different from seemingly not experiencing anything during his stereotypical behavior. His move to repeat the experience showed that he felt something and wanted more. Since I was the one who provided him with that experience, he knew where to go to get more. Jason's second response helped me know what to do to make him feel his body, to know that he had been touched by me. I held on to his hand longer the second time and added words and excitement to my voice. Jason communicated clearly without words what he needed. He and I had the makings of a relationship in our first meeting.

Session 2: First Month

Present: Mother
Jason is sitting on the couch facing Vi. His mother is observing from the rocking chair. Vi has a bottle of lotion.

  Vi: (Taking one of Jason's hands, puts lotion on his hand and arm; rubs it in slowly but firmly; massages his hand and arm in a circular motion, beginning with his hand and moving up his arm almost to his shoulder. As she begins to slide her hands down his arm, says, looking at him) Pull . . . pull, Jason. (This is the Slippery Hand game)
Jason: (Does not move his arm; no eye contact)
  Vi: (Slides her hands down to the end of his fingers and lets go) Oh, your hand got away! (Said with a surprised tone)
Jason: (Allows her to do it)
  Vi: (Taking Jason's other hand in hers and repeats game with that hand) We can't leave this hand out. It wants some, too.
Jason: (Again, does not move his arm, but passively allows the game)

46

Vi: (Taking off his shoes and socks) Let's see if these feet would like some, too. (Puts lotion on one foot and repeats the game, now the Slippery Foot game)

Session 3: First Month

Present: Mother

Vi: (Initiates the Slippery Hand game) Pull, Jason . . . pull.
Jason: (Pulls his arm through this time)
Vi: Good, Jason . . . you've got it.
Vi: (At end of hour) It's time to go.
Jason: (Sits down and puts his shoes and socks on)

Session 4: First Month

Present: Mother

Jason: (Comes in, sits down on couch, takes shoes and socks off, hands Vi the lotion bottle and holds up one foot)
Vi: (Does the Slippery Foot game with that foot)
Jason: (Holds up his other foot, as if to say, "Now do this foot")
Vi: (Does that foot)

Comments

Sessions 2, 3, and 4 show Jason is continuing with what he started in session 1. There's continuity from one session to the next. In session 2, Jason not only allowed the touching, but he began to experience some sense of pleasure in it. He did not understand the meaning of "pull." He did however, understand the meaning of it the following week in session 3. And he began to respond to the ritual I set up (taking shoes and socks off in the beginning and putting them back on at the end of the session). Jason showed that he can learn and that he can remember. He still gives very little eye contact. In session 4, Jason showed new energy. He initiated much of the interaction. He didn't wait for me to do it. What was started in session 1 started a chain reaction that has its own momentum. Now there is an adult who touches and a child who feels touched.

Parents' Report at End of First Month

Father: "We both feel excited. We're both being a lot more verbal with him, and we play with him like you did a lot more. He seems to want to be hugged and touched. Now there's no hassle about going to bed. Before it took 1 to 3 hours. He looks at us. It's quite a change. It looks like something must be going on."

47

Mother: "He sits at the table and eats with the utensils, which he never did. His wildness has disappeared." The parents' report presents evidence that Jason is transferring what he learned with me to his parents. They, too, have changed. They initiate more contact and respond to his cues. They enjoy him. Parent and child are showing signs of becoming bonded.

Jason's Behavior the Next Four Months

For several sessions, Jason always started a session with the Slippery Foot game (described in session 2). Then, around the third month, he began a new behavior—standing on my couch and jumping up and down. He did this with a lot of energy and enjoyment. I entered into this game by holding up my arms for him to jump into them. At first, he didn't get the message and ignored me. Then I would reach over and pick him up and hug him. After this, he changed the game to turning my back to him so he could climb on my back and have me walk around carrying him. If I got tired and stopped, Jason would get upset, expressed in either hitting me or butting his head into my stomach. Jason also loved to have me take one arm and one leg and swing him around and around. He would greet me at the beginning of a session by holding up one leg, which meant "Swing me." He never wanted to stop.

Comments

The examples above illustrate how the Developmental Play therapist deals with the basic behavior problem of autistic children, namely, their stereotypical behavior and their need for sameness. Jason had this tendency even when he was learning something new; for example, when he discovered how much fun it was to jump on the couch (something all young children love to do), he wanted to continue it for the whole session and without making any contact with me, either visually or through touch. My goal, in the beginning stages, was to help Jason experience me in whatever he was doing. He was not allowed to be by himself. Therefore, I made his jumping game one that always ended up with his jumping into my arms.

My focus, then, in the first four months was getting Jason used to the idea of allowing me to participate in whatever he was doing. To get him to do something new, I had to first participate in what he was already doing and then gradually change it to something new. Otherwise, his play got very boring for me and he lost contact with me. It was work to do this.

Parents' Report at End of Fourth Month

From the parents' reports, Jason is more aware of his body. "He grabs himself in the genitals and puts a pillow between his legs at bedtime. He cries with tears more. When he fell and hurt his elbow, he cried. He used to not feel anything."

Father said, "He sticks his finger in my mouth and feels my teeth. He also trusts me. At the pool, he'll let me put my hand under his back and hold him up to float."

"Jason has been waking up in the middle of the night sobbing with tears. Last night he did, and mother went in to settle him, but he wouldn't get back into bed. He hid behind the bathroom door and giggled. Father put him back into bed and held his door shut. Jason tried to pull the door open but couldn't. He yelled and banged his head on the door and then went to sleep." The parents said they lock their bedroom door at night to keep him out. At first he responded to this by defecating in his bed, but he doesn't do that anymore.

From the parents' reports, Jason is definitely becoming attached to them, especially to mother. She said he wants to be with her all the time. He wants her sole attention. When they have company, Jason intrudes and demands her attention, and this upsets her. (The teacher at school also reported a similar behavior—when she plays with another boy, Jason comes over and pushes him away.) Mother reported he had a "crying jag" once when she got angry with him. Mother said she enjoys having him in the kitchen when she cooks, and he sticks his finger into food to taste. She even let him ride on her back once while she got the whole dinner (the only way to get the dinner done, she said, and he's a big boy). Mother reported that Jason will eat with a knife and fork so long as she keeps her mouth shut and doesn't notice it. If she notices it, Jason will put them down hard and dig into the food with his hands.

From the parents' reports, Jason is more outer directed. He brings out his toys and plays with them. When they have relatives visit them, "he looks at them and studies them a long time. He used to look and then look away." He tries to do what he sees older kids do outside.

Mother said she told Jason not to do something this week, and he stopped. The teacher also reported he stopped being so noisy when she asked.

Both parents sounded pleased. Father said, "It was hard to love him before when he would hit you or not respond. Now it's easier to love him because he's so nice and he's fun. *AND it has been hard work!*"

Comments

To better understand the parents' report, compare my report (p. 48) on Jason for the first four months with the parents' report. Look at my behavior with Jason and then look at the parents' behavior with Jason. In my work with Jason, I am constantly and continually intruding into his world to make him experience my presence—making whatever he did an interaction between us. In the parents' report, it is Jason who is constantly intruding into their world. He is doing to his parents what I did to him—taking the initiative to make contact. He is doing the initiating and forcing them to notice him and be with him in one way or another. By so doing, he is also changing the way they feel about him. They are beginning to like him, at least some of the time. He is a person now and not just a thing. He is a very alive little boy who doesn't let his parents forget that he is present and that he is their son.

The changes in Jason in four months as seen and experienced by his parents are quite remarkable. First of all—and the most important—Jason shows that he enjoys being in the world. He has a good time with people and feels good about himself (his giggling, smiles, the little tricks he plays, such as hiding behind the bathroom door). It is this experience of pleasure that stimulates his bonding to his parents. He wants to continue this feeling of pleasure that he gets from being with them. It is this sense of pleasure that gives Jason the first sense of who he is and the first feeling of an organized self. Jason now has an *I* and can take charge of himself. His behavior, both with me and with his parents, demonstrates that he knows what he wants, can ask for it even without words, that he enjoys it when he gets what he wants, and he reacts when he doesn't get it (sometimes with crying).

Jason is definitely bonded to his parents, especially mother. The fact that he cried a long time when she got angry with him shows how important she is to him. He has feelings. He doesn't want her to be mad at him. He has an emotional tie to her (the definition of attachment).

Jason relates to his parents like a very young two-year-old or younger. His behavior is normal for the developmental stage he's working on. He wants his mother's attention all the time and is "jealous" if she looks at anyone else or talks to anyone else in his presence. Jason clearly communicates his feelings (happiness, sadness, and anger) through his body. He is not passive. He does something to let you know where he is.

At times, Jason's behavior shows a higher level of consciousness. For example, mother's report on his new eating behavior (using the utensils) showed that he did not want her to make a big deal of this new behavior. He wanted this new accomplishment to be *his* accomplishment, not hers. It's *his* achievement! To mother's credit, she got the message.

50

Young children discover who they are first through experiencing and becoming aware of their bodies—through pain (Jason felt pain for the first time), through touching themselves (Jason felt his genitals), and through touching and looking at others (Jason put his fingers in father's mouth to feel his teeth; using his eyes to stare at a relative). Jason is open on three levels—his body, his emotions, and his mind.

Jason could do all these things now (initiate touch, look at, laugh and cry, make demands) because there was someone there to see him, to touch him, to play with him—and Jason was ready and wanting to be seen, touched, and played with. There is a toucher and a person needing to be touched.

The Developmental Play therapist's task is to find ways to introduce new activities which the autistic child can accept. For example, cradling is an extremely important contact for all children to experience, especially autistic children.

Jason responded to my attempt to cradle him in my arms by stiffening his body. I then offered him other ways to experience cradling—being swung in a sheet or rocked in a cardboard box. I had mother hold one end of the sheet while I held the other. At first, Jason had to be picked up and put in the sheet because he didn't understand the directions, "Get in."

Session 17: 6th Month

Present: Mother

> Vi: (Gets the sheet out and spreads it on the floor)
> Jason: (Immediately jumps in, lies down spread-eagle; he looks very relaxed and has a pleased look on his face)
> Mother: (Takes one end of the sheet)
> Vi and (Sing while swinging Jason in the sheet) Rock-a-bye Jason in the tree
> Mother: top, when the wind blows, the cradle will rock; when the bough breaks, the cradle will fall, and down will come Jason and I will catch you.
> Jason: (Said what sounded like) More.
> Vi: More? Okay, you want us to do it again.
> Vi and
> Mother: (Repeats the song with the swinging)

Comments

The excerpt from session 17 illustrates how the Developmental Play therapist encourages contact by paying attention to the child's invitation for contact and by giving meaning to her sounds. Jason's new behavior was his attempt to communicate through speech and his obvious enjoyment in being with us. He feels good about himself.

Session 22: 8th Month

Present: Mother
Setting: Added to other furniture is a cardboard box large enough to hold Jason sitting in it (the cradle box); a simple jigsaw puzzle on the desk.

Jason: (Comes into the office giggling; goes over and stands on the window sill— a sign for Vi to get ready to catch him; he turns his back to Vi)
Vi: (Puts her hand on his back)
Jason: (Falls backward into her arms)
Vi: (Catches him)
Jason: (Lies limp in her arms, totally relaxed)
Vi: (Blows gently on his face)
Jason: (Blows on her face and tries to kiss Vi by touching his mouth to her cheek)
Vi: (Puts him down as his body is getting tense)
Jason: (Walks over and goes into the closet and closes the folding doors; then he opens the doors and appears. This is obviously the Hide and Seek game)
Vi: Peek-A-Boo. Here is Jason.
Jason: (Hides in closet again)
Vi: Now where has that Jason gone? He was here a minute ago.
Jason: (Miraculously appears; laughs)
Vi: Oh, there you are! (Said with delight in her voice)
Jason: (Starts to walk on the tops of all the furniture—the chairs, the back of the couch, the cabinet file, the window sill, the desk)
Vi: (Holds his hand as he does this to support him)
Jason: (Smiles; picks up lotion bottle and drops it)
Vi: (Picking up bottle) Oh, you want to put some lotion on me? (Handing him the lotion bottle; holding out her hand)
Jason: (Puts lotion on Vi's hand and rubs it in)
Vi: Thank you. (Taking the lotion bottle) Put your foot out.
Jason: (Puts foot up)
Vi: (Puts lotion on one foot and then the other)
Jason: (Goes over and looks at puzzle on the desk; touches it twice, sits in the rocking chair, and rocks for the first time)
Vi: (As he rocks, Vi touches parts of his body; he allows it) I got your nose; I got your knee. (sings) Rock-a-bye Jason, etc.

52

Jason: (Smiles; he likes this; goes to mother, says what sounds like) *Get up.* (He wants to ride on her back)

Mother: (Gives him a little ride)

Jason: (Gets the cardboard box, gets in it, looks up at Vi)

Vi: (Rocks him in the box, singing again rock-a-bye Jason)

Jason: (Won't get out of the box at the end of the session; he doesn't want to leave; he finally gets out and then jumps up on Vi, putting his legs around her waist, wanting her to carry him out of the office and to the car; he holds on to her and hugs her hard. [Now, he is also facing her instead of being behind her as when he rides on her back])

Vi: (Carries him out of the office; his hugs are so hard that she experiences them as pain)

Comments

Session 22 in the eighth month illustrates how the DP therapist supports and enhances the autistic child's new behavior that reflects trust and taking risks to explore the outer world. Jason's new behavior demonstrated that he felt safe with me and trusted me. *Trust* is the new quality, the first stage of man (Erikson, 1965).

Jason's new behavior includes the giggling (he's smiled before, but here he's added sound), wanting me to catch him when he falls (new the previous week), being relaxed in my arms for a brief time, kissing me (he doesn't know how to kiss), the hide-and-seek game, walking on the furniture, sitting in the rocking chair, looking at and touching the puzzle, saying what sounds like, "Get up" to mother, not wanting to leave at the end of the session, jumping up on me and wanting me to carry him out of the office, and the "hard" kissing he gives me at the end (pressing his mouth hard against my cheek).

Jason's new behavior expresses the realness of his attachment to me—his trust in me and his delight in being with me. He also uses that new sense of self experienced through me to make more contact with mother when he told her to "Get up." The intensity of Jason's touching (hugging me so tightly and kissing so hard that it hurts) is a reflection not only of his attachment to me but also of his need to touch hard in order to feel anything. (By the time children are two, they should know how to kiss. Jason either blows softly or presses hard on my cheek.)

On my part, I was available to Jason in everything that he did. I understood both his nonverbal and his verbal language. Two interactions need to be noted: 1) Jason's walking on the furniture was both allowed and supported. At this stage in Jason's development when he's trying out new things, he needs to feel successful. The appropriateness of his behavior is irrelevant. At this stage, he is not ready for limit setting. 2) Jason's picking up the lotion bottle and dropping it was interpreted as an intent to make contact with me. And he responded by putting the lotion on me. In other words, I gave meaning to Jason's behavior which, on the surface, had no meaning. And this meaning or intent connected him to me. Meaning and intent comes about through interaction with another.

The DP therapist interprets most child behavior as an attempt to communicate. The DP therapist helps the child experience meaning to her behavior.

Session 24: 9th Month

Present: Mother
Following a two-week break. Jason and Vi are sitting on the floor facing each other.

    Vi: (Taking one foot in her hand and touching each toe) This little pig goes to market, this little pig stayed home, this little pig had roast beef. this little pig had none, and this little pig said, "Wee wee wee all the way home."

Jason: (His lips begin to tremble and a few tears run down his cheeks, but he makes no crying sounds; stares at Vi for a long time as if seeing her for the first time; then climbs into her lap, puts his arm around her, and lays his head in her neck; lies relaxed a long time; then looks up at Vi and hugs her. When time to go, he runs into the other room and hides)

Session 25: 10th Month

Present: Mother

Jason said "apple" when he saw the apple I sliced up for him. When he hid in the closet, he said, "good-bye." He had fun imitating Vi making raspberry cheer sounds with his tongue and mouth. At the end of the session, he responded to Vi asking, "Are you going to say 'Good-bye' by looking at her and waving. (Although his words are approximations, they are definitely meant to be specific words.)

Comments

In session 24, Jason's quiet tears seemed to be related to the first break in the continuity of the therapy sessions. The fact that his behavior in session 22 showed evidence of becoming aware of his feelings of attachment to the therapist (he didn't want to go at the end, and he jumped up on the therapist and put his legs around her waist) supports this premise. His tears showed that he was aware that he missed her. Again in this session (24), he doesn't want to leave (he runs into the other room and hides). That behavior again is evidence for solidness of the attachment phase. The arousal of tears everytime the therapist did "this little pig went to market" may also have been related to a memory of it done earlier in his life (by the therapist, for one).

This emotional experience expressed in the tears also seemed connected to a past memory of being touched. This was the first time he really looked at me for any length of time. The tears helped him experience his own inner self and that self organized him to look at me and to seek nurturance from me. That greater self-organizing ability was reflected in his initiation of more words (speech sounds) in session 25 (saying good-bye when he hid in the closet).

The ability to cry, with tears and with voice, is extremely important for the child's development of her sense of self. The first crying is a call for help that says "I need something" (people, food, diaper changed, to be moved). In Jason's case, his tears expressed a feeling of some depth, an expression of an inner self. When Jason climbed into my lap and laid his head on my neck and looked at me and hugged me, he realized at some unconscious level that he needed this and that he had a right to this nurturance. He was so relaxed and at peace there that I imagined it was like coming home to him. He had been there before at some time.

The tears provided Jason with the experience he needed to be able to look, see me, and make sounds. After the crying, he looked at me as if seeing me for the first time. In Jason's case, tears preceded eye contact.

Session 29: 11th Month

Present: Mother

Mother: (Sitting next to Jason on the couch; whispers in his ear) Go get the box on the desk.
  Jason: (Brings the box to mother)
Mother: (Whispers in his ear) Touch my hand. (Not moving her hand)
  Jason: (Reaches over and touches her hand)
Mother: (Looks pleased)

Mother's Report

Mother reports that Jason wants to be with her all the time. He doesn't want her to leave him. When father drives them to school, he sits on her lap until he has to get out.

Comments

Mother's report shows that Jason is transferring his attachment from the therapist to his mother. He wants her to do the things with him that the therapist does. He would like her just to hold him when father drives them to school. That holding is exactly what he needs. This is hard for mother to do because she wants him to be more advanced—and what mother wouldn't.

Jason, however, is going through his infancy right now to pick up what he needs to grow. At the same time he is going back to get something, he is also going forward very rapidly (initiating contact, being playful, making speech sounds, learning to feel emotionally, crying). As we continue Jason's story, you will notice that, even at age 7, Jason is learning to do things very young children do—for example, finding his mouth and his thumb by sucking his thumb and the comfort from doing it.

Session 46: 16th Month
Present: Mother

In the 16th month, Jason was placed in a residential treatment facility and saw Vi only on some Saturdays.

Jason: (Looks at his hands, studies them. With one hand he pushes the four fingers together of the other hand; then he takes Vi's hand and pushes her four fingers together; then he pushes his hand [the one with the four fingers together] up under her hand; laughs, giggles)

Session 47: 17th Month
Present: Mother (three weeks later)

Today, I saw Jason go over to mother and put his arms around her. She hugged him back. He initiated a lot of contact with her, for example, taking mother's hand to help him do the puzzle. Once he said what sounded like, "Oh well." He smiled and laughed a lot today and was also more quiet and contained. He went to the toilet and urinated on his own. (He was not toilet trained a year ago.)

Vi: Put your feet on mine. (Both Vi and Jason are barefoot and standing)
Jason: (Puts one of his feet on one of Vi's and the other foot on her other foot)
Vi: (Holding him close with her arms around him, starts walking around the room with a rocking motion, singing) Riga jig jig and away we go, away we go; away we go . . . riga jig jig and away we go; hi ho hi ho.
Jason: (At first didn't know if he liked it; then he did)
Vi: (Initiates all the activities we did last time: for example, going out on Vi's porch, going to the piano, wanting Vi to make his hands play)
Vi: (Takes his finger and plays "Mary Had A Little Lamb" on the piano.
Jason: (Smiles—he likes it)

Whenever mother and I talk a little, Jason expresses his displeasure by going into the closet and shutting the folding doors, where he stays until we pay attention to him.

Comments

Since Jason has been placed in a treatment facility during the week, he sees me less often. This seemed to have the effect of "Absence makes the heart grow fonder." He initiated much more contact with mother as well as with me. He also showed three other behaviors—a lot of giggling and laughter, exploring his hands as if just becoming aware that they are part of his body (something infants do before age one), and exploring new, spatial territory (going into other rooms and my porch, outside the office and wanting to play my piano).

Session 51: 18th Month

Present: Mother
Jason is now 7 years old.

This week Jason played with the bottle and the objects on the desk: the little blocks. He put the blocks in the bottle, shook it, and tipped the bottle upside down to get the blocks out. He also, on his own, went over to the desk and worked on the puzzle (a car). When I got out my big sun hat, Jason played with it. When mother put it on, hiding her face, Jason went over, climbed up on her lap and peeked under to see her face. Mother responded by holding him tightly and by kissing him all over. At one point, Jason, sitting on the floor, turned around and just stared at his mother as if seeing her for the first time.

Today, Jason made two different sounds—one that sounds like a "yes," and one that sounds like a "no." In a clapping-our-hands game, he wanted me to hold my hands in a certain position.

Session 53: 19th Month

Present: Father

Jason: (Upon entering, looks at Vi, comes over and kisses her, looks around the room, perhaps looking for mother; he looks like he's thinking. For 20 minutes sobs loudly, tears running down his cheeks. Then he reaches out, takes Vi's hand, plays with it, and holds it close to his stomach)

Vi: (Strokes him, touching his tears) There's a tear and it's running down your cheek.

Jason: (Stares quietly at Vi for long time; later goes over and looks at book on desk, plays with it)

Vi: (Gets out the sheet for rocking him)

Jason: (Does a little dance before jumping in. This time, he sits up as we swing him; he doesn't want to stop. Wants her to play piano in other room, shown by taking her hand and leading her to the piano.)

Vi: (Plays "Mary Had A Little Lamb")

Jason: (Smiles—likes it)

Comments

Jason's behavior in the two sessions above show that he is not only bonded to mother, but he is aware of his emotional tie to mother. The evidence for this awareness is shown in his eye contact—staring at mother (staring is something healthy infants do) and in his sobbing, a new behavior (when mother is absent, he misses her). The sobbing in session 53 shows that Jason has internalized his mother; that is, he has memory of her when she's not present (the permanent object stage). His eye contact (which was very slow in appearing) seemed to follow or coincide with his ability to cry and his attempts to talk. All these behaviors emerge as both mother and child interact in a way to create a relationship. They are both the result of and evidence for the existence of a relationship.

This relationship is reflected in Jason's emerging sense of joy, of spontaneity, of just being alive (his little dances). In addition to his growing interest in people, Jason also shows increasing interest in the outer world (his exploring the other rooms outside of my office, his playing with the bottle and working on the puzzle).

Sessions 51 and 53 illustrate how the Developmental Play therapist responds to and supports the autistic child's emotional expressions and exploratory behavior. I went along with Jason's exploring my other rooms outside of the office. He is not ready for limit setting. He needs to feel success when he does almost anything on his own at this stage. His leaving my office did have a tinge of testing-me-out behavior, but I went along with it for the time being.

Session 56: 20th Month

Present: Father

Vi: (Got the sticks out, taking two and handing Jason two)

Jason: (Wants Vi's two sticks also)

Vi: No. These are my sticks and those are yours. (Pointing to his two sticks)

Jason: (Cries briefly, eyes wet but no sounds; pushes his face up against Vi's lips
        hard, wanting her to kiss him)
    Vi: (Kisses him hard, making loud sounds on his lips)
Jason: (Repeats this over and over—putting his mouth hard on Vi's cheek)
    Vi: (Sitting opposite Jason on the floor, taps his stick)
Jason: (Looks at Vi lovingly, wants her to put her stick between his toes)
    Vi: (Puts her stick between his toes)
Jason: (Makes a soft blowing sound)
    Vi: (Imitates his soft blowing sound)
Jason: (Looks at Vi, smiles—he likes it)

Comments

Jason takes a step forward in session 56, 20th month. He can handle the
limit setting which I provided (by not allowing him to take my sticks) because he
has a relationship with me now. Jason reacted first with tears, showing that he
felt the rejection and that he has an emotional tie to me. Then he recouped by
initiating contact with me—his hard kissing. It almost felt like "making-up" behavior. Then he asked me to do something for him (put my stick between his
toes), which I did. I am important enough now to Jason that he is willing to experience some pain in order to keep contact with me. This is an extremely important stage in any young child's life. It means that he can experience the pain and
still maintain the relationship.

Session 57: 20th Month

Present: Father

Jason played ball today. When told to pick up the ball, he did. When told to
throw it to me, he did. When told to hold out his hands to catch the ball, he did.
When told to throw the ball to father, he did. Jason opens the top drawer of my
desk and peeks in, then closes it. I lie on the floor and pull Jason, face down, on
top of me and we roll over. He likes it.

Session 58: 20th Month

Present: Father

Jason: (Enters room, comes over and kisses Vi)
    Vi: (Hugs him back, sticks her tongue out at him)

Jason: (Looks at her, sticks his tongue out at her. Sits studying the fingers of one hand, opening and closing his hand, watching it open and close)
  Vi: (At end of session) Time to go.
Jason: (Puts shoes and socks on, comes over and kisses Vi good-bye)

Session 61: 23rd Month

Present: Father

Jason: (Standing on the file cabinet, looking at Vi, ready for her to catch him)
  Vi: (Standing back and holding her arms up) You can jump by yourself now, Jason.
Jason: (Looks scared, but finally jumps, looks happy and pleased)
  Vi: You look happy, Jason. See, you did it!

Session 62: 23rd Month

Present: Father

  Vi: (Alone in her office; hears a knock on the door, goes to the door, opens it, doesn't see anyone, looks down, sees Jason on his knees)
Jason: (Looking up at her laughing)
  Vi: (With a little gasp of surprise followed by laughing) Oh, it's you, Jason. You caught me by surprise. You really did!
Jason: (Closes the door and repeats this game with Vi)
  Vi: (At end of session) Time to go, Jason.
Jason: (Cries, doesn't want to leave, puts his cheek on Vi's)
  Vi: (Walks down the stairs, out the door with Jason and father)
Jason: (Sitting in their car, watches Vi wave good-bye as they drive off)

Comments

Excerpts from sessions 57, 58, 61, 62 and months 20-22 illustrate how the DP therapist provides activities that help a child experience herself in contact with the therapist and how she provides activities that help a child experience herself separate from the therapist. For example, I responded to and supported Jason's kissing me at the beginning of the hour and at the end of the hour (like his Hello and Good-bye ritual). I also supported him doing something by himself by jumping off the file cabinet without holding on to me.

Jason showed growth in his ability to be influenced by an adult—doing as requested, imitating an adult, accepting my support for the jump. The most amazing behavior, in terms of cognitive growth, was his "joke" played on me. To do this required a feeling of attachment and a desire to please, a memory of what he usually does and a fantasy of doing something different (Jason kneeling at my door). It also required a memory of what I usually do and a fantasy of what my reaction might be when I open the door and no one is there. This represents enormous cognitive growth for this boy, even if he just thought of it at the moment of arrival (which is probably how it happened). It's the beginning of abstract thinking. Jason is also becoming curious (peeking in my desk drawer).

Session 65: 25th Month

Present: Father

Family returned from a two-week vacation. Father reported upon arrival that Jason had a hard time at school today.

Jason: (Comes in crying, head down, no eye contact. Pushes Vi off the couch, sits on it, cries; saliva is running out of his mouth; he picks lint up off the floor, eats it and runs out of the room)
Father: (Brings him back)
Vi: (Touching him gently on the head) I'm here to play with you, Jason.
Jason: (Gradually comes around, initiates old games, plays his jumping-off-the file game)
Vi: (Initiates the Row Row Your Boat game while sitting on the floor)
Jason: (Straddles Vi, a familiar game to him)
Vi: (Sings the song while rocking him back and forth, after which she pulls him over on top of her, holding him close, face to face)
Jason: (Allows Vi to comfort him; he begins to look at her) *At the end of the session* (Grabs Vi's hand, holding it tight, indicates that he wants her to walk him out the door)
Vi: (Walks him outside)

Session 67: 25th Month

Present: Father

Jason: (Initiates the Row Row Your Boat game, but this time he wants to roll completely over instead of just side to side; he actively does this while making singing sounds)
Vi: (Tapping her mouth, says, "Ah, Ah, Ah [like Indians])
Jason: (Imitates her) Ah, Ah, Ah. (Touches Vi's face with his mouth open; presses his face against hers so hard that it hurts her)
Vi: (Holds him while she sits in the rocking chair)
Jason: (Allows it now although he is not completely relaxed)

Comments

Session 65 illustrates how traumatic changes in routine are for autistic children. Jason had been away on vacation (trauma by itself) and had to return to school after this absence (another trauma). It was devastating. I had never seen this behavior before—the drooling, picking up lint and eating it, and being totally out of contact. Parents reported that he does this when they argue. When things get hectic at school, teachers report this behavior. I never knew he did this until now.

This session illustrates how a DP therapist helps an autistic child connect again after such a devastating experience. In session 67, Jason lets me hold him for the first time with me sitting in the rocking chair.

Session 69: 26th Month

Present: Father

Jason: (Came in smiling—tests Vi out by going out to her porch and putting his legs up on the railing; that is a no-no. He does get down and comes to the room)

Vi: (Carries him in her arms with his face up close to hers, touching his face)

Jason: (Is relaxed and allows this for a long time)

Vi: (Sits down in the rocking chair holding Jason and sings Rock-A-Bye Jason)

Jason: (Is more relaxed this time and allows it for long time; looks up at Vi, sticks his finger in her mouth and plays with her mouth as small babies do)

Vi: (Puts her finger in his mouth and massages his gums)

Jason: (Some time later gets up and goes to the door)

Vi: Not time yet, Jason.

Jason: (Comes back, sits on floor, looks sad and starts crying: then gets up and goes to door again)

Vi: Not time yet, Jason.

Jason: (Comes back to Vi, leans against her and starts crying again)

Vi: (Strokes him)

Jason: (Allows Vi to comfort him. In leaving at the end of the session, Jason looks back to see if Vi is still there)

Father: (to Vi) He has said "mama" several times at home.

62

Session 70: 27th Month

Present: Mother

Jason: (When Vi picks him up and rocks him, now he puts his arm around her; when he cries, he crawls up into her lap, plasters his front against her front and rests his head in her neck)

Vi: (Makes him into a gingerbread cookie)

Jason: (Allows all of this until time to be baked. At the end as he and mother go out, he looks back to see if mother is there)

Mother: I'm here.

Jason: (Looks around to see if Vi is still there)

Comments

Jason started his first sobbing in the 19th month. (His first tears were at 9 months, but there were no sounds—following a break in therapy.) That crying seemed related to mother being absent for the first time. In the 26th and 27th month, he did more crying, sessions where he cried nearly the whole time, but it was a quiet kind of crying that seemed to make him feel present with me. He just seemed to want to be with me in a quiet way without doing anything (laying his head against me). With the crying came eye contact and the feeling that I was important to him. He initiated kisses and hugs. When I hugged him, he would hug back; that was new. He would look at me with a definite loving look. He clearly showed over and over that he did not want to leave at the end. Even without words, this feeling was strong enough that father got it ("Jason just loves coming here"). You will see the evidence of his increasing attachment to me in the remaining sessions.

This attachment was reflected in Jason's allowing me to cradle him with his body being totally relaxed—after 2 1/2 years. Even the first games, which we still played at times, were experienced differently by him. When I did the Slippery Foot game, he would just let go and sit there looking at me with such loving looks. Another behavior that was new was his giggling, his little dances, and his feeling of joy when he arrived. These are some of the things to notice in the next sessions.

Session 71: 27th Month

Present: Mother

Jason: (Sits in rocking chair, rocks, then holds up his face to Vi to be kissed)

Vi: (Kisses him)

Jason: (Goes over to mother who is sitting on the floor: he wants her to do
    something, taking her hand)

Mother: Say Up.

Jason: (Seems to really want to be with her today: he tries again to get her to
    do something, maybe to rock the chair as Vi did. He kisses her; he tries
    to pull her up)

Mother: (Does not move)

   Vi: (to Mother) He really wants you to do something. I think you should re-
    spond.

Mother: (to Vi) He needs to be frustrated sometimes.

Jason: (Withdraws, just sits on the floor, with no eye contact)

Mother: (to Jason) I love you.

Comments

Parents of an autistic child get very excited when their child says a word or
what sounds like a word. They have high hopes now that their child will talk. As a
result, they tend to put pressure on the child to say words on command. The child
cannot do that until his spontaneous involuntary speech is more highly developed
through play and wanting to be with someone because she is having fun. If a child
hasn't begun to talk by three and that child is also autistic, the chances of her developing speech for communication is very slim. Jason, who is over 7 now, is beginning to try to communicate with "words." At his age, that is quite unusual.

Jason's emerging speech came about because I responded to his non-verbal
(body movement) communication and gave it meaning in terms of our relationship. The experience of enjoyment with me moved him to add sounds to his body
movements, and these sounds are specific. They sound more and more like "Up,
no, more, mama." At this stage, however, to demand that Jason say words to get
his needs met is asking him to do the impossible. I tested this out myself, and he
could not do it. However, you will notice that as our work progresses and Jason
feels closer to me, he uses more words for communication.

Session 73: 28th Month

Present: Mother (After Vi's Vacation)

Jason: (Hugs Vi, squeezing her very hard. Puts his face on her face. Puts his
    hand on her head, pulls her hair hard and laughs)

   Vi: Let go of my hair, Jason. That hurts.

Jason: (Continues to pull hard)

Vi: (Pulls his hair just as hard as he is pulling hers)

Jason: (Lets go of Vi's hair. Explores making lip sounds—spitting and enjoying it)

Vi: (Gives Jason paper and Crayon)

Jason: (Scribbles on two papers and looks at one of them)

Vi: (Opens the book of the Three Bears and asks Jason to) Show me the baby bear.

Jason: (Points correctly)

Vi: Show me the daddy bear? The mama bear?

Jason: (Does it. Later, says to father, who is sitting in the rocking chair) Up. (Wants father out of the chair)

Father: (Gets out of the chair)

Jason: (At the end of the session, takes Vi's hand to walk down the stairs; halfway down, says) Up.

Vi: (Turns around and walks back up with him and father, saying) Up . . . up . . . up.

Comments

In session 73, following a break in our relationship due to my vacation, Jason showed several new behaviors: 1) Pulling my hair (which mother reports he does to her—this behavior may be his reaction to my absence); 2) he does what I ask him to do (using the Crayons, pointing to pictures in the book); 3) he's very assertive with father and uses a word to tell father to get out of the rocking chair; and 4) after leaving, going down the stairs, he stops halfway, points to the top, and says "Up." Jason seemed to be getting a sense of ownership—that the rocking chair belongs to him. He used speech to communicate to father, and his message was very clear ("Up." Get out of that chair. *That's my chair.*).

This session illustrates how a DP therapist takes an autistic child's new behavior one step further. For example, when Jason said "Up" as he pointed up, I walked down and took his hand, father took his other hand, and all three of us walked back up, saying on each step, "Up. Up. Up."

Session 76: 30th Month

Present: Father

Jason: (Takes his shirt off and drops it behind the file cabinet, looks down at it, takes Vi's hand for her to retrieve it)

Vi: (Reaches down and picks up his shirt)

Jason: (Takes puzzle pieces from the desk, drops them down behind the file
cabinet, takes Vi's hand for her to retrieve them)
  Vi: (Retrieves them)
Jason: (Wants to ride on her back)
  Vi: (Allows it)
Jason: (Climbs up on her back, putting his knees on her shoulders and resting
his cheek against hers)
  Vi: (Walks around for brief time)
Jason: (Giggles, makes "talking" sounds)
  Vi: (Puts him down)
Jason: (Stands on file cabinet and stomps his feet *hard*)
  Vi: (Imitates him by stomping her feet on the floor)

No Session 81: 31st Month

Father misunderstood that Vi would not be here on this day and brought Jason
anyway.

Father: We climbed up the stairs, knocked on the door, and turned the knob—
nobody came to the door.
Jason: (Cried all the way back home)

Comments

In session 76, Jason is very active, doing what he needs to do. What he did
shows that developmentally, Jason is at about a 1 or 1 1/2-year-old level. Dropping objects behind my file and watching them drop is the behavior of a two-year-
old in her high-chair dropping food and spoons and watching them fall. Riding on
my shoulders, an old behavior of his, is also that of a young child. Stomping on
my file cabinet had a new quality—one of energy and truly feeling his body moving, of feeling truly alive and loving it. As the DP therapist, I encouraged him by
stomping my feet on the floor in rhythm with him, smiling as I did it. For an autistic child as disturbed as Jason to initiate some physical activity that makes him
feel pleasurably alive is very wonderful to see. My goal was to enable Jason to
both experience his body moving and the pleasure that accompanies it. It's a fun
thing to do! This new sense of aliveness is reflected in Jason's new behavior at
home reported by father.

Parents' Report

Father reported that Jason has learned to ride his two-wheeled bicycle. Father also reported that suddenly Jason has begun to eat. "He's eating as if food is going out of style. Now he eats everything; before only bread."

Session 81 demonstrated that Jason, in his crying reaction to my absence, has internalized me and can experience disappointment and pain.

Session 85: 33rd Month

Present: Father

Jason: (Comes in, goes out to my porch, looks around and then giggles as if he's laughing at a private joke: tests Vi out by putting a foot up on top of railing—standing on the railing is a no-no)

Vi and
Father: (Lead Jason back to the office)

Jason: (Gets in rocking chair: wants Vi to rock him hard so that he has to hold on in order not to fall out. At the end of each rock, he covers his eyes and puts his head in his arms)

Vi: Where is Jason? Jason's gone away. (Peeking under his face, finding his eyes)

Jason: (Looks at Vi; puts his arms down. This game is repeated several times; Jason enjoys this play he set up)

Father: (Sits in rocking chair later in the hour)

Jason: (Gets very angry: screams, hits father in the back hard)

Vi: (Takes Jason's hand, trying to get him to rock father in chair)

Jason: (Still angry—no response to Vi)

Father: (Gets out of the chair)

Jason: (Sits in rocking chair)

Father: (Trying to be playful, tries to slide into the chair next to Jason— three times he tries)

Jason: (Pushing father out of the chair)

Vi: (To father) Father, he's giving you a message. He doesn't want you in the chair. He doesn't know how to respond to your teasing.

Jason: (For the rest of the hour is very upset; he lies on the floor crying. He hits the floor hard [It was as if his beautiful rhythm of enjoyment had been spoiled by father, and he couldn't get it back])

Father: (Moves to hug Jason)

Jason: (Turns away from father)

Vi: Give me your hand, Jason.

Jason: (Gives Vi his hand; crawls toward Vi and puts his head in her lap; gets up and gets in the rocking chair)

Father: (to Vi) Rock it softly.

Vi: (Rocks Jason in the rocking chair very gently)

Jason: (Gets upset with Vi if she doesn't get his message that sometimes he wants to be rocked slow and soft and sometimes rough and fast, shown by butting his head into her stomach)

Father: (to Vi) Jason is getting very subtle in telling you exactly what he wants.

Vi: You're right!

Father: I was only seeing what would happen if I teased him.

Vi: And you found out. That's the way you find out. When you do something (like you did when you sat in his chair), you observe and pay attention to Jason's responses. In your case just now, he tried to push you out of the chair. That message is pretty clear. You don't need words to get it. For you, that means you have to change your view of Jason. He is not like an older child who would enjoy you doing this—playing game of chairs with you. Jason did not find what you did funny. When he smiles and wants more, he is communicating that he likes it and he likes being with you.

Jason: (Lingers at the end of the hour as if he doesn't want to leave. When the sheet is brought out for father and Vi to rock him, he goes over to the desk and looks at the puzzle before getting in the sheet. He takes Vi's hand to walk out)

Comments

The most exciting happening in session 85 was Jason's ability to be angry with father, to express this anger in a focused direct way, to accept my comfort and to pull himself together and go back to what he was doing before father interrupted his play. He could accept my help and, at the same time, keep his goal in mind. This was quite amazing for him to be able to do.

Session 86: 33rd Month

Present: Father

Jason: (Reaches his arms up to Vi, puts his arm around her, pulls her down to his level, hugs her and holds her tight)

Vi: (Picks Jason up, holds him, rubs her cheek against his) Your cheek is so soft and nice—no wonder your father likes to hug you.

Jason: (Smiles—shows he likes it. Puts his thumb in his mouth and sucks his thumb for the first time)

Vi: (Draws a face on paper on the desk and gives Jason a Crayon)

Jason: (Takes the Crayon, makes some marks on the side of the head this time as opposed to scribbling over the face as he previously did)

Vi: *At the end of the session* (Picks Jason up and cradles him while sitting in the rocking chair, sings) Rock-A-Bye Jason, etc.

Jason: *(For the first time allows himself to be totally relaxed during the cradling with Vi sitting in the rocking chair)*

Vi: (Could feel his body let go more and more until it went limp) Jason is letting me love him today.

Session 92: 36th Month

Present: Father

Jason: (Keeps pulling on my plant)

Vi: (Tells him No-No, but he keeps doing it; Vi slaps his hand with the No-No)

Jason: (Raises his hand to pull plant and then puts it down)

Vi: Good, Jason. (Gets paper and Crayon out)

Jason: (Draws a long time on the paper, scribbling)

Vi: Sit down, Jason, and I'll do your feet.

Jason: (Sits immediately, smiles, hands Vi the lotion bottle, holds up his foot)

Vi: (Does the Slippery Feet and Hand game)

Jason: (Wants his arms done over and over)

Vi: (Touching each toe) This little pig goes to market, etc.

Jason: (Soft, silent tears roll down his cheeks looking at Vi)

Vi: (Hugged him tight and kissed him noisily all over)

Jason: (Looks at Vi with that quiet, direct loving look; being totally present with her; makes sounds that sounded like he says "Happy") *When time to go* (sits motionless on the file cabinet looking very sad)

Father: (Gets the sheet and gets in it himself)

Vi: (Sings Rock-A-Bye to father)

Jason: (Still sitting, looks sad)

Session 94: 37th Month

Present: Father

Jason: (Jumps up and down on couch, distancing himself from Vi)
   Vi: (Grabs him, hugs him tightly and kisses him hard—the way he likes)
Jason: (Smiles—likes it—is present with Vi now) (Initiates the Row-Row-Your-Boat game by taking Vi's hands and sitting down)
   Vi: (Pulls him over on her stomach)
Jason: (Holds Vi close and repeats the game)
Jason: (Goes over and smells her plant instead of pulling it out. Goes and stands on the window sill and hides behind the curtains, sometimes peeking out to be acknowledged, sometimes sitting on the window sill just being quiet and hidden behind the curtain; does this a long time)
   Vi: (Gets drawing paper and Crayons out)
Jason: (Makes horizontal lines for the first time) (Once when Vi kisses him, his eyes cross)
Father: (When time to go) Put your shirt on. Time to go home.
Jason: No (Said loud and clear)

Comments

An activity initiated by Jason the last year was his standing or sitting in the window sill behind the curtain and ever so often peeking out at us. Sometimes he would sit with his feet up on the sill, and he would just quietly sit behind the curtain in a peaceful way, not withdrawn but listening to father or mother and me talk. It was not the hide-and-seek game, but rather like a baby playing in his bed while others are around. Quite nice, in fact.

Session 102: 41st Month

Present: Father (Jason was sick the past week and therefore had no session)

Jason: (Today he seems overcome with joy to be here; runs and claps his hands)
   Vi: (Initiates the Circle Time with father, Jason and her, singing) If you're happy and you know it, clap your hands, etc.
Jason: (Claps his hands, then runs out into the hall)
   Vi: Where is Jason?
Jason: (Comes walking in as if announcing himself, stands there smiling) (Goes to the door, touches the door knob but doesn't go out)
   Vi: (Gets drawing paper out)

Jason: (Starts drawing a part of a face)
  Vi: (Draws the outline of the head) (To Jason) Put the eyes in.
Jason: (Draws the eyes, nose and mouth) (At the end takes Vi's hand and wants her to go downstairs with him to the car, as if to take Vi home with him)
Father: (to Vi) Jason loves to come here.
  Vi: (Takes Jason's hand, walks downstairs with him and father, watches them drive off in car)
Jason: (As car moves away, watches Vi, waves good-bye)

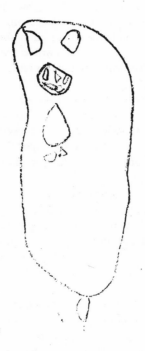

Jason's Drawing

Comments

At the time, I didn't know that this was going to be our last session. Jason's behavior, however, seemed to show that he had some awareness that it was when he wanted me to walk him down to the car and watch him and father drive off.

OVERVIEW OF JASON'S THERAPY

When I first met Jason, I remarked on his very limited self-initiated behavior and that his scarce repertory included no move toward others or behavior that appeared responsive to what others did or said. In all but physical appearance I felt I was meeting an infant; mentally and emotionally, Jason had hardly grown since infancy. I perceived that his overriding need was for the psychological development that would coalesce into a sense of self. Accordingly, as his therapist my task was to awaken the dormant seed of self that lies within the newborn human.

Because Jason was so like an infant at the beginning of therapy, I assumed total responsibility for him as any good parent does for her baby. I took the initiative; I directed all the action of the early sessions. I touched Jason, held him, carried him, chose our play. Such activities are suitable for an infant, but even more important was the effort I made to ensure that what I did would give pleasure to Jason. I deliberately sought to make his contacts with me so pleasurable that Jason would want more.

To succeed in this, I had to attend closely to Jason's body language (nonverbal communication through gesture, facial expression, tone of voice, posture, etc.). This was not easy. I had to learn what body expression showed Jason felt pleasure and what expression showed he wanted something specific from me. With a child not normally expressive and one who avoided communicating, I often, at first, had to make educated guesses.

When I observed, for example, that Jason wanted to be touched, I touched him and tried hard to make that touch a delight to him. While doing what he wanted, I also openly showed my delight in him and my pleasure in being with him. My intent was to bring Jason into a relationship with me by providing him with experiences that convinced him that relating to another person could make him feel happy and alive. Perhaps "the Godfather" would say that what I did was offer Jason a deal he couldn't refuse.

Even in the very first session, Jason intimated (by holding out his hand to me) that he wanted me to do again what apparently had pleased him, or at least interested him (my holding his hand briefly). In subsequent sessions, I made numerous much longer and closer physical contacts with him. These pleasured Jason and also led him to allow experience of his body into his awareness. Over time, he began to recognize and to own his bodily self. In this, he was taking the first step a very young child makes toward self-recognition. The fruits of the loving touches by a loving adult who saw him were that Jason came alive, that he felt his body as vigorously alive, and that he liked the feeling. It also meant he was willing to venture into using his body purposefully; for instance, he learned to play ball and to control and direct his running and jumping.

Life force, unimpeded, manifests in the young in growth. Jason began to evidence the growth he had not achieved in his actual infancy and young childhood. He began to feel pain and to cry with tears and sobbing sounds; he sucked his thumb; he learned to blow, to kiss, to look at his hands (as babies do). He used his eyes to look and stare (as babies do); he smiled and giggled and felt hunger and ate (as babies do). Of greatest importance for the development of his capacity to relate to others, he learned to trust me. (It was first apparent that he did trust me when he finally allowed his body to relax when I cradled him.) As therapy progressed, Jason matured beyond infancy. He showed this especially in his emotional development. He became capable of feeling and openly expressing a variety of emotions. These included both physical and emotional pain, sadness, disappointment, anger, joy, contentment, and love. He clearly communicated these feelings, though not by speech. He defecated when angry, drooled and picked up lint when he felt hopeless, attacked those who angered him by hitting or butting his head into them. His strong love for me shone in his facial expression and his gaze. It was a poignant, moving experience for me when Jason chose to sit with me, not moving, often with quiet tears running down his cheeks, absorbed in lovingly looking at me. An inner wisdom seemed to tell him how much he needed experiences of simply being with another in deeply felt, undisturbed communion.

The stimulus for all of Jason's growth was his bonding to me in a close, loving relationship. This bond developed and grew strong because a Developmental Play therapist provided the relationship needed for an autistic child to feel touched. Moreover, I worked to develop a similar bond between Jason and each of his parents. During the therapy sessions, I encouraged meetings between Jason and the parent who was present. I discussed with his parents how they could also see Jason in their home. Jason's parents began to understand Jason's need for bonding with them. According to his father, it was dramatically evident. He said, a few weeks after therapy began, "It's fun now being with Jason; but he won't leave us alone, and that's very draining." No doubt the bonding process was both gratifying and difficult for Jason's parents. It is hard to be available to the suddenly urgent demands for relating with an older child functioning at the level of a very young child. Yet Jason did bond with his parents, and they progressed in their ability to see him. As he met with me less often in the final 18 months of therapy, his development was sustained and furthered by his emotional bonds with his parents.

At the time therapy terminated, Jason was 9 1/2. He was a public school student in a program for handicapped children. His teachers said he was learning. Both his teacher and his fellow students liked him. Jason liked them, too, and took part in games and other school activities with them. He still did not talk. (Years later his parents told me he never learned speech). Jason did learn sign language, showing his strong desire to communicate.

Developmental Play therapy helped this autistic child to develop a sense of self. Although Jason did make many speech sounds that clearly expressed specific words, he never really developed speech. He was, however, able to relate, to feel, to express those feelings and to communicate what he wanted and what he did not want even without words. He joined his fellow human beings in the give and take of the world they hold common. All of this testifies to the effectiveness of Developmental Play therapy with an autistic child, and all the changes Jason was able to make pleased me. But, most of all, I was pleased that Jason also came to feel good about the self he became, with his giggles and his "joke." That judgment is the touchstone for enthusiastic participation in what life has to offer.

This case study shows the effect of being touched on one autistic boy, Jason, at age 6.

A Word About Tears and Crying

Along with touch, crying is a basic avenue for communication. Tears are a physical expression of the body, but crying is an emotional expression that shows a connection to someone. Crying gives evidence that you belong to someone, and the crying brings back that connection.

In addition, tears are a normal function of the body. If a child has never cried, her body is not functioning. One autistic child with whom I worked did not cry. Her tears were first expressed by her whole body. She perspired with her whole body. It was as if her whole body cried. Then she began to have a few tears just coming from her eyes. She would describe her eyes as "wet." Eventually, she could sob. Then she would say, "I'm crying."

Jason began crying, without sound at first, with just a tear or two followed by more tears. Later he cried with big sobs. All the autistic children with whom I worked did this. "Crying is an experience of the care-taking self" (Levin, 1988, p. 173).

In my work, two things preceded the emergence of the crying. The child shows she is attached to the therapist. She shows she enjoys coming. Then some event interrupts the continuity of the meetings (vacations, holiday breaks, termination). Jason's first tears came in the ninth month after a two-week break. His sobbing came after longer breaks and especially when mother came much less often and father brought him instead.

All the autistic children with whom I worked, including Jason, seemed to enjoy their crying at some level because often they would do it for the whole session. For example, they would get up to go, and I would say, "It's not time yet."

74

Then they would come back, lean against me or put their head in my lap, and start crying again. (More than one child did this.) When Jason did this, he would sit and just look at me as if seeing me for the first time. Jason's eye contact really appeared during and after his crying periods. "Only with the crying, only then, does vision begin" (Levin, 1988, p. 172).

The effect of this crying on all these children, including Jason, was to release a lot of energy to do new things. They could still cry, but they didn't cry all the time. They seemed to have a new sense of freedom—to provide their own structure (games and activities and especially exploration). Jason, for example, acted so free as he tried out different things in my office (for example, jumping off my file cabinet all by himself). He became interested in things in my office and doing things with people. He wanted to look around and explore, going into the room with the piano and out on the porch. He did this at the end of the hour, and I allowed it. For a boy who could do absolutely nothing in the beginning, he needed as few limits as possible—as does a two-year-old. During this period right after the crying, Jason tried to communicate with words. The most important effect of all was Jason's intense feeling of pure joy—his giggling, his smiles, and his joke.

From my experience with many very disturbed children, I believe that the experience of being able to cry with sound is essential for their healing. The crying makes the child aware that she has a relationship. The crying deepens the relationship, makes it more stable, and provides the conditions needed for the child to move on, as demonstrated with Jason.

A FINAL NOTE

The chapter on autism in the history of therapy recounts how difficult its treatment has been and how often it is only partially successful or unsuccessful. This remains true today when the prominent therapeutic approaches are behavior modification and pain-producing aversive and punishment techniques, the latter based on the belief that causing pain will force the autistic child to abandon her isolation and turn to her parents for comfort (Lovaas, 1971, 1977).

The Developmental Play therapy approach to the autistic child contrasts sharply with these current therapies. Behavior modification can sometimes change specific behaviors but does not promote capacity for choice and creative activity, essential functions of the self. The Developmental Play therapist further insists that pain does not lead to healthy bonding. On the contrary, the stimulus to bonding is the pleasure felt by the autistic child in the presence of a loving adult who sees her. That opens the child to relationship and its accompanying emotions, including, as with Jason, the eventual recognition and tolerance of pain. Experiencing a sense of aliveness, experiencing energy, delight, quiet and exuberant pleasure in the presence of an adult therapist and then with parents is the effective basis for bonding.

Developmental Play therapy, then, stands in opposition to pain-producing stimuli as therapeutic method in the treatment of an autistic child. Jason's treatment exemplifies the alternate Developmental Play therapy approach and puts forward its rationale.

4 TOUCHING PSYCHOSIS: DEVELOPMENTAL PLAY THERAPY WITH KENNY

Psychotic children are more advanced developmentally than are most autistic children. They can take care of themselves at a basic level and carry on the ordinary transactions of family life most of the time. They usually have excellent speech, but they don't use it to get their needs met.

Psychotic children respond to not getting their needs met by creating a fantasy world into which they withdraw. Living in a fantasy world, however, cuts them off from the real people needed to enable them to know who they really are. Their withdrawing into their own world is often accompanied by periods of explosive, destructive, acting-out, out-of-control behavior. These children have no core self—the part of the child that knows how to communicate what it needs. These behaviors describe Kenny.

KENNY, A PSYCHOTIC CHILD

At age 6, Kenny was brought to me by his parents for Developmental Play therapy. From mother, I learned that she first became concerned about Kenny (their first child) when he was two because he didn't talk. He didn't talk at three. The pediatrician said not to worry. At age 3 1/2, he was placed in a preschool class for handicapped children. At 4 1/2, he was assigned to a 15-week group Developmental Play program for eight 4-year-old boys—all very disturbed boys. Each boy had his own therapist sitting on the floor facing him who played with him for one-half hour. Each child-adult pair was assigned a specific place in the room. This one-to-one play was followed by Circle Time where the adults, each holding their child, sat in a circle and helped their child interact with the other children in activities led by the Leader. I was one of the child therapists, but I did not work with Kenny. (For further details on the DP group program, see Chapter 5.)

Although Kenny seemed to enjoy this group at times, he was very tense, hyperactive, easily distracted, and aggressive. He did considerable yelling and screaming.

At age 5, Kenny began withholding his stools. He was given enemas every other day until the pediatrician told the parents to stop. At age 6, the parents brought Kenny to me for DP therapy.

Mother said she was "desperate," that she had been to many medical doctors and that nothing helped. One of them suggested she place Kenny in a residential program. Mother added that she, herself, was an only child, that she had never been around children much in her growing up, and that she had no idea what to do with Kenny. She said she felt no love for her child, but it was evident to me that she was trying very hard to be with him. She got little support from father. (The parents have a second child, a girl, two years younger than Kenny. They seem to have no problem with her.)

When I saw Kenny at age 6, he was a handsome, blond-haired boy with a solidly built body, large for his age. When asked to list Kenny's qualities—both positive and negative—his parents described the following behaviors:

Qualities parents liked about Kenny

Mother: Can converse nicely with parent, can play nicely with sister at times, well-behaved when drawing and playing by himself, when he's doing some activity nicely with parent is intelligent, imaginative.

Father: Bright, has potential, lovable, enjoys the outdoors, interested in tools and woodworking, handsome young man, full of energy, hungry for knowledge.

Qualities parents disliked about Kenny

Mother: Whiny, temper tantrums, back-talk, uncooperative, soils pants, loud voice, rowdy behavior, fights and teases little sister, constant storm of endless talk and questions to the point that it's annoying.

Father: Sometimes rude, unreasonable and demanding, selfish, does not pay attention to directions, too much of a perfectionist, gets frustrated too easily.

The parents paint a picture of a child with high potential, a child with tremendous energy expressed in intense demand for attention and drive to be accepted. What stands out in their report is the unevenness in Kenny's behavior.

His "nice, lovable, hungry for knowledge" qualities contrasts with "rude, rowdy, back-talk, demanding, doesn't pay attention" behavior. Both Kenny and his parents experienced much frustration.

I saw Kenny as lacking a core self that begins with a bodily self. The bodily self is experienced though touch. My goal in working with Kenny was to provide him with the relationship needed for him to feel touched—to feel himself being touched by me.

The first year, I worked with Kenny and mother together. First I worked with Kenny in the session and mother observed. Then mother would play with Kenny and I would observe and/or coach her. Some of these sessions were videotaped, and mother saw these. My purpose in doing it this way was to demonstrate how to make contact with Kenny and then have her practice doing it.

This case study presents the basic work I did with Kenny the first year to help him develop a sense of self. Following the termination of work with Kenny, I worked with mother for 2 1/2 years to help her become a capable toucher.

DEVELOPMENTAL PLAY THERAPY WITH KENNY

Session 1

Present: Kenny, Mother, and Vi.
Setting: The same as described for Jason—a couch, a rocking chair, a desk and chair, and low file cabinet.

Vi: (Sitting on the couch, holding Kenny on her lap, looking at him, touching him; mother in rocking chair observing Vi and Kenny) I have to say Hello to your eyes.

Kenny: (Looking away from Vi) Hello.

Vi: Wait. I have to see if anybody is in there. Hello, Kenny. Anybody there? (Looking into his eyes as if they were windows)

Kenny: No.

Vi: Nobody home? I see the window shade is up. Let's see. (Putting her face close to his, looking into his eyes; Vi plays Knock at the Door game) (see Appendix)

Kenny: (Opens his mouth)

Vi: Oh, the door is open. Hello.

Kenny: Why couldn't we do this in the circle? (Referring to Circle Time in the DP group program he was in)

Vi: We're doing it right now. Here's your forehead. (Kissing it) Your two eyes. Your nose, lips, chin. (Touching them) And did you bring all your toes?

Kenny: All ten. Now watch. (Counts them)

     Vi: You're wonderful—the way you can count.

Kenny: I want to listen to the tape.

     Vi: Let's see if all your fingers are here.

Kenny: (Counts them)

     Vi: You are so smart. (Kissing him) Did you know you had hills and valleys in your hand? (see Appendix) (Sliding her finger down and up between each finger on each hand)

Kenny: Can I listen to the tape recorder?

     Vi: After a while.

Kenny: What are you doing?

     Vi: I'm putting some lotion on your hands and arms. Isn't that nice? Let's see if this elbow works. (Moving his elbow) Look at this. Your elbow can do all these things.

Kenny: Like poke?

     Vi: We don't poke.

Kenny: Like touch?

     Vi: Yes, like touch.

Kenny: (Interrupts Vi's doing the Slippery Hand game, knocks on his forehead with his fist) Knock Knock peep in, open the latch on the door.

     Vi: Oh, you remember that. (Continuing on with the Slippery Hand game she had started) Are you ready to pull?

Kenny: Yup. (Pulling his arm through Vi's hands)

     Vi: Keep pulling.

Kenny: (Holds up the same hand for a repeat)

     Vi: Oh, this hand says, "Do it again." (Not taking the offered hand but picking up the other hand) Would *this* one like some?

Kenny: Yes. (Starts pounding his fist on Vi's file cabinet)

     Vi: Keep pulling . . . all the way.

Kenny: (Starts pulling loose buttons off the back of the couch)

     Vi: Please don't pull those off.

Kenny: (Sings very loudly) Good morning. It's my favorite. Good morning.

     Vi: Oh, am I your favorite?

Kenny: No. Is your sister coming?

     Vi: No.

Kenny: I want to meet your sister.

     Vi: (Putting her hand over his abdomen) See if you can breathe. Push my hand out.

Kenny: (Tries to do as Vi asked)

Vi: There you go. Keep doing it.

Kenny: I want to listen to the tape.

Vi: Right now, I have to do your feet. (Massaging them with lotion)

Kenny: Oh, okay.

Vi: Were you glad you came today?

Kenny: Yes.

Vi: Would you tell me you were glad you came?

Kenny: (In mocking tones) I'm glad to come today. I can tell today is Wednesday.

Vi: That's right.

Kenny: Every Wednesday.

Vi: We used to have Developmental Play every Wednesday (referring to the 15-week DP program he was in where I was also present)

Kenny: And you were in there.

Vi: That's right.

Kenny: Your name is not Dr. Rody.

Vi: Brody is one of my names, but you can call me Vi.

Kenny: I like to call you Vi, and my Mommy calls you Dr. Brody.

Vi: (Returning to his legs; massaging them with lotion) I have to finish this leg.

Kenny: Beep beep. Can I listen to the tape recorder?

Vi: Right now I'm doing your feet. Can you feel me touching your toe?

Kenny: No.

Vi: You can't? (Looking at it: touching it) Hello Big Toe.

Kenny: Go down in the valley (see Appendix).

Vi: Go down in the valley? Here we go. (Sliding her finger up and down between his toes; repeats with other foot) Down in the valley, over the hill, and then it goes right up your leg, over your head, around here and down to your toes. (Moving her hand over his body)

Kenny: (Imitating Vi's hand movements with gestures in the air and Vi's words) Down in the valley, up in the valley, round in the valley, come back. (His movements are random; they do not fit his words)

Vi: Close your eyes and see if you can tell where I am touching you. Where did I touch you?

Kenny: On my knee.

Vi: That's right. (Kissing him) Did you feel it that time? Oh, you're looking at me.

Kenny: Do it again.

Vi: Okay. This is a hard one. (Touching his chin) Where did I touch you?

Kenny: On my mouth.

Vi: What's this? (Touching it) It's your chin.

Kenny: On my chin.

Vi: (Kissing him on his chin) Now close your eyes. I'm going to give you a real hard one and no peeking. (Touches his thumb)

Kenny: My thumb.

Vi: Oh, you're wonderful. Now are you ready? This is going to be so hard. Are you ready?

Kenny: Yes.

Vi: (Touches his big toe)

Kenny: My toe.

Vi: Which toe?

Kenny: (Points to big toe)

Vi: That's right. (Kisses him) You are superb.

Kenny: I'm superb. (Laughing) The trombone, the trombone. (Pushing against my shoulders hard) I'm going to do Hills and Valleys on your toes.

Vi: Gently, gently! You can do it on my hands.

Kenny: (Taking Vi's hand and moving his finger between her fingers) Up in the valley, down in the valley, up in the valley. (His movements do not fit his words; i.e., on "up" he's going down) Let me do it to your toes.

Vi: I haven't made a gingerbread cookie boy yet. (Placing him lying down across her lap) (see Appendix)

Kenny: Do it with gingerbread flour and take a little shorter [sic], just make a tiny one. I'm ready. (Lies quietly across her lap)

Vi: We mix the dough. (Gently massaging his body)

Kenny: Just a tiny cookie.

Vi: For a tiny boy.

Kenny: For a tiny Vi. And it was my birthday. I had a tiny cookie and a V for Vi.

Vi: And now I'm mixing you up. I take out my rolling pin and smooth you out. (Gently rolling her arm over him from head to toe) Now I take my cookie cutter and make your head (outlining it with her hand), and here's your shoulders, arms, hands fingers, body, legs, feet and toes. (Outlining his whole body)

Kenny: (Hears a truck outside; makes noise of truck) The truck goes all around your room.

Vi: (Continuing) I'm making this toe, and the next one, and the next one, the next one, and the little one that said wee wee wee all the way home.

Kenny: A cherry for my buttons . . . and my eyes, my mouth, whipped cream for hair.

Vi: Now I put you in the oven. (Leaving him on her lap as if her lap were the oven; makes SHHH sounds) Here is the heat.

Kenny: I'm done.

Vi: Oh, you're not done. Feel how nice it is here. (Slowly moving her hands over his body from head to toes) Are you done?

Kenny: Yes. (He doesn't move, lies very still, his eyes trance-like; slowly sits up)

Vi: You can sit quietly too, like this. (to mother) Notice how quiet he is. When he's in that quiet place, just let him be there.

Mother: He's not as still with me.

Kenny: I do good with Vi and I'm not good with you. (Said quietly)

Mother: I said you're not as still.

Kenny: I know.

Mother: I didn't say *good*. (slightly hostile tone)

Vi: (to Kenny) You can do it with your mother, too. It's nice to have Mother do this with you too, right?

Kenny: Right. Are we almost finished?

Vi: I have to take you out of the oven and taste you. (Kissing him on his hands and face) You taste so good. You're yummy.

Kenny: Do my legs, arms, waist. Don't eat this. (His belly button) Okay. That's decoration.

Vi: I'm going to let you be with your mother now.

Mother's work with Kenny:

Mother: (Holds Kenny on her lap as she sits in the rocking chair)

Kenny: You're going to rock me, and then I can draw.

Mother: Hello Kenny. How's my boy today?

Kenny: (Has gotten a pillow and put it under his head; he is lying there quietly with thumb in his mouth. He begins to close his eyes)

Mother: Let's see if you have any kissable spots. (Starts kissing him fast and loudly) They're coming back like polka dots.

Kenny: I don't like your arm under me.

Mother: Oh, excuse me. I'll put it here.

Kenny: (Snuggles into the pillow, sucks his thumb)

Mother: (Starts kissing him again) Look at those kissable spots. They're coming out again.

Kenny: (Loud voice) Don't do it. . . no more . . . no more.

Mother: (Continuing) I didn't get these.

Kenny: (Loud voice) Can I . . . can I . . .

Mother: You smell like . . .
Kenny: Can I play with that football? (a toy football in room)

At this point, Vi interrupts and says to mother that she doesn't have to work so hard, that she could just be quiet and really look at Kenny and see where he is. She could just quietly rock him and both be quiet.

Mother: (Rocking Kenny and chanting in a soft voice) Rock, rock. It's so nice to rock. It's so nice to feel you. It's so nice to hold you. You can relax.
Kenny: Rock fast . . . rock fast.
Mother: You can rest after a busy day at school.
Kenny: I don't want to. I can't see the words. (Of a saying on the wall)
Mother: (Chanting) Comfy, cozy.
Kenny: (Pinches her)
Mother: You don't pinch. You don't need to pinch. (No anger in her voice)
Kenny: Bite.
Mother: No biting and no pinching. (Said more firmly) You can bite the pillow. That's fine.
Kenny: I'll bit you then.
Mother: You don't bite. We kiss and hug. (Hugs him) My goodness, that mouth is wide open. I see the door.
Kenny: I'm going to close it. Put your finger in there. (Teasing tone)
Mother: Oh, my goodness.
Kenny: (Yelling) Put it in there!
Mother: (Hugs and kisses him)
Kenny: (Yelling) Put it there!
Mother: I'll put a kiss in there.
Kenny: (Softer voice) I want the pillow the other way.
Mother: How's that?
Kenny: (Opens mouth)
Mother: The door is open wide. Are you welcoming me in?
Kenny: (Soft voice) Yes. Come in.
Mother: Oh, a kiss went in there. (Kissing him on the mouth)
Kenny: (Yells) *Don't! Stop it!*
Mother: Oh, I put all my kisses in there.
Kenny: (Screaming) Stop it, Mommy!
Mother: (Kissing him) All my kisses went in.
Kenny: (Yelling) Mommy, they're breaking the dishes.
Mother: Breaking the dishes? (Laughs, kisses him) I though they were unbreakable dishes.

Kenny: (Makes crying sounds) They're breakable. Now they're broken.
Mother: Now I'll put them all back.
Kenny: Now can I get up? (Said calmly)
   Vi: Yes. And here is drawing paper. You said you wanted to draw.
Kenny: I'm writing my name and smiling face [sic]. It's going to be a long time before I finish.
   Vi: You don't want to leave?
Kenny: I don't want to leave, because I like you.
   Vi: Thank you. I like you, too.

Mother's reaction to observing Vi play with Kenny:

It's so different from anything I've seen before (laughing and smiling). I have to think about it a little more. If somebody asked me how I would describe it . . . it's different. I see where it gives a personal contact . . . that you normally don't have in everyday life . . . by the massaging and the lotion . . . the rocking. It's more personal contact than in day-to-day life. You don't know how little personal contact you have. There hasn't been that much contact. You know I feel like I have some with my children, but not that great amount . . . concentrated time . . . specific time set aside for it. Mine is just kind of here and there . . . you know, during the day, but it's not concentrated like that. I think I understand what you're doing behind it.

Comments

These verbatim excerpts from session 1 illustrate how a DP therapist said Hello to a psychotic, very unfocused boy—how she enabled him to experience his body being touched by her and to feel contact with her through touch.

1. *The DP therapist paid attention to Kenny's cues.* For example, Kenny turned away from Vi when she said Hello to his eyes, and he didn't seem to feel her touches. He constantly tried to distract her from what she was doing. Kenny moved away from contact. Kenny tried to control, but what he did when he tried to control was not organized and was out of sync with what Vi was doing with him. Therefore, as she worked with Kenny, she saw that he could not use touching as a way to experience his body until he experienced limits.

2. *The DP therapist set limits for Kenny.* Limit setting is not always a "No" or "Stop that" or "You can't do that." With Kenny, Vi set limits in a subtle way—by ignoring his distracting and controlling behavior and bringing his

attention back to feeling his body being touched by her. She did this over and over again. In doing this, she created boundaries for Kenny. He didn't have to do anything but be with her in the present and experience his own boundaries. She set limits through touch.

3. *The DP therapist used massive doses of touch to bring Kenny's awareness to his body*—awareness that his body is being touched by Vi, that his body has feelings. Vi held Kenny on her lap, counted fingers and toes, looked for kissable places on his face and hands, played focused body-contact games involving hands (The Slippery Hand and Hills and Valleys games), face (Knock at the Door game), and the whole body (The Gingerbread Cookie game). See Appendix for DP games.

What the DP therapist learned about Kenny from session 1: Kenny is a child without a sense of self, without an "I." He has no boundaries. He cannot separate what is *not* he from what *is* he: he cannot distinguish stimuli that come from inside him from stimuli that come from the outside. For example, as Vi touched parts of his body in making the gingerbread cookie, Kenny heard a truck outside, made the noise of the truck and said, "The truck goes all around your room." He seemed totally unaware that Vi was touching him. He could not shut out outside stimuli and be present with Vi. It was hard for him to stay focused on anything—even his body. His behavior had a psychotic quality.

At first, Kenny could not respond to anything Vi said or did. What he initiated had nothing to do with what Vi was doing. He tried to get her angry, but this was not a conscious act. He just seemed to need to control her.

Kenny also had problems with language, although his speech was excellent. Sometimes he just said words that did not fit the gestures he was making. He could not play the Knock at the Door game because he could not imagine himself in space and time. He could not feel his body being touched in the present.

One thing is clear: talking does not help Kenny. It only makes him feel less connected. He cannot relate through language because he lacks the experiences that give words meaning. Touch and holding is the avenue to meaning and relationship for Kenny.

By the end of this session, however, Kenny was able to feel himself being held by Vi. He let go of his need to control and just lay relaxed in her arms, with thumb in mouth and eyes nearly closed. He was also able to respond to Vi calmly with a relationship statement: "I don't want to leave because I like you." He began the hour with no sense of who he is. He ended it with the ability to allow himself to be touched and held. He had the beginnings of a bodily self.

Mother's work with Kenny: Mother had a hard time, but I'm not sure she experienced it that way. Her time with Kenny began with Kenny telling her what to do ("Rock me") as he lay in mother's lap with a pillow under his head, which he had put there. She didn't respond to him. Instead, she introduced something else ("How's my boy today?"). Kenny then got himself comfortable with a pillow, put his thumb in his mouth and closed his eyes. Mother didn't get his message again— his desire just to be quiet and relaxed with her. With her loud, noisy kisses, she disturbed his peace. He tried at first to ignore her, but she continued to do it. Eventually, he resorted to yelling at her, "Don't do it . . . no more . . . no more!"

· At that point, when I tried to coach her, it didn't work. Kenny's peace was already disturbed. She paid no attention to his continued screaming. From then on, both mother and Kenny dealt with each other from a fantasy place. Their talk about the "broken dishes" was very strange and had a psychotic quality. It was as if both were in a strange land and neither one was aware of it. They couldn't find "home" because they've never been "home." They were out of touch with each other.

That this "personal contact" through touch felt very foreign to mother was expressed both in her reaction to observing Vi play with Kenny (p. 83) and in her own work with Kenny. It became obvious from this session that mother was never going to be a capable toucher for Kenny until she herself learned to experience herself touched.

Session 7

Present: Mother, Kenny, Vi, and person videotaping. Family had been on vacation for two weeks.

Vi: (Cradling Kenny in her lap) I haven't seen you for a while. Let's see if you are all here. (Placing her face close to his and her arm around him) Here are your eyes. (Touching them) Here are your ears. (Touching them)

Kenny: (Turns his head away)

Vi: You're with me right now. (Turning his face toward her: putting her cheek next to his) Let's see how this cheek feels.

Kenny: (Pulls away; no eye contact) Ow.

Vi: Have you got any new teeth? I see two holes in your nose. Can you breathe? (Putting her hand on his stomach)

Kenny: (Breathes; puts thumb in his mouth)

Vi: Oh, you're wonderful. (Hugs him)

Kenny: (Pulls away) Why you taking pictures? (Referring to the videotaping)

Vi: You know. We've done that before. (Stroking his cheek) You've been
      out in the sun.
Kenny: (Looks away)
Vi: I haven't rocked you in a long time.
Kenny: (Looks up at ceiling)
Vi: (Holding him closer) Let's see if you have any kissable places.
Kenny: (Closes his eyes; sucks his thumb)
Vi: There's one. (Kissing his hand)
Kenny: (Pulls away; grins and laughs loudly; kicks with one foot) I'm going to
      break your ceiling. (In loud voice)
Vi: (Ignoring his remarks; continuing) Is there one on your ear?
Kenny: (Loud, silly laughter that he can't seem to stop) I'm going to break your
      ceiling down.
Vi: (Attempts to distract him by tapping on his mouth as he's yelling)
Kenny: (Just yells louder)
Vi: (Pulls him close to her and holds him tightly with her face against his)
      I'm going to rock you right now. (Sings) Here is Kenny, here is Kenny,
      etc.
Kenny: (Fights it, whines, continues his silly laughter and yelling)
Vi: You haven't said hello to me yet. You can scream all you want to. I'm
      going to hold you right here. (Said firmly)
Kenny: Let go of my hand!
Vi: Stop pulling away, then. (Loosens her hold on him)
Kenny: (Relaxes, puts thumb in his mouth)
Vi: This is more like it. I haven't seen you for a while, and you haven't said
      hello yet.
Kenny: (Lies quiet for a few moments) I got to go to the bathroom. (Goes to
      bathroom, returns and wants mother and Vi to go look at his BM)
Vi and
Mother: (Go to bathroom and return)
Vi: (Resumes holding Kenny)
Kenny: (Lies quietly sucking his thumb, looks as if he's planning something,
      something mischievous judging from the grin on his face; laughs) I'm
      going to break your. . . (Stops himself)
Vi: (Picking up bottle of lotion) I think you need some lotion. (Does the
      Slippery Hand game with him).
Kenny: I'm going to slip away from you, and I won't come back! (In loud voice)
Vi: Are you mad because you didn't see me for two weeks?
Kenny: Yeah, Yeah, Yeah. I'm mad. (Bellows it out)

Vi: Did you have a good time on vacation?
Kenny: Yes.
Vi: Tell me that.
Kenny: Yes.
Vi: With mommy and daddy.
Kenny: Yes. (Gets silly—out-of-contact laughter)
Vi: Are you testing me out to see how bad you can be, to see if I still like you?
Kenny: (Giggly; kicks Vi)
Vi: (Stopping him by holding his leg) We don't kick. (Holds him tightly; his head is on her shoulders)
Kenny: (For few moments lets Vi rock him without fighting it) (Yells) I'm going to draw on your wall.
Vi: (Continues singing) Rock-a-bye Kenny, etc.
Kenny: (Although his body is still, from the expression on his face, he seems to be planning some mischief)

Comments

In session 7, Kenny had a new task to master; namely, to learn how to reconnect after an absence (family vacation). After an absence, everyone requires a little time to get reacquainted. Kenny had a hard time.

Kenny showed his difficulty at the beginning by turning away from the therapist and then by getting silly and lashing out with "I'm going to break your ceiling; I'm going to slip away from you, and I won't come back; I'm going to draw on your wall." He couldn't seem to stop himself.

To help him experience his body by being held, I picked him up and held him tightly. He responded with a very loud, "Let go of my hand." When I loosened my hold on him, he became quiet and relaxed for a few moments. Then he said he had to go to the bathroom. Upon returning, he wanted his mother and the therapist to go and look at his BM. (This request shows his developmental level of functioning.)

What the therapist did. Only two things the therapist did seemed to help: when she put her hand on his abdomen and told him to breathe, and when she held him tightly and he yelled, "Let go of my hand." In those two places he relaxed, lying quietly with his thumb in his mouth.

These quiet moments, however, did not last, and the other touching games that had worked before didn't this time. He would let me put the lotion on him, and he would lie still during the cradling at the end; but I could tell by his face and the feel of his body that he was not letting me in at all. He was busy thinking up something mischievous.

This session points out that no matter how you touch or hold a child, he may not allow himself to feel the touch; no matter what you do, nothing works (or it feels that way to the therapist).

Kenny's new behavior. One thing was positive, however. Kenny felt more alive. Kenny's usual pattern is to respond to people by distracting them—his way of controlling them. When he does that, he is not feeling anything. It's his usual habit. In this session, however, Kenny's shouting made him feel the energy in his body. He also experienced himself being out of control. Yet, at the same time, he was not punished. At one point, he did show some self-control, indicating some awareness of his behavior, when he stopped himself in the middle of his sentence ("I'm going to break you . . .").

This session shows how fragile Kenny's inner structure is. His behavior shows the effects on it by a change in the ordinary routine of living (going on a vacation and missing his therapy sessions). This change totally wrecked the little internal structure he had. Yet, Kenny gained a lot from the experience of this psychotic break, as will be seen in session 10.

Session 10
Present: Kenny, Mother, Vi.

Kenny: Why you got that poster on your wall?
   Vi: I like it.
Kenny: You going to change it every day?
   Vi: I'm going to be with you right now. (Picking him up and holding him on her lap, sitting on the couch)
Kenny: We going to have Circle Time?
   Vi: I heard you were at camp today. Did you have a good time?
Kenny: Yes.
   Vi: Who did you play with?
Kenny: This was the first day. Tomorrow will be #2 and tomorrow will be #3 [sic]. (Begins to talk faster, not looking at Vi) It started to thunder and they told us to get out right away.
   Vi: I have to say hello to you now. (Turning his face toward her)
Kenny: Why you got shorts on?
   Vi: You've got shorts on, too. Let's say hello to your eyes. (Touching them gently) Hello, nose (Touching it)
Kenny: (Covers his mouth)

90

Vi: Oh, your mouth has gone away. Now you are looking at me. Where is your mouth? Is it in your ear? Is it in your other ear? (Looking in each ear)

Kenny: (Uncovers his mouth)

Vi: Now your mouth has come back. Something is in there.

Kenny: Teeth.

Vi: And something else.

Kenny: Tongue.

Vi: Right. (Looking at his feet) Your feet are wet and full of sand (Carries him to the bathroom; washes his feet and dries them) Look in the mirror. Who is that?

Kenny: Me.

Vi: And who is me?

Kenny: Kenny.

Vi: (Brings him back into the room and shows him how to stand on his head, holding his feet against the wall) Put your hands down. Feel your feet against the wall?

Kenny: Yes.

Vi: (Counts to see how long he can do it)

Kenny: I can do somersaults. (Smiles) (Does one forward and one backward)

Vi and
Mother: (Clap)

Vi: Do that again! You have to push hard with your feet to get over. (Kenny does it) Come back here to me now. (Sitting on couch, takes him on her lap)

Kenny: (Leans his head against her shoulder, sucks his thumb, looks up at Vi, relaxed)

Vi: You're so quiet. (Without touching him, chants softly) I see your eyes, I see your nose, I see your mouth, I see your cheeks, your cheek is so soft. (Puts her face close to his cheek)

Kenny: Can I take that picture home? (Pointing to picture on wall)

Vi: No, it belongs to me.

Kenny: When you don't need it anymore, will you give it to me?

Vi: No, because I'm going to leave it there. When you go home, you can make a picture for your wall. Right now, I'm going to paint a picture of you. (Taking her finger for the paint brush, touches every part of his face; names and describes each part) And this is a little boy and his name is Kenny. (See Portrait Game, Appendix)

Kenny: I'm supposed to meet my teacher at the diving board. I swam at the shallow end.

Vi: (Continues portrait game) And here's your backbone, and your arm, and your elbow, and your arm goes down like this (touching every part). And you have something on your hand (a green X). What does that mean?

Kenny: That means I go to the diving board.

Vi: Oh, that's what it means.

Kenny: This hand (with the X) is dangerous.

Vi: And this finger? (The finger looks bruised)

Kenny: It means I "axelenity"...

Vi: Accidentally, you got a bruise?

Kenny: Yes, and don't touch no fingers. It'll hurt.

Vi: I better kiss that part. (Kissing bruised finger)

Kenny: It's all my fingers. Don't touch that one.

Vi: Oh, this little finger would like to be touched.

Kenny: You can't touch them. I told you. (Yells) Don't touch them!

Vi: As I am rocking you, I feel how soft your cheek is. I haven't given you a butterfly kiss (see Appendix) in a long time. (Brushes her eyebrows on his cheek) You're looking at me. You're so quiet. And it's nice to hold you like this.

Kenny: Aren't we going to do Circle Time?

Vi: No. We're not doing that.

Kenny: Why? (Yells) I want Circle Time.

Vi: Because I like being with you like this. (Continues as before, talking in a monotonous, hypnotic rhythm and tone regardless of the subject) And here's your hair. We don't do the same thing every time. Look at all the somersaults you did today, and look at that ear. It's got lines in it. Let's see if there's a sound in there. Can you make a sound?

Kenny: (Hums with her and gently taps his mouth as Vi had once done to him)

Vi: You're so nice today. I like being with you.

Kenny: I'm going to make a picture just like that one (one on the wall). Would you hang it up?

Vi: You bring it. I'll hang it up. (Continuing in her monotonous voice) Oh, these are nice fingers. They like to be touched.

Kenny: (Yelling) It's dangerous. See!

Vi: It's not dangerous. I'm not going to let those fingers do anything bad. I'm not going to let them hurt anybody.

Kenny: (Pointing to his right hand, talking in calm voice) This one is okay.

92

Vi: This one is good.

Kenny: And this one is bad (left hand).

Vi: One is good, and one is bad. I see. What can we do to make this hand good?

Kenny: Put a Band-Aid on it.

Vi: Oh, that's a wonderful idea! Here's a Band-Aid. (Pretending to have one and pretending to put it on). And I'm putting it on your hand. Maybe if I kiss it, too. (Kisses his hand)

Kenny: (Yelling) You get a real Band-Aid.

Vi: We can have a pretend Band-Aid like this. (Touching him)

Kenny: It's a real cut . . . a real Band-Aid.

Vi: Where is the cut? (He does not have a real cut)

Kenny: Right across here (pointing to his palm), up to my thumb and all around in a circle.

Vi: We got to fix this one up (the "bruised" finger)

Kenny: A big Band-Aid.

Vi: (Moving her fingers around his hand and in between his fingers, talking in a sing-song voice) One around here and one in between here, etc.

Kenny: (Lying very relaxed; not talking)

Vi: You're so quiet and lying here so nicely—wonderful.

Kenny: Will you give me something for being good?

Vi: Yes. I will give you something.

Kenny: What?

Vi: (Kisses him all over) You taste so good.

Kenny: Give me a rainbow.

Vi: I'll make you one, right here. (Making one on his face) I like it this way. You taste so good. How many kisses shall I give you?

Kenny: Zero.

Vi: Only zero—after you did all those somersaults? I think you're worth five kisses. (Kisses him)

Kenny: No. Zero. (Doesn't resist the kissing now)

Vi: And you turned the bad hand into a good one.

Kenny: It's not better yet. It'll take a while.

Vi: You're letting me hold you.

Kenny: It'll take four weeks.

Vi: So you'll be coming at least four weeks.

Kenny: (Is rubbing Vi's back very gently, giving her some love pats, touching her hair) (Not talking)

Vi: Oh, that finger came around for a kiss. (Kisses it) It was rubbing my back, and now it's touching my hair.

Kenny: When are you going to get a hair cut?

Vi: When did you get one?

Kenny: A long time ago.

Vi: Your hair is beautiful. (Touching it)

Kenny: Don't touch it. It's got oil in it.

Vi: Oh, that won't hurt anything.

Kenny: It's hot oil. It will burn you.

Vi: What will we do to make your hair so I can touch it?

Kenny: Put a Band-Aid on it.

Vi: (to mother) Have you got any Band-Aids?

Mother: (Pretending to look in her purse) I've got a lot of Band-Aids. (Hands one over to Vi)

Vi: (Pretending to put Band-Aid on Kenny's head)

Kenny: And one more.

Vi: Mother, do you have any more?

Mother: (Hands Vi a pretend one)

Vi: (Puts it on Kenny's head)

Kenny: (Lying in Vi's arms so quietly, really feeling her touching him) You got one for the back, Mommy?

Mother: I should have brought the whole box. (Hands Vi one)

Vi: (Puts it on the back of his neck and kisses it)

Kenny: You got a giant one, Mommy, for my middle?

Mother: Oh, yeah. Oh, boy. (Hands Vi one)

Kenny: (Smiles, laughs) Yeah.

Vi: Look, it goes clear to your toes. (As she moves her hands from his middle to his toes)

Kenny: Don't cover my eyes.

Vi: I won't. I'll just do the sides of your head.

Kenny: Now take the big Band-Aid off. It feels better now.

Vi: It's better. Okay, are you ready? I'm going to peel it off. (Pretending that it is sticking over his whole body) Oh, can you feel it pulling off? I got it off. (Tosses it over to mother to put in the waste basket)

Kenny: And my hand is better. Throw that one away.

Vi: (Rubs it off)

Kenny: For real.

Vi: We got rid of that X sign that said you're dangerous. (Kisses place where X sign was)

94

Kenny: Oh, oh! The thumb is dangerous. You got another Band-Aid?

Vi: (Puts Band-Aid on the thumb, thereby giving the thumb a massage)

Kenny: Now take my head Band-Aid off. (After Vi takes the Band-Aid off, Kenny wants to talk into the tape recorder)

Vi: (Taking the mike and speaking into it) Ladies and gentlemen. This is Kenny we are interviewing today. Kenny, what can you tell us about yourself?

Kenny: I can do somersaults, and I am 6 years old.

Vi: What do you like best that you are doing with me?

Kenny: Rocking.

Following this, Kenny had his session with mother. She held him as she sat in the rocking chair. Mother reviewed what he had done that morning in getting ready for camp, adding how pleased she was with him. Kenny, in turn, said in a coherent way, without any of his out-of-contact silliness, what he had done at camp that day. Then Kenny and mother each drew a picture. It was important to Kenny that mother put a "sun" and "smiling faces" in her drawing. At the end:

Vi: (To Kenny) Looks like you're really happy today.

Kenny: Yes.

Vi: Look at your mother and say it.

Kenny: (Not looking at mother) I'm happy today.

Comments

Kenny's interactions with Vi in session 10 support the theory upon which Developmental Play therapy is based: namely, that children who experience caring touch from an adult who knows how to touch will grow, develop, and heal earlier traumas. In this session, Kenny began not only to allow himself to be touched, but he began to experience himself being touched by Vi, to experience the touching as pleasurable, and to ask for it. Kenny has met the basic goal of DP therapy.

Kenny's behavior demonstrates how touch is the basic ingredient children need to stimulate growth. Once Kenny got to the place where he could allow Vi's touching, he became a different child. He could engage in a dialogue with her. In this dialogue, however, he participated as a much younger child. The child that he became was a two- or three-year-old—the way he played with Vi's hair, his peek-a-boo game with his mouth, sucking his thumb, his request for mother and Vi to look at his BM (in session 7), his inability to separate fantasy from reality (saying it makes it so), and his delight in experiencing being touched in the Band-Aid game that he created.

Kenny's growth started at the place where growth had stopped. He went back to this earlier period to pick up and bring forward what he had missed so that he could move on. One of the experiences he had missed was being touched by a capable toucher.

Kenny's behavior also demonstrates the ongoing quality of the growth started by the touching relationship. Once the child picks up the earlier stage needed for growth, she moves at the same time into a later stage. For example, Kenny made a "giant leap" in session 10 when he assessed his own growth using excellent language and abstract thinking: "It's not better yet. It'll take a while. It'll take four weeks."

Experiencing the earlier stage freed Kenny to be more mature. Kenny could cooperate with Vi, could accept some suggestions from her to help him provide his own structure. There were moments where Vi and Kenny worked together to build their relationship. In other words, Kenny could utilize Vi as a *"You"* for her to help him find his *"I"*. And that was a true dialogue. (See Buber, p. 26.)

Kenny was much more quiet. Instead of using talk to control the outer world, he used it to express wants and needs that came from inside him. In this session, Kenny had a breakthrough wherein he separated from himself what was not him. In that moment when Kenny suddenly experienced Vi's touch as pleasurable—expressed in his asking for a Band-Aid for his "dangerous" thumb—he separated fantasy from reality, thought from body feelings. At that moment, Kenny *knew* that he was pretending, knew that he was using an old behavior to get something new—to get Vi to touch him more. He delighted in his discovery. And so did Vi! Kenny has a core self.

Kenny's behavior in session 10 demonstrated the three stages through which children progress during Developmental Play therapy: 1) Learning to allow tactile contact and.to experience it as pleasurable; 2) behaving and experiencing themselves as much younger children; and 3) behaving and experiencing themselves as children at a later stage—even more advanced than their chronological age. In Kenny's case, all three stages appeared within one session.

The DP therapist's work with Kenny: The DP therapist has three tasks in working with a child: 1) To provide the child with the conditions needed for her to feel touched; 2) to respond to the child's invitations for contact in a way that helps her create her own structure for growth; and 3) to support the child's feeling good about herself.

1. *Vi continued her touching and holding Kenny.* In the Band-Aid game he created, he received what amounted to a total body massage—once

when Vi put the Band-Aids on his body and once when he asked her to take them off. Touching was required to do both.

Vi invited Kenny to contribute to finding a way that his body could be made safe to touch. Vi used his Band-aid idea (a metaphor for healing) as an avenue for providing him with touch.

Vi has been touching Kenny for several weeks, but it is in this session that he truly experiences her touching him. His asking for more and more speaks for his awareness of the pleasure. The pleasure makes him aware of his body, how much fun it is to be with Vi, and that he has a self.

In this session, Vi added her voice to her holding—chanting in a monotonous, sing-song, hypnotic rhythm and tone. That was extremely effective. She ignored all his distractions and just continued her monotonous tone. Kenny stopped talking, put his thumb in his mouth, and lay in her arms in a trance for a few moments.

It was Vi's consistent and persistent touching that enabled Kenny to experience his body. Experiencing his body being touched enabled him to feel real. His fears of destroying or being destroyed vanished. He began to live in the real world. Kenny himself said that it was "for real."

2. *Vi responded to his cues and invitation for contact.* In this session, Kenny had something to say to Vi. She responded to his saying that one hand was bad by asking him how that hand could be helped. He could answer coherently ("Put a Band-Aid on it"). From that, he created the whole wonderful Band-Aid game. He wanted more "Band-Aids," and Vi responded. He asked to speak into the microphone. Vi furnished the structure for this by making it an interview of Kenny. Again, he responded to Vi's questions coherently: "I can do somersaults and I am six years old." And, he liked the "Rocking" best. By responding to Kenny's invitations for contact, Vi enabled Kenny to speak for himself.

3. *Vi helped Kenny to feel good about himself.* First, she made Kenny feel safe with her by protecting him from being overwhelmed by his destructive fantasies. Vi said, "I'm not going to let them (his fingers) hurt anything or anybody." Because he was enabled to feel safe, Kenny could ask for his whole body to be touched. Vi helped Kenny do something with his body (stand on his head), and this gave him the idea of turning somersaults, for which he received applause from mother and Vi. Vi expressed delight in his enjoyment of being touched more and more—all over. She also gave him the opportunity of defining himself ("I can do somersaults and I am six years old") and saying how he felt ("I'm happy today").

Session 18

Present: Kenny, Mother, Vi. At the beginning of this session, mother worked
with Kenny. He is sitting on her lap.

Mother: Are we going to play some records?
Kenny: Yes.
Mother: Are we going to play some of my records? Oh, boy! I can play some of
        mine. Okay, let's turn the record on. Let's see what kind of song is on
        there. (Singing) Jingle bells, jingle bells. I must have gotten my Christ-
        mas records out. (Continues singing)
Kenny: (Yells) No Christmas records. (Pushes her away)
Mother: (With tinge of anger in her voice) Wait a minute. Got to treat my re-
        cords gently here. Let's try this record. (Pretending to take one out)
Kenny: What one?
Mother: I don't know. My records are all mixed up. (Sings) You are my sunshine.
Kenny: No, not that one.
Mother: You don't want that one, either?
Kenny: No. (Begins silly, out-of-contact laughing)
Mother: (Singing) How much is that doggie in the window.
Kenny: No, not that one.
Mother: My gracious. Let's try this one.
Kenny: (Laughing) Okay.
Mother: (Singing) Rain, rain go away.
Kenny: No, not that one.
Mother: Oh, no. (Little laugh)
Kenny: (Silly giggle)
Mother: My records are all mixed up. I don't know what I'm playing.
Kenny: Do it.
Mother: (Starts rocking and singing) Rock-a-bye baby.
Kenny: No, not that one. (Giggling)
Mother: Those are my lullaby records. Let's try this one. (Pretending to pick out
        another record)
Kenny: (Laughing and silliness increases)
Mother: Oh, my goodness. (Singing) Mary had a little lamb.
Kenny: No, not that one. (Laughing)
Mother: Those are nursery rimes.
Kenny: Oh, let's try the back then.

Mother: Okay. Let's see what's on the back. (Pretending to look, sings) Little boy blue, come blow your horn, the sheep's in the meadow, the cow's in the corn.

Kenny: Okay. (Said calmly without laughing)

Mother: (High-pitched voice, with tinge of frustration) I wasn't finished yet.

Kenny: Well, I don't care. Now, what else you got? I better look.

Mother: (In resigned tone of voice) Well, here's one right here.

Kenny: Yeah. Just sing it. Turn it on. You got yours all mixed up.

Mother: (In mildly resigned tone) Oh, they just got mixed up. (Sings) It's a small world.

Kenny: (Loudly) No, not that one.

Mother: Oh, no. . . Let's try that one.

Kenny: Oh, yeah.

Mother: (Singing) A B C D E F G.

Kenny: No, not that one. Come on. Go go. (Being silly)

Mother: (Singing) Good night, Kenny.

Kenny: (Loudly) Not that one. Put it off. I got one. Just wait a minute. I'll just pretend.

Mother: (With angry tone) Those are my mother's. She would not like you to play with her records. Nhn nhn (meaning *No*). Definitely not.

Following this, Kenny told mother they were going to play hide and seek. Kenny would hide his shoe while mother closed her eyes.

Vi suggested that Kenny himself hide, then mother try to find him. Kenny got more and more giggly and out of contact. Stopping this game, Vi told Kenny it was time to draw (Kenny likes to draw) before the session ended. Kenny and mother sit at the desk, each one doing a drawing.

Kenny: You want me to draw nothing?

Mother: (With angry tone) You're supposed to draw about today.

Kenny: (Looking over at mother's drawing) What is that?

Mother: (Angry tone) You'll find out when we tell each other about our pictures.

Kenny: (Drawing) Can I draw anything I want to?

Mother: Mhm. Mhm. (Yes)

Kenny: I'm going to draw everybody's name that was bad today.

Mother: We were bad? I thought we were good. Who was bad?

Kenny: Vi was bad so she goes to the time-out place. (Drawing it)

Vi: I've got to go to the Time-Out room?

Kenny: Yes. Right there.
   Vi: What did I do that was bad?
Kenny: You pushed me. You have to go to the isolation room. Right here.
        (Points to drawing) Your name goes on the Sad side.
   Vi: Did you get put in the isolation room today?
Kenny: No. Mother is bad, too, and she gets a check. One person was good.
   Vi: Was that person you?
Kenny: Yes. Kenny goes on the happy side. I'm going to draw on the back.
   Vi: It's time to go now. Put your shoes and socks on. That was very good,
        your drawing.
Kenny: Thank you.
   Vi: You're welcome. Let's put the crayons back.
Kenny: (Marks Vi's desk up with crayons and laughs; continues doing it)
   Vi: (Slapping his hands) We don't do that! (With angry tone) Stand up.
        Let's put your socks on.
Kenny: (Yelling) I want to see my mommy's picture.
   Vi: You started writing on my desk and didn't listen to me. What's this all
        about—you writing on my desk?
Kenny: It's magic. (Silly; giggling)
   Vi: It's not nice, and I don't like it.
Kenny: (Writes on the desk again; giggling)
   Vi: (Grabs his hands) Stop it! I mean it.
Kenny: (Tries to do it again; half laughing; half crying)
   Vi: (Continues holding his hands) I don't want you to do that. I want you to
        put your socks on.
Kenny: (Screaming) I mean it right now.
   Vi: (In calm voice) That's right. I do mean it right now.
Kenny: (Starts for desk again)
   Vi: (Stops him, carries him to the couch, starts him putting on his socks,
        helping him)
Kenny: (Yelling) And I'm going to put you in jail ... if that's the way you act.
        (Calmer voice) I'm going to put you in jail. The next time I come here,
        I'll put you in jail. (Starts to get up)
   Vi: Wait a minute. I'm not through tying your shoe yet.
Kenny: (Sits calmly while Vi finishes the shoe tying)
   Vi: (Said calmly) You didn't like it when I got mad at you.
Kenny: (Loudly) Yes, I did! Didn't you hear me laugh? Now let me go.
   Vi: Tell me good-bye.
Kenny: (Looks at Vi; pauses) Good-bye. (Said calmly)

Vi: (Hugs him) Good-bye.
Kenny: (Allows the hug)

Comments

Session with Mother—lack of structure: Mother relied on Kenny to provide the structure ("Are we going to play some records?"). She tried hard to please Kenny but only got rejection. She became frustrated but never expressed it directly. Toward the end of the session, when she and Kenny were drawing, mother began to experience her anger but only expressed it feebly by her tone of voice. Kenny, on the other hand, forced into the adult role, is totally unable to handle it. He got sillier and sillier, more and more out of contact. Drawing, which he likes to do, helped to organize him; but when he asked his mother for instructions on what to draw, she answered with an angry voice. Kenny responded to her anger, drawing mother and Vi in a school setting where they have to go to the "isolation" room because they've been bad.

The interaction between mother and Kenny had the quality of two babes lost in the woods. They were in no-man's land. Since the content of their interaction was based on fantasy (playing imaginary records), there was no way that it could be checked out in reality. Even in their imaginary play, neither of them responded to the other's feelings directly. Mother did finally feel her anger, but she could not own it. She projected it onto her mother ("Those are my mother's. She would not like you to play with her records. Nhn, nhn. Definitely not.").

Closing time with therapist; structure provided: When it was time to say good-bye at the end of the session, Kenny showed his typical falling-apart behavior. That is, he threw things and started to tear up the room. I was not able to catch him quickly enough to stop him from marking up my desk, but when he did that, I expressed my anger and set limits—both verbally and physically. At first, Kenny could not respond appropriately to my anger or my verbal limit-setting. He was like a two- or three-year-old who continues to do the very thing forbidden because he cannot help himself. Because he could not control himself, I picked him up and removed him from my desk to the couch. There I put his shoes and socks on. I was calm but firm with him, enabling Kenny to express his anger directly and in an organized way ("I'm going to put you in jail if that's the way you act"). Following this organized response, Kenny was very present and aware of me. In his response to my statement that he didn't like it when I got mad at him, he shouted, looking directly at me, "Yes, I did." That behavior and those words showed Kenny was present, and in his body, and in touch with me. He left the session calm, organized, and together.

101

Kenny's behavior with mother and with Vi support the DP theory that:
1) The child who feels his body touched by an adult who knows how to touch,
who controls the activities (and sometimes the child, when needed), and who sets
limits will develop a core self demonstrated in organized behavior; 2) children deprived of this basic touching relationship will not show this development.

Mother did not provide a touching relationship, control activities, or set limits. Even though she held Kenny on her lap as she sat in the rocking chair, she
did not touch him. Kenny, though sitting on mother's lap, did not feel touched by
her. There was no toucher and no one touched.

When Vi provided Kenny with these DP conditions, he became organized,
expressing his anger directly to Vi physically and verbally. He recaptured the
sense of self he had previously gained and moved ahead.

Session 25

Present: Kenny, Father, Vi (after holiday break)
Father held and played with Kenny at the beginning of the session. Kenny gave
Vi a little Christmas tree ornament to hang on her lamp. He is restless and cries a
little. Father's way of responding to this behavior is to make fun of Kenny in a
hostile way by saying, "I'll call the teacher and have her put your name on the
"Baby Side" (a practice in Kenny's school). Father laughs as he says this. Vi then
works with Kenny.

Vi: (Looking at Kenny) Is that a new shirt? (Puts him on her lap)
Kenny: Yes . . . No.
Father: It's a schmertz shirt. (Teasing)
Kenny: It's an old one.
Vi: Well, it's been a long time since I've seen you. And it's really nice just
holding you like this. Remember how we used to do this? (Touching
him, starting at the top of his head) Put your head down. That's right.
And there's your nose and I can see your eyes, and your nose goes like
this and your cheek goes like this, and your little dimple there and
there's a tooth—it's just nice holding you like this and being quiet. And
your arms go down like this, and your nose has two little holes right
there.
Kenny: (Moves around)
Vi: We have to get comfortable here. There.
Kenny: I'm not comfortable. (Starts crying—real crying) I can't see.
Vi: (Putting her cheek next to his)
Kenny: (Starts fighting, pulling away, pushing Vi)

Vi: Stop it! You're making me angry.

Kenny: (Crying) I'm sorry, Vi.

Vi: Okay, then, sit down with me. I'm not hurting you. I'm just holding you.

Kenny: I need a Kleenex.

Vi: (Hands him a Kleenex)

Kenny: (Crying hard with tears)

Vi: I haven't seen you in a long time.

Kenny: Can I be on your shoulder, Vi?

Vi: Yes, you can be on my shoulder, like this. (Putting him in upright posi-tion with his head on her shoulder) Just put your head down and see how nice it is. (Soft voice) Okay. I can feel your cheek. That's nice. (Vi feels him relax) You're such a nice boy, and I really like you, and I wouldn't send you back to the "Baby Side" because I like you and it's okay if you cry.

Kenny: (Crying softly)

Vi: I can feel your backbone right here. I can feel your ear against mine. And you have so many kissable places. There's a kissable place right there, and one on your shoulder, on your arm, one on your elbow, one on your hand, one on your fingers.

Kenny: (Quiet, making little baby-like quiet sounds such as infants make lulling themselves to sleep)

Vi: (Singing) Like a ship in the harbor, like a mother and child, like a light in the darkness, I'll hold you a while. We'll rock on the waters; I'll cradle you deep; and hold you while angels sing you to sleep. (Cris Williamson Song, *The Changer and the Changed*) I haven't held you for such a long time. You smell so nice. You taste so nice. (Kissing him)

Kenny: You didn't have to worry about any Christmas.

Vi: Were you wondering what I was doing at Christmas?

Kenny: No. (Said quietly)

Vi: It was nice of you to bring me a present.

Kenny: I didn't wrap it.

Vi: I like it just the way it is. Were you sad because you didn't see me for a couple of weeks?

Kenny: No. (Said quietly) It was fun putting up the decorations.

Vi: What's it like being back with me?

Kenny: Nice.

Vi: (Plays Knock at the Door game, touching his face) Knock at the door, peep in, lift the latch, walk in. Oh, the door is open. (Kenny's mouth) Here is a side door. (His ear) Is there a sound in there?

103

Kenny: (Hums)
    Vi: (Chanting) I hear a sound in there.
Kenny: What's that on the floor? (Some string)
    Vi: Oh, that's nothing to bother about.
Kenny: (Lays his head on Vi's shoulder)
    Vi: Oh, you put your head down on my shoulder. That's so nice. (Sings)
        Come in the evening, and
        Come in the morning
        Come when you're looked for
        And come without warning.
        Kisses and welcome
        Will be here before you
        And the oftener you come, dear
        The more I'll adore you.
        Happy was my heart
        From the moment I met you
        Never will the day come
        When I can forget you
        Happy is my heart
        When you say that you love me
        May the light from your eyes
        Ever shine from above me.
        Come in the evening
        And come in the morning
        Come when you're looked for
        And come without warning.
        Kisses and welcome
        Will be here before you
        And the oftener you come, dear
        The more I'll adore you.
        (an old Irish song)
Kenny: (Just lies there during the singing as if in a trance. At the end of the
       song, he is still quiet, not talking)
    Vi: (Looking at Kenny) This looks like Kenny. (Touching him)
Kenny: (Soft little laugh)
    Vi: I got to make a gingerbread cookie out of you.
Kenny: Oh, no. (Objects)
    Vi: (Beginning the Gingerbread Cookie game—see Appendix)

I mix the dough up like this. (Massaging his body) Then I take my cookie cutter out and cut out your legs (going around each one), put your shoes on, put your knees in, and then I do the next one. Then I put your fingers in, your ears, and then I put your eyes in, and your nose. Have you got any raisins in your pocket?

Kenny: A red gumdrop for my nose.

Vi: What for your lips?

Kenny: Raisins.

Vi: Okay.

Kenny: Oh, you forgot the holes in my nose and my nose.

Vi: Okay.

Kenny: And raisins for my mouth and eyebrows.

Vi: That's right. And coconut for your hair.

Kenny: I want some whipped cream.

Vi: Okay. We better bake you first. (Pretending to shut the oven door over him as he lies in Vi's lap, which serves as the oven) Now you're cooking. SHHHH. Here comes the heat. SHHH. (Slowly moving her hand over his body for the heat)

Kenny: (Quiet)

Vi: I don't think you're done yet.

Kenny: (Knocking on the oven door)

Vi: Are you done yet?

Kenny: (Laughing) No. (Covers his eyes)

Vi: Now you've gone away.

Kenny: (Puts his hand over Vi's eyes)

Vi: Now you've made me go away.

Kenny: (Peeking through his fingers at Vi)

Vi: You see me. Peek-a-boo.

Kenny: (Covers his eyes)

Vi: Now you made me go away.

Kenny: (Laughs; uncovers his eyes)

Vi: Now you made me come back. Now I have to put the "whipped cream" on. (Spreads the "whipped cream" all over the top of him; does it slowly to help him relax and experience his body; when done, said) Now you can do your drawing.

Kenny: (Slowly gets up, goes to desk and gets paper and pencil and starts to print words. When he misspelled the word Christmas (he recognized it), he starts to cry.)

Vi: What's the matter?

Kenny: I didn't want that letter, Vi.
    Vi: It's okay if you make a mistake. Everybody does.
Kenny: I want to get rid of it.
    Vi: Why don't you just cross that letter out and change it?
Kenny: No. (Crying hard)
    Vi: I tell you what you do, cross this out . . .
Kenny: (Crying as if his heart will break) It won't do any good, Vi. I messed up.
          Give me a new paper.
    Vi: You can do it right here.
Kenny: (Crying) I messed up.
    Vi: It's okay if you messed up.
Kenny: I don't want a messed up paper, Vi.
    Vi: Put your "c" right here. You don't have to be perfect.
Kenny: I do . . . I do. (Solves the problem himself by tearing the paper in two.
          On the clean half he writes, with Vi spelling for him, "I am happy.")

Drawing time: Father and Kenny are sitting side by side at the desk, each working on his drawing.

    Vi: (To Kenny, looking at his drawing) Very nice, Kenny.
Father: (Looking at Kenny's drawing) He makes nice decorations.
Kenny: A candy cane.
    Vi: Very good. It's time to stop now. You can finish it at home.
Kenny: No. (Objects, then immediately catches himself, says quietly) Okay, you
          can throw this away (his messed up paper).
    Vi: You want to hear what Daddy says about his drawing?
Father: (Pointing to his drawing) Here's the rocking chair and Daddy, and
          Kenny all relaxed with his arms around Daddy and his head is on
          Daddy's shoulder. He looks so relaxed and happy.
    Vi: (To Kenny and pointing to father's drawing) What are you saying to
        Daddy here?
Kenny: I don't know. (Sing-song tone)
    Vi: If you had to make it up, what would you say?
Kenny: I . . . am . . . happy.
    Vi: I am happy, Oh! (Delighted tone)
Kenny: (Starts printing these words on father's drawing)
Father: Wow, wee!
    Vi: (to father) Do you have an answer to that?
Father: (Turns to Kenny and kisses him) I love you.

Vi: (Pointing again to father's drawing) Now what is Daddy saying back to Kenny?

Kenny: (Watches father print)

Vi: Kenny, what does it say?

Kenny: (Reading) I . . . love . . . you. You . . . may . . .

Father: (Helps Kenny) Make . . .

Kenny: Make me happy.

Vi: That deserves a hug.

Father: (Hugs Kenny)

Vi: Now you tell Daddy about your picture.

Kenny: Okay. (Pointing to his drawing) That's my stocking. My name's on it. It says Happy Xmas.

Father: Wow!

Kenny: I have to finish it.

Vi: You can take it home to finish it. You going to say good-bye to me?

Kenny: Good-bye, Vi.

Vi: (Gives both Kenny and father a good-bye hug)

Kenny leaves at the end of the session without his usual falling apart and throwing things. He walks out like a "normal" child. Both Kenny and father feel good about themselves at the end.

Comments

Changes in Kenny: The two greatest changes in Kenny were demonstrated in his responses to Vi's limit setting and to Vi's cradling him. Kenny used the limit setting to create his own boundaries, to shut out irrelevant stimuli— for example, his response to Vi saying, "Stop it" was "I'm sorry, Vi," followed by "I need a Kleenex" and "Can I be on your shoulder, Vi?" Vi's limit setting enabled Kenny to provide his own structure.

Kenny's response to the cradling also enabled him to create his own boundaries. Lying there quietly in Vi's arms as if in a trance for such long periods of time (for him) showed that he could let go of his need to control and could trust Vi. In so doing, he became aware of his body and the pleasure of being held. His attention had shifted from the outer world to his inner world—to actively experience the enjoyment of feeling his own presence in a safe place with another. Kenny was much more quiet. His constant talking stopped.

Vi's consistent and persistent limit setting and cradling over time is paying off. Kenny is moving. He showed behavior not seen before:

1. His sobbing. He has learned to really cry—feeling his body and feeling his emotions related to Vi. Crying is an important body-felt experience.
2. His peek-a-boo games with Vi. These games represent the omnipotent phase of infancy where the child feels the power to make the mother appear or disappear.
3. Bringing Vi a present. This behavior shows Kenny's ability to invest in another person—an investment needed for growth (called attachment in Object-Relations theory).
4. Kenny's ability to stay focused without falling apart: his sticking to his request for a clean sheet of paper when he made a mistake. He not only stayed focused with Vi (who, in this instance was not really understanding him), but he stayed with it long enough to solve the problem himself-without Vi. This behavior showed Kenny's intense desire to do something right.
5. His feeling good about himself. ("I'm happy")
6. His inner control. When he started to "lose it," he caught himself and was able to bring his attention back to what we were doing.
7. Abstract thinking. Vi asked him to respond to the figure of himself in father's drawing (father drew himself holding Kenny). To answer that, Kenny had to imagine himself there in the drawing.
8. An intense interest in giving form to feeling and ideas on paper. He always liked to draw. Now he wants to know how to write words.

My contribution to providing the conditions he needed for this growth was probably the addition of my voice to the cradling. The constant, monotonous, sing-song, hypnotic chanting and singing I did, regardless of what he was doing, caused him to relax into his quiet, trance-like place. And once there, he stayed there. This chanting was also a form of limit setting. Once I started it, he fell into it in a short time. The chanting helped him experience his core self.

These sessions cover a time period of eight months, but this included time out for summer vacations and Christmas holidays.

Session 35 (the next to last session)
Present: Kenny, Father, and Vi.

Vi: (Looking at something in Kenny's hand) Did you bring me something?
Kenny: Yeah, A flower. (Very soft voice)
Vi: Let's see it. Does it smell?
Kenny: I don't know. (Hands it to Vi)

Vi: (Smelling it) Oh, it does. That's beautiful!

Kenny: I found it in the plaza. (His energy is quiet and soft, relaxed, compared to the loud, raucous quality he used to have)

Vi: Well, thank you. That is very nice.

Kenny: How many days do I have?

Vi: How many days do you have left?

Kenny: Yes.

Vi: One more.

Kenny: I have to do more work on my diploma. (He talked about this last week— making himself a diploma for ending) My mother made a diploma last week.

Vi: Yes. Last week Mother made one for you.

Kenny: I could do one next week with Nina (his sister). The whole family could come and then there would be five people.

Vi: You'd like the whole family to come on the last day.

Kenny: Yes.

Vi: So what are you going to put on your diploma?

Kenny: We're going to run out of time.

Vi: I don't think so. Maybe we should put on it that you discovered you had a lot of kissable places. Like here. (Kissing him on the cheek)

Kenny: No. (Said calmly) Let's do it on the floor. How about Row, Row Your Boat? (See Appendix) We'll put that on. (Removes shoes)

Vi: Okay. You're taking your shoe off.

Kenny: Yeah. I'm taking my shoes off and we'll do something. I don't remember. Do you remember? I don't remember all of them.

Vi: What do you remember?

Kenny: We could do an interview here. I'll take my socks off. (Lies on stomach, on floor)

Vi: (Also sitting on floor) Let's see your feet. Oh, your feet are warm. Come over here. (Moving him beside her) You have kissable places on your feet. (Kissing foot)

Kenny: (Gives her a mild kick)

Vi: Don't kick. I don't want you kicking me.

Kenny: It tickles.

Vi: That tickles? Turn over so I can see your face.

Kenny: No.

Vi: All right. Then I see your back.

Kenny: Pretend that's my face.

Vi: Pretend that's your face?

109

Kenny: (Starts getting into a box nearby)

Vi: Leave that alone. Right now, you're here with me. Here's your face. (Outlining his face on his back) Oh, he's gone to sleep. He's lying on the floor on his stomach, with his thumb in his mouth and his eyes are closed. So we'll just start at the top of his head and go down like this. (Touching him on top of head and moving down to his feet)

Kenny: (Turns over, face up)

Vi: Oh, he's waking up, or maybe he's dreaming about what he's going to do on the last day. Is that what you're dreaming about? Now, he's moving over and he's covering his eyes and he can't see me anymore. Can you see me with your eyes closed?

Kenny: No.

Vi: See if you could. Close your eyes.

Kenny: I can't.

Vi: Well, try. Close your eyes.

Kenny: I can't.

Vi: (Putting him on her lap)

Kenny: (Pulling away; whiny tone) Let me lie like this.

Vi: You know we always start by me holding you a little bit.

Kenny: I'm tired.

Vi: Well, if you're tired, I will hold you.

Kenny: (Starts to whine)

Vi: Oh, for heavens' sake.

Kenny: (Louder) I don't want to.

Vi: All right. Here we go. (Cradling him)

Kenny: (Whining) I don't want to.

Vi: (Holding him) What will I put on your graduation diploma?

Kenny: I don't know. We can interview. (Becomes immediately calm)

Vi: We can interview right now. Ladies and gentlemen. I am interviewing Kenny. How old are you now? I think he's counting on his fingers. He has his eyes closed.

Kenny: Nhn, nhm. (No)

Vi: Oh, you're not counting.

Kenny: I'm sleeping.

Vi: And he's thinking about . . .

Kenny: I'm not thinking about anything.

Vi: Oh, all right. You can just be here and not have to think about anything . . . (Quiet moments)

Vi: The first thing you said today when you came in was how many days? Right?

Kenny: Right. One more, and that's today.

Vi: (Not really hearing him) So how you going to say good-bye to me on that day?

Kenny: I don't know. (Starts hitting Vi's couch and laughing)

Vi: What is your hand saying when you do that?

Kenny: (Keeps on hitting it)

Vi: You know what your hand is saying? It's saying, "I don't want to stop."

Kenny: Mhm, mhm. (Yes) (Changed it to) No. (Calm)

Vi: I don't like it that we're going to stop.

Kenny: No. (Keeps on pounding couch with his fist)

Vi: I don't like you because we're stopping.

Kenny: No. (Said calmly, still pounds)

Vi: What is it saying, then?

Kenny: Nothing. (Still pounding) (Loudly) I'm going to break your couch! That's what it says! (Laughs; shows some anxiety)

Vi: That's what you used to do; that's what you used to say. If you're mad at me, you can tell me directly. So tell me you're mad at me.

Kenny: (Stops pounding; quiet)

Vi: It's okay to tell me you're mad.

Kenny: (Silent but listening)

Vi: Are you saying to yourself, what am I going to do on Mondays when I don't go to Vi's?

Kenny: No. (Said quietly)

Vi: Do you know why I'm stopping?

Kenny: No.

Vi: Shall I tell you?

Kenny: Yes.

Vi: I'm stopping seeing you because you're getting so grown up, you don't need to come anymore.

Kenny: Uh, uh. (yes) Do we have to do special time anymore?

Vi: You're doing so well that you can have special time with your mother and father. You don't need special time with me.

Kenny: (Crying voice) I don't want to stop special time.

Vi: You don't want to stop special time?

Kenny: (Calmly) I do want to stop special time.

Vi: Well, that's what we said.

Kenny: Are we going to stop special time?

Vi: Yes.

Kenny: I want to know why you put me three days to come instead of one day?

Vi: Because I thought you needed some time to say good-bye.

Kenny: I could say good-bye right away.

Vi: You could, but I thought you needed that much time.

Kenny: I don't.

Vi: So you're ready to go.

Kenny: Right. And your last gift was the flower.

Vi: This flower that you brought today was my last present?

Kenny: Yes.

Vi: So this is my good-bye present. That's nice of you to do that.

Kenny: I might pick another flower if I can.

Vi: Where did you find this one?

Kenny: When I went on a nature walk. I found it today.

Vi: You must have been thinking about me. Well, I will miss you when you don't come anymore.

Kenny: Uh, uh. (Yes)

Vi: You've done so well that I'll have to give you five gold stars right across your forehead. (Touching his forehead as she pretends to stick the gold stars on)

Kenny: Could we? I'll sing you a song.

Vi: All right. Why don't we sing it right here?

Kenny: No, because we can't tape it.

Vi: You can hear it right from here.

Kenny: No, I can't. (Starts crying)

Vi: Are you going to cry again? (His whiny crying)

Kenny: No. (Said calmly; stops whining)

Vi: You know what I like about you?

Kenny: What?

Vi: You used to get into trouble here, and now you can stop yourself.

Kenny: Why didn't you give me a whole week?

Vi: Well, it is a whole week. From here until next Monday is a week.

Kenny: But I thought you were going to give me all through May.

Vi: You mean you want to come longer than this?

Kenny: Yes.

Vi: Well, tell me. Say "I would have liked to have come longer."

Kenny: I would . . . Why don't you come to my house? Could you come to my house on Tuesday? You could see my sister, mother, father, grandparents, and I have three friends.

Vi: So you have friends that you can play with.
Kenny: But they don't live there. They live somewhere else.
Vi: Do they come over and play with you?
Kenny: Evan does.
Vi: (Touching his bare feet; still sitting on Vi's lap) Your feet are so warm. It's really nice holding you, just being here like this, isn't it? And we don't have to do anything.
Kenny: (Gets mirror and looks at himself)
Vi: You got a new tooth coming there, and you're getting real handsome.
Kenny: (Sweet little laugh) Yeah, but my buck teeth.
Vi: (Looks at his teeth) Now you go over and let your Dad hold you.
Kenny: I don't want to.
Vi: You always spend some time with your Mother or your Dad.
Kenny: (Whiny voice) I don't want to spend time with my Dad today. (Clear, calm voice) It's so special. You said there was only one more day so we don't have to do that. We just do Vi. I don't want to do Mommy, I don't want to do Daddy on the last day.
Vi: So what do you want to do on the last day?
Kenny: I want to play on the last day and gonna talk on the last day.
Vi: You just want to be with me today?
Kenny: YUP!
Vi: Well, go over to your Dad and say to him, "I just want to be with Vi today." So he'll know what your plans are.
Kenny: Okay. (Looks at father) I want to be with Vi today.
Vi: Give him a hug and two kisses first.
Kenny: I'll give him three kisses. (Goes over and kisses Dad; starts to return to Vi)
Vi: Wait a minute. He has to give you some back.
Dad: I got to give you some back.
Kenny: Oh, yeah.
Dad: (Kisses him)
Kenny: (To Dad) Give me three.
Dad: (Gives him three kisses) Thank you for telling me that.
Vi: (To Kenny) Now look at your Dad. Say to him, "That was nice."
Kenny: (To father) That was nice.
Dad: (Smiles) You're welcome.
Kenny: Now I can make my poem up. That's going to take some time. I might write it.

Vi: I tell you what you do. You sit on your Dad's lap and sing your song and it'll go on here (the tape recorder) while I get the paper.

Kenny: Okay. That would be fun.

Vi: You're really good at making up songs.

Kenny: Okay.

Father: You think it through first before you start.

Vi: Well, sometimes, you just have to start.

Father: (Counting) One, two, three, go.

Kenny: I'm not ready.

Vi: Well, take your time.

Kenny: I'm almost ready. Okay, I got it. It's only a short song. (Chants) You are my spring . . . Wait a minute . . . This year is spring and there's a lot of pretty flowers. April is here and it's kind of cold for the weather, and the flowers.

Vi: (Plays his song on the tape recorder so all can hear it)

The good-bye part of the session: Kenny is sitting at the desk with father, who is writing what Kenny dictates to put on his "diploma."

Kenny: Vi, I am graduating from . . .

Vi: From coming here?

Kenny: Yeah. I'm glad I was at Vi's. (Reads what father wrote, adds) to spend time. I like . . . before I like Vi . . . (Reading, and then adds) to play with her. Then how much I like to. . .

Father: Now where are we going? (To Kenny)

Kenny: I really like her . . . today.

Father: Now we better say something about good-bye and tomorrow, huh?

Kenny: I say good-bye to Vi. (to Vi) What's the date of our last day?

Vi: May 2.

Kenny: (Adds May 2 on his diploma)

Father: Who's going to sign this diploma?

Vi: (to Kenny) I think this is between you and me. You and I should sign it.

Kenny: Yeah. Just me and Vi sign it. (They both sign)

Vi: Would you like to read it now?

Kenny: (Reads it very well)

Vi: Time to get ready to go.

Kenny: Can I have some paper to take home?

Vi: Here's some paper to take home. Are you going to say good-bye to me?

Kenny: Good-bye, Vi. (Jumps up on her, putting his feet around her waist)
        Could you carry me to the door?
Vi: You have to put your shoes on first.
Kenny: (Laughing and enjoying this; still has his feet around Vi) Vi can put one
        on and Daddy can put the other one on. I hope Vi wins. (While being
        held, father and Vi put his shoes on)
Vi: (Carries him to the door, big as he is)

Comments

Session 35 illustrates how the termination process in DP therapy helps the child to integrate and give form to her growth. It also illustrates how the DP therapist provides the conditions the child needs to do it.

What stands out in session 35 is Kenny's goal-directed behavior—his ability to provide his own focus throughout the session and his ability to use the therapist as a helper. Everything Kenny did or said was organized around the Goodbye theme.

To begin with, Kenny brought the therapist a flower. (He gives her something by which to remember him and to show his love for her.) This act was immediately followed by asking, "How many days do I have?" Then he brought up the idea of working on his "diploma," which he had started the previous week.

Following this, Kenny became a little unfocused or perhaps seemed to be struggling with something. He moved quietly from one thing to another. He asked to have his whole family come on the last time. He lay down and was quiet. He didn't want the therapist to touch him. Once he started to kick the therapist. (He was told that was not allowed.)

Then the therapist took charge and picked him up and held him while doing the "interview" he wanted to do. The therapist became the interviewer and simply described what she saw Kenny doing or thinking. When the therapist said, "And he's thinking about . . .," Kenny said loudly, "I'm not thinking about anything."

When the therapist said, "How are you going to say Goodbye to me on the last day," Kenny started pounding the couch with his fist. The therapist said, "What is that hand saying?"

In his answer—"I'm going to break your couch. That's what it says!"—he experienced real anger. Unlike previous outbursts, this one was real because he connected his words to his body (pounding the couch with his fist). The way he said it and the way he looked at the therapist showed that Kenny was aware that he felt angry—for the first time. He not only felt the anger, but he was also aware that he felt it when he answered the therapist. The anxiety he experienced after he said it speaks for this awareness and the depth of his relationship with the therapist. Kenny had used these same expressions in earlier sessions, but they were not connected to his body. They were just words.

Thus, what Kenny was doing during this interim period, when he didn't seem to know what to do, was really taking time—some quiet time—to allow his feelings about the termination to emerge. First, these feelings started to emerge when he rejected contact from the therapist, when he would deny he's thinking ("I'm not thinking about anything") and when he tried to kick her. He could really experience the anger in his voice and in his body when he answered, "That's what it says" as he pounded the couch.

Although Kenny had begun to experience anger in session 18 when the therapist moved him away from her desk, that anger was a reaction to what the therapist did to him. This time, his anger was a reaction to his own inner feelings—the fears around termination.

This episode in session 35 is another example of how a felt bodily experience connects the child to her feelings and makes the child aware of her feelings and her connections to the adult. It helps the child experience not only her body but also her relationship with the adult to whom she is attached.

Following this outburst, Kenny quieted when the therapist said that he could tell her that he was mad. He cried a little, saying that he didn't want to end "special time," why can't Vi go to his home, and "why do we have to stop after three sessions?" The therapist asked him about friends at home.

At this point, there was too much talking. (The therapist did some of it, too.) To bring Kenny back to experiencing himself as real, the therapist touched his feet while holding him and saying, "Your feet are so warm. It's really nice holding you, just being here like this. We don't have to do anything." Kenny responded by picking up the hand mirror and looking at himself. While he's looking at himself, the therapist said, "You've got a new tooth coming there and you're getting real handsome." Kenny was very moved by being noticed and responded with a sweet little laugh, adding, "Yeah, but my buck teeth." He was able to take in the therapist's love, at least for a moment.

This interaction again shows the power of the touch to refocus the child (and the therapist) on the issue; namely, helping the child be present in the moment—experiencing herself feeling. Kenny stopped his constant talking and questions and focused his attention on himself when he was touched by the therapist and when he looked at himself in the mirror. At that point, there was a dialogue between child and therapist.

Kenny again took charge of himself when it was time for him to go and be with father. He said what he wanted. "I don't want to do Daddy on the last day.

We just do Vi." He did, however, agree to sit on father's lap as he made up his song, which was taped, and to accept father's help in filling out his "diploma."

Kenny's Poem

You are my spring.
This year is spring,
And there's a lot of flowers.

April is here,
And it's kind of cold
For the weather and the flowers.

And His Diploma

"Vi, I'm graduating from coming here. I am glad I was at Vi's to spend time. I like before, I like Vi, to play with her. How much I like you. I really like her today. I say Goodbye to Vi."

Endings were always difficult for Kenny. In this session he ended it by creating a community with the three people there: a family with a mother, a father, and a child. He did this by spontaneously jumping up on Vi, putting his legs around her waist, asking Vi and father to put on his shoes from this position, then asking Vi to carry him to the door. (And she did.) He enjoyed it, and so did they. In doing this, Kenny was creating a memory to take with him and inviting others to share this moment with him. By remembering this act and this image, he can calm himself. (Other children in this book also dealt with the last sessions in the same way. See Jason, Chapter 3, and Mira, Chapter 5.)

Overall, Kenny certainly did some very deep work. As the therapist, I was moved by his ability to hang in there the whole hour.

In light of the fact that in the beginning Kenny could not use words at all as a relationship tool, his verbal output (his "song" and his "diploma") is quite remarkable. Again, this shows how touch provides the foundation for language and cognitive development. He moved from the concrete into the abstract. His "song" is a metaphor that describes his relationship with the therapist and his feelings about termination ("It's kind of cold for the weather and the flowers").

117

Conditions the Therapist Provided

1. I allowed him to be a two-year-old when he needed to be. He was really relating to me although as a younger child. This is not regression but a return to an earlier stage to bring back some experience needed to move forward (Levin, 1989, p. 55). For example, Kenny's jumping up on me at the end of the session and wanting father and me to put on his shoes represents a time when a child needed to be carried and nurtured, a time when the child is omnipotent. Kenny needed to experience this, to ask for something and have it granted without question. To an observer, this would be seen as very inappropriate behavior for this age boy. For him, he was only being where he needed to be. That he did it at all is amazing. It showed that he felt safe to do it. That this big boy had so much enjoyment requesting two grown-ups to do this changed the whole energy and feel of the Goodbye for all three of us—Kenny, father and me. This is why I granted his request to be carried to the door regardless of his weight. That is what I did to enable him to feel touched.

2. I supported Kenny's shift toward being quiet, just letting me hold him or sit close to him. At the same time, I made him feel my presence by describing in a sing-song way what I saw him doing or what I thought he was thinking. He loved this. His initial response to the holding in the beginning of therapy was to fight it and try to distract me by constant talking and questioning. Now he clearly experiences it as pleasurable and organizing. Whenever I sensed him getting lost or not knowing what to do, I would return to focusing him on his body. It had the effect of organizing him, and he could then go on.

3. I continued to set limits, but Kenny did not require as much limit setting because he could calm himself. I also used more verbal limit setting because he could hear my voice. After a period of body contact, I would direct his attention back to the work when I thought he was ready.

4. I helped Kenny get in touch with his anger by returning him to his original focus relating to the termination ("How many days do I have?"). Although he said the same thing in earlier sessions ("I'm going to break your couch"), he was in a different place when he said it this time. Hence, I responded differently. Instead of stopping him as I did before because he was out of contact, I allowed him to go with it this time because he was beginning to experience his body and his anger. Instead of stopping him, I focused his attention on the meaning of his gesture ("What is your hand saying?"). He was able to answer.

This is an example of the therapist shifting her focus as the child becomes more organized and present—for example, responding differently to the same behavior because the child is in a different place.

5. The most exciting thing I did in this session was helping Kenny do what he wanted to do. He provided most of the structure in this session. He had a plan, but he needed help to carry it out. He wanted to make something concrete that would represent and give form to his experiences with me. I helped him do that (his "song" and his "diploma").

6. Lastly, I helped Kenny and Daddy communicate with each other. I modeled for father to show him how to relate to Kenny.

The Role of Touch in the Separation and Goodbye Process

This session illustrates how touch furnished Kenny with the foundation he needed to experience and express his feelings about the parting and his ability to give form to these feelings in his poem and his "diploma." The therapist provided him with touch (holding him) when he got too far afield with too much talking, thereby losing his sense of self. Kenny himself utilized body action to feel his anger, and touch (when he spontaneously jumped up on Vi and asked her to carry him to the door) to experience himself asking for what he needed and to experience pleasure. In other words, the touch provides the foundation for the development of later functions and a centering or meditation function to keep the child aware of her inner self.

Session 36: The Last Session

Present: Kenny, Mother, Vi, and Lena, who operates the video camera. Kenny already knows her. Mother reported Kenny got a headache as he was coming up the stairs to my office.

     Vi: (Sitting on couch holding Kenny, who was in considerable pain) So today is our last day. Right?

Kenny: Mhm, mhm. (yes)

     Vi: Well, the first thing you said when you walked in was "today is our last day."

Kenny: Why you got the stool there?

     Vi: So Lena can sit on it.

Kenny: Where did you found it?

     Vi: (Touching him) Does your head hurt right here?

Kenny: No. It hurts down here. (Showing Vi)

     Vi: Will it help if I kiss it?

Kenny: No. (Quiet voice)
   Vi: It won't?
Kenny: The only thing you can make it in is medicine. Maybe a bone is broke.
   Vi: You think one of your bones is broken?
Kenny: Yeah. They could take an X-ray of it to see if it's broken.
   Vi: Maybe it just needs a little loving.
Kenny: No, it doesn't. That won't help either. (Said quietly)
   Vi: That won't help either?
Kenny: Uh, uh. (negative)
   Vi: Well, you're lying here. It's just nice being here with me like this. Right?
Kenny: Mhm, mhm. (yes) (Long silence)
   Vi: Does your head hurt here?
Kenny: No. All around here. (Touching his face) Now it's over here.
   Vi: Your hurt keeps moving around.
Kenny: (Makes crying sounds; looks in pain) I don't know what to do.
   Vi: Just lie still here with me and see if it gets any better. (Stroking his head)
Kenny: (Crying) I don't think it is.
   Vi: You don't think so. Well, you can just be here with me and we don't
       have to do anything on our last time to be together. Right?
Kenny: Right. (Quieter) I wanted to. . . (Cries and rubs his head; his eyes are
        swollen)
   Vi: It hurts on top of your head, too?
Kenny: (Crying harder) Yes, all over here. (Pointing)
   Vi: Are you hurting because you have to stop today?
Kenny: No. (Calm voice, quieter) I don't know when it started.
   Vi: What could I do to make it better?
Kenny: (Crying voice) I don't know . . . (Silence)
   Vi: Maybe if I sang to you a little.
Kenny: No, that wouldn't help.
   Vi: Why don't you close your eyes and just lie still for a minute?
Kenny: (Crying) That won't do it, either.
   Vi: I wonder what would make it better? . . . (Silence) Just nice being here
       and not doing anything, right?
Kenny: I want it to be better before supper time.
   Vi: It better be better before supper time. Maybe it will be.
Kenny: It might not be. (Crying)
   Vi: Would you tell me "I'm not feeling very good right now"?
Kenny: No. (Loud voice) It hurts. (Crying voice)
   Vi: Let me see if I rub it if that helps. (Rubs his head)

Kenny: No, that won't help.
   Vi: Maybe if I kiss it. (Kisses his forehead)
Kenny: No. (His voice lighter)
   Vi: Maybe kissing you down here.
Kenny: That doesn't help either.
   Vi: Well, maybe here. (Kissing him)
Kenny: That doesn't help it. (Less crying)
   Vi: Well, just lying here will be just okay.
Kenny: That doesn't help it. (Crying more) What am I going to do?
   Vi: What do you want to do?
Kenny: (Crying) I want to get rid of this!
   Vi: Okay, why don't you lie down like this. (Moving him so that he's lying across her lap)
Kenny: (Loud) No . . . No. That won't help it. (Strongly objects)
   Vi: Well, do you have an idea?
Kenny: (Pausing to think) No. (quiet voice)
   Vi: I have an idea.
Kenny: No, that won't help either.
   Vi: (Laughing) You haven't heard what the idea is yet.
Kenny: That won't help either.
   Vi: I haven't told you what the idea is yet.
Kenny: What is it?
   Vi: (Laughing) You were thinking of something, and then you said that won't help. What were you thinking of?
Kenny: Nothing.
   Vi: You looked at me and you thought of something, and then you said that won't help either.
Kenny: That won't help.
   Vi: Well, we could just be here and not do anything. (Stroking his face)
Kenny: Yeah. (Quiet voice)
   Vi: All right. (Massaging his head)
Kenny: (Crying). I want to feel better. (Hears Vi's answering phone ringing) You better answer that or you'll be in big trouble. (Yells) Tell me who it is.
   Vi: I'm here with you right now. How are you going to say good-bye to me today?
Kenny: I don't know. (Quiet voice)
   Vi: Well, it looks like you're doing it right now . . . just being with me and we don't have to do anything. You're squeezing my hand right now.

Kenny: Yeah. I was going to bring you a flower, but know what . . . there's no
more flowers in the plaza . . . store, so I just . . . didn't bring anything.

Vi: You did bring something.

Kenny: What? Who?

Vi: You brought Kenny. You brought yourself.

Kenny: I wanted to bring something for you. I didn't bring a thing for you.

Vi: The flower you gave me last week lasted all week and it's still good.

Kenny: Yea!

Vi: (to mother) Would you be willing to go and get that flower in the other
room and bring it here. (Looking at flower mother brought in) (to
Kenny) It was nice of you to think of me like that.

Kenny: And I knew that flower would stay healthy all through the year . . . all
through May and it will die at the end of May. (His speech here is good,
with excellent enunciation)

Vi: It will die at the end of May?

Kenny: Maybe before that.

Vi: (Looking at his flower) See, it is still there. It lasted all week.

Kenny: I'm glad it did. I was going to bring you another one so it wouldn't be so
lonely—so it would have a friend. Maybe you could put some fertilizer
on it to keep it growing so it won't die ANYTIME!

Vi: Thanks, Kenny, for thinking of me.

Kenny's session with mother:

Vi: Go over to your mother now and ask her to hold you.

Kenny: (Goes over to mother, gives her a kiss, wants to get down and draw)

Vi: It's time to be with your mother now. (Mother is in the rocking chair)

Kenny: (Crying) I told you on the last day we didn't have to do this. We didn't
have to do this. I'm so mad.

Mother: I heard you tell Vi you wanted to be with Mommy. (He did earlier)

Kenny: I do not want to.

Vi: It's kind of nice being with Mommy.

Kenny: (Calmer, but starts being provocative by playing with the mike cord)
What is this?

Mother: (Firmly said with a tinge of anger) You know what that is.

Kenny: (Stops playing with it) (to Vi) How much you hold—you held me?

Vi: I held you nearly half an hour.

Kenny: I'll let Mommy do that—35 minutes.

Mother: That sounds like a good idea.

Kenny: Will that take all night?

Vi: You'd like to stay here all night?

Kenny: Yeah. I want to stay all night with you. Could I do that?

Vi: Well, you really had a good time here, and it's hard to say good-bye.

Kenny: Mhm, mhm. (Yes) Let's not do nothing, Mommy.

Mother: We don't have to do anything. We can just rest.

The two talk about the birds in pictures on the walls. They were doing well until Kenny does his old stuff of provoking her. He pulls on the mike cord.

Mother: (Said clearly with anger) I don't like that Kenny . . . yanking on that wire.

Kenny: That's not really important.

Mother: It's important to me. Just leave those wires alone! (With anger in her voice)

Kenny: I hate you! I'm going to close my eyes.

Mother: I see an eyebrow right there. And I see an ear.

Kenny: (Covers his ear)

Mother: There's a nose.

Kenny: (Looking over at Lena) Why is she doing that?

Mother: So she can see you.

Kenny: I remember her. She was at our school. (True)

Lena: (The video operator) Yes, I was there.

Vi: Tell your mother what you did with me.

Kenny: No. I just want to sit quiet and do nothing.

Mother: That's one of the things you did with Vi was sit quietly.

Kenny: I'm doing it again. I want to wash my feet again. (What Vi had done in earlier session)

Vi: You said you wanted to sit quiet with your mother.

Kenny: I wanted to wash my feet again.

Mother: (He is lying across her lap with his head on a pillow—mother is sitting in the rocking chair. She takes one of his feet in her hand) Well, let's see. (Smelling his feet) They still smell pretty good. MHM, MHM. You know, they smell like Cashmere Bouquet soap.

Kenny: (Laughs; looks at her)

Mother: That's what they smell like. (She hands him his foot) Can you smell the soap?

Kenny: Does that one smell better than the other one?

Mother: I don't know. Let's see. (Smelling other foot) I think this one smells more, doesn't it? (Moving that foot over to him)

Kenny: (Smells other foot) Mhm, mhm. (Yes)

Mother: Okay, you see which one you think.

Kenny: (Smelling his foot) That one.

Mother: (Delight in her voice) Yeah. I think so, too. Wait, I can only do one at a time. Mhm. That one smells most.

Both: (Laugh)

Mother: We'll have to try that with our soap.

Kenny: I have an experiment to try at home on plants. You know what? You could put water in one of them and then leave one dry and see which one grows the fastest.

Mother: Which one do you think?

Kenny: The one with water. You know what? You could put a big cover over them and then you could see what happens when the plants don't have no sun.

Vi: (to mother) Tell him how good he is.

Mother: You're a scientist.

Kenny: Mhm, mhm. And I do good on reading. My head feels better!

Vi: Do you know what made your head feel better?

Kenny: (Silent)

Mother: What is Vi saying to you?

Kenny: The quiet time.

Vi: (to mother) I think he needs a couple of kisses for all his good answers.

Mother: Here's one for school and here's one for the plants.

Vi: Thank her for the kisses.

Kenny: Thank you.

Mother: You're welcome anytime. Thank you for your kisses.

Drawing time at end of session:

Kenny: (Sits at desk, talks as he draws) This is Florida, and this is where Vi lives, and this is where I live.

Vi: Put your name on it now. Time to stop. (Gives him some Magic Markers for a good-bye present because he likes to draw so much)

Kenny: (Initiates hugging Vi. He kisses her.)

Vi: (Hugs him back firmly)

Comments

The way the child handles the good-bye sessions is a measure of the child's growth. For example, does the child fall apart at the end? Or does she use her relationship with her therapist to create new ways of being to create her own world and to experience a sense of independence?

The last two sessions that focused on the termination was an integrating and moving experience for both Kenny and myself. In the next to the last session, Kenny reviewed and relived his past experiences with me, including expressing anger at having to stop. Then he integrated these experiences by giving them form—his poem and his diploma. He defined for himself and for me what the relationship meant to him. In that session, he really worked on separation, on saying good-bye.

In the last session (36), Kenny allowed himself to be there—to be present with me without any agenda. He just brought himself as he was along with his migraine headache, which he let me see. The intensity of his physical pain made him really experience his physical body. I just stayed present with him without interpreting except once ("Are you hurting because you have to stop?"). It was just a quiet, close time together.

When I directed Kenny's attention to thinking about good-bye, his concentration on telling me about the plant he wanted to bring seemed to relieve some of the pain. His concern that I might be "lonely" expressed in terms of plants showed his new ability to feel both for himself and for others. He became aware that his "head was better" and attributed this to his "quiet time" with Vi. At the end, he created his own anchor, that is, a reminder of his happy experiences here. He did this by drawing a map of where he lived and where Vi lived. He took it with him. He walked out healed (even from his headache), organized, and calm.

Mother's work with Kenny: The first and last sessions included sessions with mother and Kenny. Comparing their interactions in these two sessions, both mother and Kenny showed considerable improvement in their ability to relate to each other. Both had moved out of their psychotic fantasy world. Both related to each other in the here and now. Mother made up a touching game to which Kenny both responded and enjoyed—very new behavior for both of them. When Kenny tried his old provocative behavior, Mother set limits and expressed anger. Kenny also expressed anger directly ("I hate you"). They didn't really deal with their anger, but they both experienced and expressed it. She also helped Kenny stay focused. (When Kenny said, "My head feels better," Vi said, "Do you know what made your head feel better?" When Kenny didn't answer, mother said, "What is Vi saying to you?" Kenny said. "The quiet time.") In session 36, mother provided some structure for Kenny.

To arrive at this more contactful approach, mother progressed through three stages. First, she imitated me—doing the body work and kissing Kenny. This did not work because she felt awkward and uncomfortable. Then she did it her way. That didn't work, either, although she put a lot of energy into it. She did, however, experience some frustration even though she did not share it with him. Because mother could feel her tension, the interaction between her and Kenny was more direct and less in a fantasy world. Eventually (session 36), mother found her own way of using touching, holding, and limit-setting. This worked. Kenny and she "met." They had a dialogue. They shared both their anger and their pleasure with each other. She really touched him. He felt touched by her.

OVERVIEW OF KENNY'S THERAPY

When I first met Kenny in therapy, I became aware at once of his total inability to communicate with me on any level, verbally or nonverbally. Yet he had excellent speech, sometimes using very advanced words for his age. His speech was all the more remarkable because his parents first sought therapy for him on the basis that he didn't talk, even at age 3.

Kenny could neither provide his own structure (stating something he wanted to do) nor accept the structure I provided (touching and holding him). He responded to all contact by trying to distract me, by directing my attention to something outside of us. He did not experience me touching him even when I was holding him. He did not experience my presence. For him, it was as if I did not exist. It was also as if he did not exist. A psychotic world! And that was the world in which Kenny and his mother lived. In session 1, mother showed her total inability to provide any structure for Kenny because she wasn't experiencing her existence, either. She was living in the same world as he.

I understood Kenny's inability to relate as a reflection of his defective bonding with his parents. He needed someone to provide the conditions needed for him to experience himself being touched and to know that he was being touched. He needed to experience his *body self*.

My goal in working with Kenny was to enable him to experience his body through being touched by me. My work with Kenny shows the organizing effect of touch and limit-setting on behavior. Even in session 1, Kenny experienced quiet moments of being held by me while sucking his thumb. By the end of the session, he was able to answer me in a calm voice (instead of yelling) with a clear coherent sentence, "I don't want to leave because I like you."

I was very surprised at his statement coming so early in the therapy and also coming after so much resistance to being touched. His statement, however, does indicate that he had a moment of awareness of the pleasure of being held and being touched.

In the following session (session 7), Kenny reacted to this new awareness with intense resistance to being touched, both verbally ("I'm going to break your ceiling down; I'm going to slip away from you and I won't come back; I'm going to draw on your wall") and physically (kicking me). The intensity of Kenny's resistance to being touched was due in part to a break in the continuity of his therapy due to the family vacation. It was also due to his beginning to really experiencing something, experiencing his body. This was new, and he didn't know what to do with this new feeling of aliveness. In the following session, Kenny shows that he is learning what to do with it. The resistance was like a last-ditch stand before letting himself surrender and enjoy it.

In the following session (10), Kenny showed two major changes: 1) He invited physical contact. He asked that his whole body be touched all over in the Band-Aid game he initiated; 2) He allowed himself to be the two-year-old (emotionally) that he was. (This was not regression; it was where he was—where he needed to be to start growing again.) He played peek-a-boo games. He also demonstrated that he was experiencing the lack of boundaries and the magic thinking of young children; for example, he said that it was "dangerous" for me to touch him because I might get hurt. For young children, saying or thinking something makes it happen. When I used my "magic" ("I'm not going to let those fingers do anything bad"), he relaxed and surrendered to total enjoyment of having his whole body touched. He couldn't get enough. He also used words to describe his new state: "My hand is better" and it's "for real." Lastly, he began touching me in a loving way (stroking my back). Kenny expressed love toward me first through touch.

About this time, Kenny exhibited another early childhood behavior—the difficulty shifting from one setting to another with short notice. Kenny never wanted to end the session. When it was time to go, to say good-bye, he would completely fall apart—yelling, throwing things, marking up my desk, tearing up things. Once I saw this coming, I would grab him, hold him, put his shoes and socks on, and move him out.

Session 18 records exactly what happened in one of these episodes, which did turn out well in terms of his growth and in terms of my learning. When I said, "Time is up," Kenny marked on my desk before I could get to him to stop it. I expressed my anger, and that made him worse—he was even more set on marking up my desk, but he was really out of control. My picking him up and holding him while I put on his socks and shoes calmed him. When I said that he didn't like it when I got mad at him, he could say calmly but firmly, "I'm going to put you in jail if that's the way you act. The next time I come here I'm going to put you in jail." Kenny, however, left at the end of the session calm and together. After this, Kenny was able to end a session without falling apart.

This episode was significant because, for the first time, Kenny was experiencing an adult being angry with him. Mother never expressed her anger directly. Mother simply complained. With me, Kenny experienced the real thing. I was really angry for a moment, and that was when Kenny totally lost control, crying and fighting me to get to the forbidden desk. The healthy thing was Kenny's ability to express anger back to me. I was a model for him. This experience changed his behavior forever.

Following this episode, Kenny showed a remarkable shift (demonstrated in session 25) from being outer-directed to being inner-directed. He showed an awareness and inner control of his behavior not heretofore present. He could catch himself in his inappropriate behavior and use my simple way of reminding him. Most of all, he had a great urge to accomplish something and do it well; for example, putting his thoughts into written words which he asked me to spell. Even when I didn't understand that he wanted to do something right in his life, he found a way to get his need met without me (when he tore his paper in half and wrote on the clean half). Instead of throwing things and yelling at me, he could really experience his frustration with himself expressed in deeply felt crying—a very healthy sign. He expressed how he felt in written language ("I am happy"). Kenny also moved into the abstract thinking realm when he could respond to my request to tell me what Kenny is saying to father in father's drawing. (Father drew a picture of himself holding Kenny.)

For a boy who began with such unfocused, aggressive behavior, this ability to stay focused on a goal he himself created, to ask for help and to express his feelings speaks well for this child's future.

This shift toward inner direction stood Kenny in good stead for the task of dealing with the termination. In the last two sessions, Kenny not only experienced his body but also his attachment to the therapist. Most important, Kenny was able to experience pain—when he expressed his anger and when he had a migraine headache in the last session.

In the beginning of treatment, Kenny did not feel much of anything—either in his body or emotionally. In one way, Kenny was like autistic children who do not experience physical pain. The autistic children with whom I worked never got physically sick until after they were able to form a relationship. They needed a relationship to be able to experience physical pain.

The child's ability to experience pain, both physical and emotional pain, comes out of a relationship in which the child experiences pleasure, safety, security, and trust. Without this kind of a relationship, the child cannot experience any pain because she has no inner or outer support to do so.

Kenny not only felt the pain in his body, but he certainly was aware of that pain. His crying and his anger made him aware of the caring part of him and of the importance of his relationship with the therapist. For example, in his not wanting the flower to be lonely, he revealed this caring part of himself to the therapist. He could love and allow himself to be loved.

Accompanying this growth in awareness of the feeling-self was Kenny's growth in the cognitive realm—giving form to the feeling-self through his "song," his "diploma," and his verbal language.

With his emerging core self, Kenny could define his own boundaries. This ability was well demonstrated in the way he ended the last two sessions: 1) when he spontaneously jumped up on the therapist to be carried and got the touch he needed, and 2) when he created a visual image in drawing his map showing where *he* lived and where *the therapist* lived to assure himself that each, though apart, still existed.

Summary of the Therapeutic Process and the Role of the Therapist

This case study shows the organizing effect of touch on the behavior of a six-year-old psychotic boy. Although the therapist did other things besides touch, such as limit setting and supporting Kenny to empower himself, it was the touching and holding that started the growth process and that became an integral part of everything he did later.

In Kenny's therapy, the therapeutic relationship went through four phases. In the beginning, Kenny gave me no cues and made no contact with me. I used touching games and cradling as a way to enable Kenny to experience his body being touched by me. At first, he did not feel my touch even when I held him. I was like a parent providing Kenny with what he needed when he was incapable of asking for it. What he needed was a body-self. The touching led him to experience his body.

The second phase came when Kenny allowed me to touch him. At that point, I had something from him to which I could respond. I held him for quite long periods of time, chanting in a sing-song mode. He would lie relaxed, with eyes half closed and thumb in his mouth. He accepted something from me. We had a dialogue.

The third phase came when Kenny became aware that he liked being touched. First he fought this awareness. He had panic reactions to being touched because his body was "dangerous" and would hurt anyone touching it. Again, I took charge. Like the fairy godmother, I banished his fears with a wave of my wand. That freed him. He then became insatiable for touch. He initiated all kinds of touching games (Peek-a-Boo) that two-year-olds play. At this point, all I did was to respond to his invitations and requests. I played his two-year-old games with him.

The fourth phase came when Kenny knew how he wanted to use his relationship with me. I just helped him do better what he wanted to do, like print words and write what he wanted to say. I backed off and was much less controlling. I waited for cues from him, and he would put out very clearly what he wanted—to be noticed for something he did well. (At this stage, Kenny really used me for a *"you"* so that he could be an *"I"*). I also gave him space to experiment with being oppositional, a behavior he seemed to be trying out. It was Kenny's show. I was more like a teacher or friend than a parent.

As the therapist, I contributed to Kenny's growth by providing him with the conditions needed at two different periods. In the beginning, he needed to experience his own physical existence through being touched. I provided that touch experience for him through the cradling, holding, touching, and singing. The quality of my touching and singing provided him with a consistent and constant presence which Kenny had to experience sooner or later. Every time Kenny got out of contact through acting-out behavior or through trying to distract me, I refocused him on feeling his body being held or touched by me. I provided what was needed to create a relationship through touch—the dialogue of touch. In the first period, the therapist did most of the work. That is, the therapist put out what was needed and, sooner or later, Kenny responded to her.

In the second period—when Kenny was eager to use his relationship with the therapist to fulfill his own needs—I stepped back and gave him space and the opportunity to do his thing. In other words, at this stage, Kenny provided his own structure and the therapist responded to him. It is very important for the child that the therapist let go of her attachment to the child; that is, let go of the need to take charge in the way that was necessary in stage one. The therapist takes charge in a different way: she needs to be more of a witness for the child. The therapist has to be just as present to be a witness as she was before.

The therapist's experience: As his therapist, I experienced being with Kenny as very stimulating. I had to be very present every minute in order to enable Kenny to experience himself being touched by me. I had to experience his energy in order to help him experience it. In spite of his distractibility and his aggressive acting-out moments, I sensed a quality of sweetness in him and a genuine desire to learn. When he began to experience his inner self, I felt a lot of love coming from him.

What the therapist learned about herself: Working with Kenny was a two-way street. I learned from him as he learned from me. Kenny made me see how rigid and controlling I am sometimes. For example, when Kenny wanted a clean sheet of paper after he had made a mistake, I could have allowed that. Making the best with what you already have was my issue. Telling him he doesn't have to be perfect was not at all helpful. In spite of me, Kenny was able to start on a clean slate without my help. In reality, he made do with what he had (by tearing the sheet in two). Children are such wonderful teachers if you can listen and pay attention!

The therapist's work with Mother: The therapist also provided Kenny with the conditions he needed to be seen, heard, and loved at home by working with mother separately from Kenny. Having her play with Kenny under my supervision during his session did not work even though she did show considerable improvement. She needed something for herself first.

Mother needed to experience her inner child before she could be a mother to Kenny. Like Kenny, she needed to experience her body, to cry, to learn to be present. For example, in one session mother said, "I don't know why I start to cry every time I come here." Later on in her therapy, she reported feeling very excited about Kenny winning some honor at school. In sharing it in her hour, she experienced an inner feeling of love for her child for the first time. From then on, she began to be aware of Kenny's reaching out to her. She actually saw his love notes to her pinned on the refrigerator. In the end, it was mother's growth in her ability to see her child that made it possible for Kenny to see himself.

Follow-up

During the time mother was being seen, Kenny was seen briefly by a male therapist, Anthony Quaglieri (who did DP therapy with him), after which Kenny returned to see me for three sessions.

Postscript

At this writing, Kenny is fifteen years old and attends a private high school. Mother said he was very good in science and art but had a hard time in reading and math. She said he likes school. (Kenny never had to be in a school for emotionally handicapped children.) Mother said he talks to two girls on the phone two or three times a week. He doesn't go out with them but does talk to them regularly. He and father belong to a model rocket club. Kenny designs and makes rockets, and they launch them once a month. Mother said Kenny's Christmas decorations were so beautiful that she said to him, "Kenny, you are really good."

SUMMARY OF PART I

WHAT WAS LEARNED FROM THESE TWO CASE STUDIES

These two case studies illustrate the effectiveness of the Developmental Play therapy approach in working with individual children who are too disturbed to benefit from the group program. They not only define the principles of Developmental Play but the process by which these principles are implemented.

THE CHILDREN

Although the two children, Jason and Kenny, had different behaviors, they had one thing in common. Neither experienced their physical bodies; hence, they had no body ego, the basic requirement for developing a core self. Neither had an attachment relationship with their parents, the primary relationship needed for the child to discover his inner self. Neither could relate to anyone. Both boys were age six at the time therapy was initiated. Many therapists would have considered it too late to do much to change their behaviors.

CONDITIONS THE THERAPIST PROVIDED

First, the therapist did what was needed for the boys to experience the life in their own physical bodies. She did this through touching and holding. In order to feel their bodies, they had to feel her presence through feeling themselves being touched by her. This presence was a quiet, relaxed but consistent and persistent presence that was always there. It was the quality of the energy and the vibration in the touch and her presence that the child's body picked up and took in. The child's body and the therapist's body communicate through the quiet energy that flows between them. No words are needed. The child's body shows the awareness of this condition by becoming relaxed, just feeling its own energy. The child is not passive.

The child's body is becoming aware of itself. This quiet, relaxed body response, like a trance, was seen in the body responses of both Jason and Kenny.

In other words, the therapist took charge. She did not ask Jason or Kenny if she could touch them. That would have made no sense at all, since neither of them had a core self that could make a "Yes" or "No" decision. Even though Kenny had excellent speech, his speech was not used to create a relationship. The therapist took charge by seeing and touching them in a way that made them feel seen and touched.

The therapist paid attention to their responses to being touched. How they responded guided her in her next move. For example, when Jason pulled back when the therapist first took his hand, she said, "Pull, Jason, pull." Even though he didn't understand that command, she gave him something to which he could respond, and eventually he did understand. When Kenny said that the therapist could not touch his hand because his fingers were "dangerous," the therapist heard the panic in his voice. She became his protector, saying that she would not allow his fingers to hurt anyone. From then on, Kenny could not get enough touching. In other words, what the therapist did made Kenny feel seen, safe, and understood.

The two case studies show that the therapist was consistent and persistent in providing the conditions needed for the child to experience his body. At the same time, the therapist listened to the two boys to find a touch and a holding that was acceptable and pleasurable. For example, when Kenny was out of control and the therapist held him firmly, he yelled loudly, "Let go of my hand." The therapist did let go with the words, "Stop pulling away, then." Kenny became quiet and organized. This is an example of the therapist both listening to the child and, at the same time, providing him with limits.

When Jason and Kenny did show signs of having an inner self, the therapist gave them space to allow that new inner self to come out and express itself. The therapist simply helped the two boys do better what they were already doing. For example, when Jason went over and stood on the window sill with his back to the therapist, she got the message that he wanted her to be ready to catch him. When Jason hid in the closet and then opened the door and suddenly appeared, the therapist responded excitedly with "Peek-a Boo, there you are!" In other words, the therapist responded with excitement to what Jason did and gave his behavior form and meaning. Jason had so much fun playing these games that, like all young children, he wanted to play them over and over. In the case of Kenny, the therapist responded to his request to spell certain words for him as he wrote down his thoughts. Now that Kenny had a core self, he could use his speech for communication. At this stage, the therapist no longer needed to do all the initiating. The boys did that now, and the therapist simply responded to what they put out.

The last condition the therapist provided was a container for all the deep and intimate feelings these boys experienced. They both had periods of heavy crying with tears. The therapist simply held them or sat quietly with them, often with neither saying anything but yet being present with each other. These were the conditions supplied by the therapist.

THE CHILDREN'S PROCESS IN LEARNING TO RELATE TO THE THERAPIST

The stages in learning to relate were exactly the same in the two boys. In some instances, the boys did exactly the same thing even though Kenny was further along than Jason. Jason related primarily through the dialogue of touch. Kenny added verbal language to the dialogue of touch. Both boys progressed through the following steps:

1. Learned to relate by allowing themselves to be touched.
2. Showed pleasure and awareness in being touched.
3. Invited and asked for touch—the beginning of a core self.
4. Created their own touching games and activities.
5. Created games and activities to get themselves noticed and seen.
6. Planned ahead of time what they were going to do in the session.
7. Showed delight and enjoyment; played jokes on the therapist (Jason).
8. Began to experience the therapist less as a parent and more as a playmate or friend.
9. Experienced feelings of physical pain: Jason, when he burned his hand on the stove at home; Kenny, when he came with a migraine headache. This behavior was new for both boys.
10. Experienced disappointment or anger: Jason, when father took his chair; Kenny, when the therapist brought up termination.
11. Allowed themselves to cry deeply with tears and crying sounds. Jason spent several sessions leaning against the therapist and just crying while looking at the therapist. Following the crying sessions, Jason showed much more eye contact.

   The ability to experience pain, anger, and unhappiness is extremely important because it means the child has a core self that can handle it and also a relationship that will support her. It is the experience of pain that enables the child to experience her caring and loving part. Many disturbed children never cry because they do not have an attachment relationship that serves as a container for these feelings.

12. Experienced intimacy with and caring for the therapist. For the first time, Jason allowed himself to completely relax in the therapist's arms. Kenny brought the therapist a flower and was concerned she would be lonely after he left.

13. Related through language as well as through touch. Jason began saying a word now and then. Kenny began using his speech for communication purposes. Kenny also created a "song" that expressed his feelings about the relationship.

14. Demonstrated the ability to empower themselves to create what they needed to say Goodbye. Both boys did exactly the same thing: each, in his own session, spontaneously jumped up on the therapist and asked her to carry him to the door. In doing this, they created an image and a memory that can be recalled when needed—the image of closeness, security, and love. Kenny also created a visual image—a map showing where he lived and where the therapist lived.

15. Most of all, experienced themselves as happy, and enjoyed doing what they did.

At the end of treatment (Jason—three and one-half years; Kenny—one and one-half years), both boys had a core self—Jason at the level of a three-year-old and Kenny at the level of a five or six-year-old. At the end of treatment, the therapist worked with Kenny's mother for two and one-half years. She did not work with Jason's mother.

APPLICATION

The fact that the Developmental Play approach is designed to provide the basic conditions needed for the development of the core self makes this approach applicable for nearly all children at some time or another.

Children With Attachment Problems—Autistic, psychotic, the physically and sexually abused, the acting-out violent child who kills, and the ADD (Attention Deficit Disorder) or ADHD (Attention Deficit Hyperactive Disorder): These children show that they are lacking in the ability to experience their own physical bodies. They need to experience themselves being seen and touched in order to become aware that they have an inner or core self that guides them.

The Attention Deficit Child. Kenny had all the behaviors of the ADHD child: disruptive at school, short attention span, almost no organizational skills, hyperactivity plus impulsive explosive behavior, poor social skills (inability to relate at all except in fantasy). Kenny was never on medication, however.

The current behavioral approach to the treatment of ADD children does not address the issue of the defective core self.

Instead of making demands on the ADD child to behave in certain ways, teachers—and especially parents—need to give the ADD child something to respond to such as noticing him, touching him so that he can feel his own existence and has something to respond to. His presence must be acknowledged by seeing and touching. The current treatment focuses on the behavior and not on the experiences of the child.

The Abused Child. Because of their abuse, these children do not own their bodies. Their bodies don't belong to them. Much of the work with sexually abused children focuses the child on telling her story. The child cannot do that until she has a relationship. Relationships with young children begin with touch. Just because a child had bad touching doesn't mean that she shouldn't learn to experience caring touch. In fact, most young children welcome a caring touch provided the adult is really present, sensitive, and finds ways to make the touching acceptable and pleasurable. The child will guide the therapist if she is present in her own body and feels the quality of the energy in the child. Then it will be right for the child, and the child can begin to own her body, to feel more complete, and heal.

The MPD (Multiple Personality Disorder) Child or Adult. The MPD individual has created different personalities as a way of protecting herself from the memory of earlier abuse. The Developmental Play focus on helping the child experience and be aware of her bodily feelings can be very effective in helping the MPD person to become one integrated self. Being present in her body now through being seen and touched results, if done appropriately and sensitively, in new feelings of aliveness and pleasure. These experiences enable the child (or adult) to experience the pain of the trauma.

The Acting-Out Destructive Child. These acting-out killer children are basically psychotic. They have no inner core or structure to guide them. Everything they do is a reaction to something outside of them. They simply do to others what was done to them. They need to be physically restrained but not in a punitive, demanding, or hostile way. They already are used to experiencing their bodies through violence. Here, the therapist works with these children by touching and holding them. You forbid them to hit you by holding them so they cannot. Then you proceed to focus their attention on feeling parts of their bodies in a gentle way, their hands or face, for example. In fact, the younger acting-out children respond very rapidly to this treatment. They start relaxing almost immediately, begin to ask for it, and begin to become organized. Lastly, they begin to enjoy themselves in an authentic way.

Not all children need a lot of touch. For those who do (and that's most of the above), touch is extremely effective. There is no substitute.

Normal Children. Even normal children can benefit from and need some touch. A little touch helps to center and focus a child. Touch helps the normal child to acknowledge and experience the beauty of her own existence. From that place, the child can do almost anything.

PART II: PUTTING DEVELOPMENTAL PLAY THERAPY
INTO PRACTICE

5 THE DEVELOPMENTAL PLAY GROUP PROGRAM

The Developmental Play group program (DP) is an intervention program based on touch for young children and a training model for play therapists and therapists. It is designed for six children (preferably ages three to six); six adults, each of whom is paired with a child; and a Leader or Trainer. The program meets weekly for three-hour sessions and runs for a set number of weeks (usually twenty). The sessions are divided into two parts:

1. One hour with the children: one-half hour of one-to-one child-adult play and one-half hour of group time, called Circle Time. This is what we will look at in this chapter.
2. Two hours of supervised training for the adults: one hour before they meet the children and one hour after the children leave. We'll discuss training in Chapter 6.

The one-to-one child-adult play and the Circle Time are designed to meet the children's needs at two different stages of growth: the attachment stage and the separation stage. Learning to create a relationship with one adult (the one-to-one child-adult play) is followed by learning to relate to peers (Circle Time). Hence, each part of DP has its own specific goal that guides the activities for that part. Each of these two parts has a beginning, a middle, and an ending or termination. These three "time-zones" furnish boundaries that both guide the course of events and give the child freedom to do what she needs to do in each part.

THE LEADER

The Leader takes charge of the training sessions before and after the children's hour, leads the Circle Time activities, and is present during the one-to-one part to help any adult who needs assistance with her child. In most cases, the Leader is also responsible for setting up the whole program—negotiating with the administration, selecting the children, finding the adults, meeting with parents, and setting up preliminary training. To do all that well requires training and several years of experience.

Developmental Play is a very intensive and focused play therapy. Although it looks simple, it is very difficult to implement. Therefore, if you want to be a Leader of a Developmental Play group, do it in your own creative way, but get training before you start and regular consultation after you begin. To be a really effective Leader requires working on yourself in order to understand yourself, the adults you are training, and the children with whom they are working (see Chapter 6).

The Developmental Play group program, when done well, has a family atmosphere. Both the children and the adults have the opportunity to experience the intimacy of a one-to-one relationship and the excitement of learning to relate to peers within a larger group, the family unit.

The DP Leader must be aware of more than just running the meetings. Let's take a closer look.

GOALS

First, you must define *your* purpose in wanting to lead a DP group. What are *your* goals? What do you want to get out of it? What do you hope to give to the group of children and adults under your care? Where can you get training?

THE SETTING

Determine where you can hold the sessions. Try to find a room with a rug on the floor, if possible. You need a place where children are available, children who need a program like DP. If you are a teacher, a school counselor, a teacher in Headstart or day care, or a therapist in a hospital setting, you already have a place and the children. This past year, a preschool director asked me if I would lead a DP group in his agency for six four-year-old children if he found the adults. If you don't already work in an agency, this is another possibility.

THE CHILDREN

For your first experience leading a DP group, select ordinary or less disturbed children. These children respond well to Developmental Play right from the beginning. They will reward you for your efforts, and their behavior will also serve as a guide for assessing the growth of more disturbed children.

Developmental Play has been effective with children up to age twelve and even with early adolescents. At the present time, however, Developmental Play is geared toward younger children, ages three to six.

THE PARENTS

Parents must sign statements giving permission for their children to participate in DP, even when it is an approved program for the school or day care facility. In addition, I always invite the parents to a preliminary meeting in which I explain DP to them and give them some idea of what we do in the program. With a few DP groups, I have run a series of four or five parent meetings to give them the "touching" experiences of DP. Unfortunately, this does not happen very often, as many parents are either unable or unwilling to attend meetings to work on themselves, even when it is free. At the end of every program, however, I do insist that parents come to a final meeting or at least fill out a questionnaire assessing the changes they experience and see in their children.

THE ADULTS

The adults who are to be the children's partners (therapists) can be almost any willing person dedicated to helping children with the energy to devote the time needed in this program. They may be highly skilled mental health professionals or experienced teachers and school counselors. Or they can be parents, graduate students, or undergraduate college students. They can even be available and interested people in the community, such as housewives with extra time or senior citizens.

The skill level of the adults in each of these three groups varies considerably, but the effect of doing DP on both the adults and the children has been very positive. The common factor in all three groups is the dedication of the adults to the children and the fact that the adults are aware that they also get something out of it: a clearer sense of who they are.

PART 1: THE ONE-TO-ONE CHILD-ADULT PLAY

THE TOUCHING DIALOGUE

The goal of the one-to-one play is to provide the conditions the child needs to experience her own body. This experience begins through the awareness of being touched by the adult partner. What the adult partner does is *touch, see, and respond*. To do this, however, means that the adult has to know how and when to touch; that is where the training comes in (see Chapter 6).

The adult takes charge and initiates the *touching dialogue* so that the child understands from the beginning that touch is a safe avenue through which she can communicate. This touching dialogue can begin, for example, with a simple Hello-handshake or a touch of the hands. In the touching dialogue, there is no

141

demand that the child do, say, or feel anything specific. The child is not asked to do anything. The child's body-response to the touch will tell the adult if the child is experiencing the touch. For example, the child may pull her hand away or smile and offer the other hand (see Chapters 1 and 2).

THE SETTING

The six child-adult pairs meet in the same room. Each pair has her own space marked out by a mat or blanket. The two sit on the blanket, facing each other. Except for the blanket and a bottle of lotion, no props (such as dolls or toys) are used. Three limits are spelled out in the beginning: (1) the child is not allowed to run around the room; (2) the child must remain on the blanket with her partner; and (3) the child is not allowed to hurt herself or the adult partner.

INTRODUCING THE CHILDREN TO THE DEVELOPMENTAL PLAY PROGRAM

The children are introduced to the DP program as a group through a Circle Time activity led by the Leader. This activity is designed to give both the children and the adults the opportunity to meet each other.

The children are seated on the floor, between the adults, in a circle. First, the Leader tells the children about the program, then gives them the opportunity to experience what it might be like through a game called Pass-the-Child. Each child gets five minutes with each adult as she is passed around the circle from adult to adult.

The five-minute *getting acquainted play* consists of holding the child on the lap and simply looking at and noticing the child—looking at her hands, counting her fingers, and doing the same thing with the feet and toes, provided the child wants to take her shoes and socks off (many children do).

Snacks are served at the end. The Leader tells the children that they will have a playtime every Monday (or whatever day is agreed on) and that one of these adults will be their "play partner."

After the children leave, the Leader helps the adults choose the child they want to work with (see Chapter 6). The one-to-one play begins the following week.

THE FIRST ONE-TO-ONE MEETING: SAYING HELLO

The adult greets her child at the door, walks her over to their section of the room, and the two sit down facing each other. The first thing the adult does is to look at her child and get a sense of how she is. You, the adult, pay attention to the child's cues. For example, the child comes in, sits down, and immediately takes off her shoes and socks. You would respond to that by saying something like, "Oh, you remember doing that last week when you were here. You're all ready to go. That's nice" (touching the child's feet).

At some point in the first session, the adult partner needs to tell the child that she, the adult, has chosen her and that they will be playing together every Monday (or whatever day) for twenty weeks (or whatever the number) and have the child count on her fingers that number. The adult tells the child her name (what she wants to be called) and asks the child her name. The adult already knows the child's name, but it's important for the child to speak her name—to listen to the sound of her voice as she says it. Listening to her own voice helps the child experience herself and begin to know who she is.

Thus, in the Hello exchange—their first meeting—the two learn each other's names and the purpose for their being together. In addition, they have a feel for each other. They have experienced each other's presence.

WHAT DO YOU DO AFTER YOU SAY HELLO?

After you say Hello, you help the child feel seen by noticing her: "Did you know that your eyes are blue?" A young child often responds by covering her eyes with her hands. That act can start a peek-a-boo game: "Where did your eyes go? They were here a minute ago." Or, touching her hands, "Where did Sally go? She's gone away. Her hands are here, though," and so on. Eventually, the child usually removes her hands from her eyes and you say, "Oh, there you are. I see you now."

The adult helps the child feel seen through touch. With a light touch on the child's hand, say, "You brought your hand with you today." The child may respond by offering the other hand, or she may withdraw the hand that was touched. In either case the child is giving you a clear message. No words or interpretations are needed.

In the above examples, the adult partner (DP therapist) is simply helping the child experience her presence through bodily feelings so that she can say Hello in whatever way she needs to. (For other examples of how to say Hello or meet a child for the first time, review Chapter 2: The Structure of Developmental Play Therapy.) The following case study presents one example of what can happen with one child-adult pair in a DP group.

MIRA AND VI: A CASE STUDY OF ONE DP CHILD-ADULT PAIR

This particular DP group consisted of five child-adult pairs. Mira, age four, and myself, Vi, were one pair. These children came from a day care center and were not referred children. Nevertheless, several in this group showed that they needed special attention, and Mira was one of them. Mira's mother wanted her to be in the DP group because she constantly fought with her six-year-old sister. She also said that Mira had been a very difficult baby.

When I observed Mira in the day care classes, I saw her as a very controlling child. She constantly called attention to herself by loud talking and telling others what to do. In the introductory meeting with all the children, where we played Pass-the-Child, Mira told Mary, the Leader, how to run the circle.

This DP group met for sixteen sessions. The following case study illustrates the dialogue of touch as it was expressed in the one-to-one—(1) the three parts of the Hello process (beginning, resistance, attachment); (2) the Separation process; and (3) the Goodbye process (negative feelings, positive feelings, celebration)—and the dialogue of touch as it was expressed in the Circle Time.

THE HELLO PROCESS, PART I: BEGINNING

Session 1
Scene: Mira and Vi sitting on their mat facing each other.

Mira: (Taking off shoes)
   Vi: Oh, you're taking off your shoes already.
Mira: Yeah. (Looking around)
   Vi: You can see everybody has a partner.
Mira: (Hands Vi part of a newspaper she had brought with her)
   Vi: Did you want to show me something?
Mira: I'm going to take it home.
   Vi: Well, thank you for showing it to me. (Returning it to her)
Mira: (Pointing to Mary, the Leader) She doesn't have a partner.
   Vi: She doesn't have one because she is the Leader. And I chose you for my
        partner. Is that all right with you?
Mira: (Mumbles something)
   Vi: So your name is Mira, and my name is Vi.
Mira: I know that. I saw you. (Last week)
   Vi: I saw you, too, and I said, "I am going to play with you."
Mira: I like to play. (Looking around the room) Is there toys in here?

144

Vi: No. We're not going to play with toys, but you and I are going to play. (Taking her hand and lightly touching her finger) Here's a finger and here's another finger.

Mira: (Shows Vi a little mark on her finger) Look at this.

Vi: My goodness. I'll have to kiss it. (Kisses her finger)

Mira: It still hurts.

Vi: It still hurts? I guess I'll have to put another kiss there.

Mira: It still hurts. That's because I pulled my skin off.

Vi: Poor little finger. (Taking out a small bottle of lotion and putting lotion on her finger)

Mira: Is that something I can keep?

Vi: No, but it's something to put on your little finger.

Mira: (Watches Vi intently)

Vi: There. Does that make it feel better?

Mira: Mhm. (yes)

Vi: Is there another finger that needs some?

Mira: Nhn. (no)

Vi: So this is our first time to be together, so hello.

Mira: Hello. (Said quickly) Do you have some cavities?

Vi: (Laughs) Let's see if you have some. (Looking at her mouth)

Mira: My mom has some. Let me see yours.

Vi: I don't think I have any. Let's see how many teeth you have. (Counting her teeth)

Mira: (Touching her front tooth) *I can feel it.*

Vi: Is it loose?

Mira: Not yet. (Looking at her hand)

Vi: Looks like you could use some lotion on that hand.

Mira: Yes. (Watches intently as Vi puts lotion on her hand; wants to put her finger in the bottle to get the lotion)

Vi: It looks like a little callous here.

Mira: (Interrupting) Can you put it on here?

Vi: Let's put it all over like this.

Mira: (Hurriedly) Put some on this hand. (Holding it up)

Vi: (Rubs the lotion on her hand and arm up to her elbow) Let's see if you can pull. Oh, it's slipping.

Mira: (Smiles as her arm and hand slip through Vi's hands) (See Appendix)

Vi: So let's do . . .

Mira: (Interrupting) No. Put it here. (The lotion)

Vi: (Playing the Lotion Game on the other hand) (See Appendix) Let's see if this hand will slip.

Mira: (Pulling her hand through Vi's hands) Can you see my teeth?

Toward the end, Mira gets distracted by what the other pairs are doing and wants to do what they are doing.

Vi: Well, we can do our things. I can count your freckles. (Initiates the Knock at the Door game) (See Appendix) Let's see if anyone is home. Knock at the door. (Taps Mira's forehead) Peek in. (Puts finger under her eyelash) Lift the latch. (Touches the tip of her nose) And walk in. (Touches her mouth) Anybody home?

Mira: Do it again.

Vi: (Repeats game)

Mira: (Opens her mouth)

Vi: (With excited voice) Oh, there *is* someone home! Here's a cheek. (Touching it) Is it kissable?

Mira: Yes.

Vi: (Kisses her cheek) Is there another one?

Mira: No.

Vi: Which one is kissable?

Mira: (Turning her other cheek toward Vi, points to it)

Vi: (Kisses it) Is there another one that needs kissing?

Mira: The eye does.

Vi: (Kisses her eye) Another one?

Mira: No.

Vi: Is your face there?

Mira: (Turns her face away from Vi)

Vi: I can see the back of your head.

Mira: (Turns her head back with her face toward Vi)

Vi: Oh, there's your face. Hello.

Mira: I want to lie down.

Vi: How about me holding you. Is that all right?

Mira: (Allows cradling)

Vi: (Softly chants the names of the parts of her body as she touches them; sings Brahms Lullaby) It's time for Circle Time now. (Brings Mira to the Circle to join the others)

Circle Time

Scene: Five adults are sitting in a circle, each holding a child. Mary, the Leader, is singing a Hello Follow-the-Leader song, a song that says "Hello" to each child and her partner.

All five children are having difficulty responding as the Leader guides them to relate to each other through simple contact activity, such as saying "Hello" to another child by touching her. Mira, however, stands out—she is very loud and controlling and demands attention. She makes noises, laughs inappropriately when others are talking, and has nothing to say when it's her turn to talk.

At cradling time, however, Mira allows Vi to hold her. Lying in Vi's arms, she looks up and reaches up to touch Vi's hair.

At the end, when Mary invites the children to ask their partner for a hug, Mira says, "I don't need one."

Comments

In Part I of the Hello Process, Vi initiated a touching dialogue to allow Mira to experience her body through touch. Through this touching dialogue, Mira experienced her own physical presence and existence and also experienced her adult partner's physical presence and existence. Vi took charge by providing the seeing and touching activities they did together.

Mira also took charge. She made the opening move by taking her shoes off. She remembered that the children had done this the week before in their introductory meeting and used it now to invite that pleasurable contact again. Then she looked around the room for Vi to define the role of the people there. By looking around the room for toys, she found out she wouldn't be playing with toys. When Vi told her her name, Mira said she already knew her name. Out of the blue, she asked Vi if she had any cavities. At Circle Time, when Mary suggested the children ask for a hug, Mira said, "I don't need a hug."

Thus, in this first session, Mira presented herself as a take-charge, competent child who already knows everything and doesn't need anything. Yet, in the group session that followed the Circle Time, her take-charge behavior didn't work, although she tried hard. She could not utilize the group experience at all. She did, however, feel secure sitting in Vi's lap during the group time, and from that place, she felt safe.

Mira's take-charge behavior in session 1 reveals how Mira experiences her world and how she copes with it. She does not experience herself as seen, touched, or heard. She does not experience herself as noticed or valued. She does not feel that she exists. She has to take charge to get seen. All her energies are outer-directed in an effort to get someone to see her. She does this by constantly calling attention to herself in loud, abrasive ways. That's the way she gets some attention. Her hyper-acting-out behavior at home did get her mother's attention, with the result that her mother did do something—she enrolled Mira in the DP program.

Mira's controlling behavior is a reflection of her lack of a solid core self—the part that organizes her from the inside out.

Vi helped Mira begin to develop this inner self through touch, through just feeling her own body and how nice it is just to be held and touched and not have to do anything but enjoy it. No matter what Mira did, Vi always came back to touching or holding her. Mira not only accepted the touch, but she invited it ("Do it again. Put some [lotion] on this hand. Can you put it on here?"). Although she clearly controlled how much touch she would allow, she always came back for more after saying no. Mira was always in control of how much touch, but she gradually began to let go of some of this need to control and would allow herself to be touched for longer periods of time (the cradling).

In summary, Mira's behavior in session 1 shows her to be a very bright, energetic child with excellent speech. However, she shows a clear developmental lag in the parent-child attachment process and a lack in the sense of self.

As the DP therapist or adult partner, I experienced a very strange kind of energy in this first session. It was as if Mira were a ghost. She didn't seem to be there, to be real. When I picked her up to put her on my lap, she seemed almost weightless. She didn't seem to have a body. Even when I touched her, I sometimes wasn't sure if she felt it.

Session 2

Scene: Mira and Vi sitting on floor facing each other.

Mira: Did you bring your purse?
   Vi: Why?
Mira: The lotion.
   Vi: Oh, you remembered that. You want that again. I have to say Hello to you first. What shall I say Hello to first?
Mira: My eyes.
   Vi: (Gently touching each eye) Here's one eye, and here's another. You're leaning up close. Oh, this finger wants to say Hello.
Mira: What's Shawn doing? (Pointing to Shawn, another adult partner)

Vi: He's just watching because his partner, James, isn't here today. Shall I kiss this finger? (Touching the finger)

Mira: Yes. (Holding up her baby finger) (With her baby-sounding voice) I want to lie down. (Lies on her back, with her head away from Vi and her feet almost in Vi's lap; looks at Vi; looks around the room) I want to play with Bea. (another adult) I don't like to play with you. (Shows Vi the lotion bottle)

Vi: Now you are showing me the lotion.

Mira: I want to put it on.

Vi: (Holding the bottle) Put your finger in. There, you got it. (Vi plays the Slippery Hand game with her) (See Appendix)

Mira: (Laughs) That hurts. You hold it too tight.

Vi: I didn't mean to hurt you. Show me where on your hand, your arm.

Mira: (Pointing to book shelves in room) What's that up there?

Vi: Those are books. (Moving her back on the mat)

Mira: I want a drink.

Vi: You can get a drink later.

Mira: I took a drink with my hand. I want to sit up. I don't want to lie down now.

Vi: You can sit up. You want me to help you?

Mira: (She turns over and lies face down this time)

Vi: (Touching parts of Mira's body gently and chanting) Hello to your feet; Hello to your leg; Hello to your back.

Mira: Why do we have to play here?

Vi: (Continuing as before) Hello to your neck.

Mira: (Yells back to another girl who yelled; speaks with whiny voice) You're hurting my back.

Vi: Sit up and let me see your back. (Touching it)

Mira: (Giggles) It tickles.

Vi: (Picks her up, cradles her [she allows it], sings Rock-A-Bye Mira and chants) It's so nice to let somebody hold you like this. I have this beautiful little girl. Her name is Mira. You were the one I picked to play with.

Mira: (Lifting her head and looking around) Is he doing his homework? (Pointing to the adult whose child was absent)

Following this, Mira has a period of screaming—some in response to another child and some not.

Vi: (Cradles her again, chanting her name, and so on)

Mira: (Raises up) I got some scratches. Will you put some (lotion) on this?

Vi: Put your fingers out.

Mira: Let me do it. (Puts lotion on herself; has another bout of her screaming)

Later in the session:

Mira: (Covers her eyes with her hands)

Vi: Where has Mira gone? (Touching her) This feels like her hair. This feels like her ear.

Mira: (Peeks out from behind her hands)

Vi: Oh, Hello Mira.

Mira: Shut up, Vi. (Said softly)

Vi: You said my name.

Mira: (Starts hitting and kicking Vi)

Vi: (Grabbing her feet) Kicking and hitting are not allowed.

Mira: (Moving her legs in Vi's hands) This one goes this way, and this one (the other leg) won't go that way.

Vi: Do I have to kiss it?

Mira: Do ten kisses.

Vi: (Kisses her knee while she counts; touching the other leg) Now this one is stuck again. What does it need?

Mira: Six kisses. Other one needs seven kisses.

Vi: (Again kisses as she counts)

Mira: (Looking around) I want to see everybody.

Vi: You'll see everybody at Circle Time.

Circle Time

In the cradling, Mira relaxed, closed her eyes, and sucked her thumb. Then she opened her eyes, briefly looked around, then turned back to Vi and closed her eyes and snuggled. When the Leader asked the children what they liked best, Mira said, "Nothing." During snacks, Mira would not share her cracker with Vi (Mary had asked the children to do so), but when Vi offered Mira some of hers, she said, "Thank you." At the end Vi hugged her without asking her permission. She liked it.

Comments

Session 2 shows that Mira has made a definite shift toward a relationship. Compared to session 1, this meeting shows an awareness of both a pleasure in being with Vi and some kind of tension or discomfort. She shows a beginning inner directedness that wasn't there in the first session. This emerging inner self is struggling with, "Do I want to be in relationship to Vi or don't I? When I am with her, I like it, and at the same time, I want to get away. When I move away from her, I want to be with her. I'm trying to decide what to do." None of this is conscious on her part, but her body and behavior communicate this.

This session is an exciting one to study because it shows the beginning stages of a new behavior—learning to trust and relate to a new adult. It is like watching a flower unfold before your very eyes. In this session you can study how a child uses body language to communicate feelings, needs, and thoughts. Language begins with the body, and Mira's behavior in this session illustrates this.

Mira's in and out, back and forth behavior—between being present and allowing contact and not being present and pushing Vi away, between allowing Vi to touch and cradle her and screaming—expresses through body language how hard it is for her to decide what she wants.

Mira began the session by asking for the lotion—inviting contact. After a few moments of contact, she moved her body away from Vi and at the same time maintained contact with Vi (her feet are almost in Vi's lap). While she's doing that, she's looking around and saying she wants to play with another adult ("I don't like to play with you"). While she's saying that, she's holding up the lotion bottle, inviting contact. She responded to the contact (the Slippery Hand Game) by saying Vi "hurt" her, yet she never responded as if Vi had hurt her. They seemed to be just words that stopped the game or what they were doing. Mira also interrupted her contact by hitting and kicking Vi, wanting to leave the scene (get a drink), and focusing her attention on the others in the group, telling Vi to "shut up." None of these behaviors, however, had much energy in them, including her request for a different partner. Her words do not fit her actions. While inviting contact with Vi, she is saying, "I don't like to play with you."

In terms of body language, Mira used the word "hurt" a lot. She used it in reference to Vi ("You're hurting my back") and in reference to herself (a finger hurts). When she said something hurt, it seemed to mean she wanted Vi to touch it, kiss it, or put lotion on it. When she said Vi hurt her, it seemed to mean that she *felt something*, especially some discomfort, or perhaps that she was losing control, but she never gave any evidence that she felt a physical hurt. After she said that Vi hurt her, she would return to either asking for touch or allowing Vi to provide it. For example, when she said that Vi hurt her back, Vi said, "Sit up and let me see your back," touching it. She responded with giggles, saying, "It tickles."

In this session, Mira never refused any touching initiated by Vi. Yet, as soon as she began to experience some pleasure in it, she immediately turned it off by distracting herself, saying Vi is "hurting" her, screaming, and so on. Then, as soon as she moved away from contact with Vi, she would move back, invite, and accept contact.

A careful study of the transcribed session shows that Mira made progress in her ability to relate. She contributed to the relationship by creating a game which required a response from the therapist. Her "stuck-knee" game was a metaphor that defined her problem: she is stuck and to get unstuck, she needs to be touched (kissed). She needs to be loved. She asked to be touched again when she said, "I got some scratches. Will you put some lotion on this?" In the third cradling, during the Circle Time, she was like a baby with her mother. Mira just closed her eyes, sucked her thumb, and experienced herself and Vi. In those moments, she experienced her core self. She was at peace with herself.

Some psychologists would have labeled Mira an Attention Deficit Disorder (ADD) child. That label only describes behavior. It does not tell us what the behavior is communicating, what the child is experiencing, or what the therapist is experiencing when working with her.

As the DP therapist (or Adult Partner), I experienced Mira as more real and also much more difficult to follow in session 2. She kept interrupting the flow of her work. She kept changing her mind as to what she wanted to do. Yet she had more energy. She was less dead. And it took a lot of energy from me to keep up with her and to know what to do. For example, when the cradling didn't seem to work the first time, I didn't know what to do. So I did it again, and that time it did work.

Much later, I began to appreciate the depth and meaning of what Mira had accomplished in that second week, especially her ability to express her needs concretely (through touch) and abstractly (through metaphors) at the same time.

THE HELLO PROCESS, PART 2: RESISTANCE

Part 2 of the Hello process represents the stage in which the child actively resists getting involved with the adult. The child's growing attachment to the adult stimulates this resistance and is expressed in the resistant behavior. Her chaotic-like behavior is saying, "I don't know what to do with this experience I'm having." (See Chapter 6 for the therapist's part at this stage.)

Mira's behavior in session 3 illustrates this stage very well. The relative ease with which she shifted in and out of contact in session 2 changed in session 3 to a very active, aggressive resistant behavior. As the DP therapist, I was unprepared for the intensity of her oppositional behavior in the beginning of that hour. (This session was videotaped, so I was wearing a microphone.)

Session 3

Scene: Mira enters room, puts her hand out to Vi, and then withdraws it. She runs around the room, yelling at another child. Mary, the Leader, picks her up and delivers her to Vi in their designated play place. Vi helps Mira sit down.

Mira: (Whiny voice) *Let go of me*! I'm going to tell my Mommy on you.
    Vi: You know what you did? You put your hand up for me to take the minute you walked in. Let's see that hand.
Mira: (Touching microphone on Vi's neck) Why you need that on? (Calm voice)
    Vi: So they can hear what we say. (Taking her hand) Was this the hand that said Hello to me?
Mira: (Hits Vi lightly)
    Vi: (Stopping her hand) No hitting.
Mira: I can hit if I want to.
    Vi: Let's see which hand. (Taking her hand)
Mira: (Pulling her hand away with a negative "eh" sound and pouty face; kicks)
    Vi: No kicking.
Mira: (Yells) Shut up. (Yells louder) Shut up.
    Vi: Can you do that again?
Mira: (Repeats it softly)
    Vi: (Touching her finger) Has this finger still got its sore on?
Mira: (Pulls her hand away, with whiny sound)
    Vi: I haven't said Hello to you yet.
Mira: (Holding her hands behind her back)
    Vi: Well, did you tell your Mommy you had a good time with me?
Mira: No. (In a clear, not whiny voice)
    Vi: Did you tell your Mother I put some lotion on your finger?
Mira: No. (Pulling away) I told her, "I hate you."
    Vi: You did? (With surprised tone)
Mira: Yes. (said calmly)
    Vi: Well, look at me. Is it my eyes you hate? You're not looking at my eyes.
Mira: (Gives Vi a brief look with a smile, then turns her face away, starts whiny crying sounds)
    Vi: (Lightly tapping her mouth) Can you make a sound?
Mira: (Pulls away, starts screaming)
    Vi: You're good at making noise. Let's see your tongue.
Mira: (Screams, lying on back, facing Vi)
    Vi: Are there some teeth in there?
Mira: (Closes her mouth tightly) Nhn-nhn. (Meaning no)

Vi: There aren't any teeth in there?

Mira: Uh-uh. (Negative) (Covers her mouth)

Vi: Your mouth has gone away.

Mira: (Screams, covers her mouth; whiny voice) Mommy, I want to sit up.

Vi: Well, you can sit up.

Mira: (Sits up, comes close, sits on Vi's lap facing Vi, puts her arm on Vi's right shoulder)

Vi: Oh, you're going to put your arm around me.

Mira: (Quickly removes her arm as if she had been touching a hot stove, whines)

Vi: We could do it like this. (Puts her in straddle position facing Vi; starts to sing "Rock-A-Bye Mira")

Mira: (Hits Vi mildly, screams)

Vi: (Continues singing)

Mira: (Continues screaming)

Vi: (Stops singing and looks at her) Every time we come together, I'm going to rock you a little bit.

Mira: (Spits into the microphone)

Vi: Oh, do that in my hand. (Holding up her hand toward Mira)

Mira: (Spits into Vi's hand and enjoys doing it)

Vi: Okay, see how that feels when I do it to you. (Taking her hand)

Mira: (Pulling away)

Vi: You want to do that in my hand again?

Mira: Yeah. (and does it)

Vi: Can I do it on your hand?

Mira: (Screaming) No.

Vi: Do it on my cheek, then. (Pointing to her cheek and leaning toward Mira)

Mira: (Does it and smiles)

Vi: You did a good one! It's my turn now. (Taking Mira's face in her hands)

Mira: (Pulls away)

Vi: (Holding Mira's face, does a "buzz" on her cheek)

Mira: That's not a good one!

Vi: Do it on my cheek.

Mira: (Does it on Vi's cheek) That was a good one!

Vi: Let me do it on your hand.

Mira: (Screams, pulls away)

Vi: All right, we'll cradle. (Putting arms around her; she's still sitting straddle to Vi; Vi starts to sing)

Mira: (Raises up and pushes her hands hard against Vi) You're hurting my neck.

Vi: (Stops singing, looks at Mira) Your neck?

154

Mira: You're choking me.
 Vi: Where is your neck? Is it back here? (Touching her neck)
Mira: (Starts to cry a whiny, pseudo kind of crying)
 Vi: My goodness! Are you going to cry? You can cry if you want to. If you are
     going to cry, I guess I'll have to rock you.
Mira: (Pulls away and whines)
 Vi: (Gets lotion and starts putting it on her hands—one of her favorite things)
Mira: (Hides her hands under her back; lying down)
 Vi: Where did your hands go? They're playing hide and seek. Are they under
     your head? (Looking) Are they under your nose? (Looking)
Mira: (Laughs)
 Vi: Are they under your ears?
Mira: (Laughs)
 Vi: Are they under your knees? Are they in your mouth?
Mira: No.
 Vi: Are they under your bottom?
Mira: Yes. (Bringing them out)
 Vi: Oh, there they are!
Mira: (Laughs, then hides them)
 Vi: Are they under your bottom?
Mira: (Spits)
 Vi: (Starts to put lotion on her hands)
Mira: (Whiny voice) I don't want any.
 Vi: You said it made your finger better last time.
Mira: (Whiny voice) I want my foot like this. (Putting both legs on same side as
     she sits in Vi's lap)
 Vi: Well, you can have your foot that way. (Helping her move it)
Mira: (Whiny voice) I want my socks off.
 Vi: (Taking her socks off) Say, "Take my socks off, please." Look what's
     there! A toe. Look, there's another toe! And another toe! You're looking
     at your toe. Here's another one.
Mira: (Sits up, leans forward, and says, "Poop" in Vi's face)
 Vi: (Ignoring this) Here's another toe. (Touching it)
Mira: Ouch! You're hurting my toe. (Immediately gets up to leave)
 Vi: (Grabs her arm and turns her back to Vi) What did you do to that little toe?
Mira: (Grabs a sock to throw it)
 Vi: (Takes the sock, puts it behind her) We're not going to throw socks. Let's
     see if all your toes are here. (Starts counting) Can you count?
Mira: (Whiny voice) I don't want to count.

Later in the session:

Mira asks for the touching games we had played in the first two sessions: the Slippery Hand game and the Stuck-Knee game she herself had initiated in session 2. When I said, "Do you want to do the Stuck-Knee game for Circle Time?", she enthusiastically said, "Yes." When asked how many kisses it needed (to get unstuck) she said, "A million." The other knee needed "Ten kisses." She responded, however, to these contacts first with loud giggles and then with ear-splitting screams. She did these earsplitting screams many times. At that point, I put Mira in my lap with her back to me and held her tightly while we played the Row, Row Your Boat game. In this game, I say to her, "I have to hold you tightly so that you won't fall out of the boat." She began to like this game and relaxed, saying, "Do it again." At the end of each boat ride, I turned her around and cradled her. Each time I repeated this game, she allowed the cradling for a longer period of time.

Mira: Be careful.
  Vi: I'll be gentle. (Continues her chanting)
Mira: (With quiet, non-whiny voice) Stop hurting me.
  Vi: I don't mean to hurt you.
Mira: (Whiny kind of crying that feels different)
  Vi: Okay. You're feeling so bad. I'll just hold you. (Sings "Rock-A-Bye") (See Appendix)
Mira: (Singing with Vi) Da da da da. (Gets restless, pushing away)
  Vi: Well, let's turn around and do it this way. (Moving her from straddling Vi to being held in cradled position)
Mira: No, I want to do it this way. (Reversing which end is her head)
  Vi: (Singing "Rock-A-Bye, Mira" and Brahms "Lullaby"; continuing by chanting) I like Mira; I like to hold her. I'm rocking her just like this up in the tree. She has her eyes, she has her little nose, she has her mouth and her teeth, she has her hands and her fingers, she has her shoulders and her elbows, she has hands and her fingers, she has legs, she has feet, she has toes, she has a bottom, she has a stomach, she has her back, she has her hair, her teeth. She has her thumb in her mouth, she has her fingers, she has her teeth. She has her ears, she has her eyes. And this is so nice, singing to you. Rock-A-Bye Mira in the tree tops. When the wind blows, the cradle will rock. When the bow breaks the cradle will fall and down will come Mira and I will catch you. And I like Mira, and I like to hold Mira. (All this sung or chanted very slowly in sing-song repetitive way)

Mira: (Throughout Vi's singing Mira was in a trance, eyes closed, sucking her
    thumb, without any movement for several minutes)

Comments

Session 3 illustrates how the DP therapist or adult partner stays present and
sets limits during this oppositional stage. In setting limits, Vi was not making
Mira do or say anything. Vi was simply noticing her and touching her, as she had
in the previous two sessions. Vi also supported her to do things she initiated or
wanted to do. No matter how hard Vi tried, however, nothing seemed to work.
Limit setting also consisted of not allowing Mira to leave the mat or hit or bite
Vi, all of which she tried to do. No matter what Mira did, she could not get rid of
Vi. Vi was always present.

In spite of the intensity of her oppositional behavior, however, Mira did experience moments of enjoyment, which she shut off when she became aware of
them. For example, she put her arm around Vi, but the moment she became
aware that she was doing it, she removed her arm. She enjoyed making "a raspberry" on Vi's cheek, saying, "That was a good one." Mira is becoming aware of
having two experiences at the same time—that she enjoys being seen and
touched and that she is resisting allowing herself to experience it. Mira is not yet
conscious of this, but her body is communicating it very clearly.

Mira, on the other hand, was not opposing the therapist all the time. In the
latter part of the session, she asked to do the touching games including her Stuck-
Knee game. Yet she couldn't maintain these games for more than a few seconds
before breaking out with loud giggles and then earsplitting screams. It was as if
she didn't know how to respond to being touched in these games because it was
so new. Perhaps the touching was too much for her. Perhaps she was afraid of losing control. One thing was clear. She was lacking a core self which organizes and
takes charge of her behavior. She had no inner model to guide her.

I responded to this chaotic behavior not by withdrawing the touching, but
by presenting it in different forms and in small amounts, always working toward
the cradling to help her experience her body relaxed and quiet. To give her the
feeling that she was in control, I always stopped when she asked me to do so even
though that didn't seem to help her be happier. It gave her a respite and also
gave her time to become aware that she wanted to be touched. I tried out different things from my repertoire of touch until I found something she could like.
What worked well was my Row, Row Your Boat game. Holding her tightly in my
lap pretending to keep her from falling out of the boat as we rocked turned out
to be something she liked and also something in which she felt my body and her

body. Through this game, she allowed the cradling for longer and longer periods of time.

Finally, at the end of the one-to-one time, Mira allowed herself to be totally relaxed in the cradling—to let go of her need to control and be in a trance (eyes closed and sucking her thumb), while Vi sang and chanted. She repeated this behavior during the cradling in the Circle Time cradling (see Mira in Circle Time).

Mira in Circle Time

(To learn what Mira did in Circle Time, turn to pages 225-230 and return to this page.) Compared to the intensity of her resistant, oppositional behavior in the one-to-one, Mira did quite well in Circle Time. She cooperated and followed the Leader's direction even though she was demanding to be the center of attention all the time. She was a little smart-alec when she blurted out, "I touched myself" (as she touched her knee). Yet, she was right on with what she said. To be in touch with one's self and with others is the focus of the Developmental Play.

When Mira was given attention (as opposed to when she demanded it), she didn't know what to do with it (example, Trick Time). She became very nervous. She relied upon her therapist (this, after all her resistance to the therapist earlier) to decide what to do and to guide her through it. She was totally unable to respond to the Leader when she tried to show her how to curtsy.

When Mira was given attention by the therapist, Mira could accept it. The only time she was quiet in the whole Circle Time was during the cradling. She was totally relaxed as she was in the one-to-one cradling a few minutes earlier. However, the minute the cradling ended, she started talking and yelling.

Mira described herself as not needing anything and not willing to give anything ("I don't want to give her a hug. I don't need a hug"). However, she did hug all the children at the end (when it is all over and no one is particularly noticing her). At the end of the first three weeks, her behavior does show the beginnings of a new self.

Overview

This session is remarkable for Mira's movement from almost total resistance to contact in the beginning to total acceptance and trust at the end. Two things especially stand out: First, the role that the dialogue of touch played in bringing about this transformation. Second, the body language (hitting, pulling away, allowing cradling) Mira used to communicate her part in this dialogue. In the beginning, Mira initiated the action through touch, and Vi responded to her. In the latter part of the session, Vi initiated the action through touch, and Mira responded to Vi. In other words, in the beginning of the hour, Mira did much of the initiating with all her acting-out behavior, and Vi was kept busy responding and trying to contain her. In the latter part of the hour, Mira could accept Vi being the initiator and respond to her. Through this dialogue of touch, Mira's core self began to emerge.

As for my experience as the DP therapist (or adult partner), I was totally exhausted at the end, both physically and emotionally. I was unprepared for the intensity of her oppositional behavior. She moved so fast from one thing to another that I had no time to think about anything. I had to respond immediately in seconds. I felt her energy and her aliveness in this intensity. She was not a ghost anymore. She was really present. At the end of this hour, I neither liked her nor disliked her. I was just drained. At the time I didn't think I had done anything, but later I realized that some wonderful things had happened. *One thing was clear: By the end of this session, Mira and I both knew that we had begun a relationship!* By the end of session 3, Mira had entered the stage of trust.

THE HELLO PROCESS, PART 3: ATTACHMENT

Part 3 of the Hello process—becoming attached—completes the Hello process. This is the basic trust stage. The child lets go of her need to control and lets herself just enjoy being a receiver. She experiences an "emotional tie" to the adult now. She has an attachment relationship.

Session 6

Mira began the session by taking her shoes and socks off and saying, "Do you remember the knee is stuck?" (Lying on the floor facing Vi)

Vi: Yes, I do. What does it need?
Mira: Ten kisses. (Holding up her two hands)
Vi: (Kisses her knee ten times and tries to move her leg)
Mira: (Leg doesn't move) It don't work.
Vi: What do I need to do?
Mira: Give it two kisses.
Vi: (Kisses her knee twice; reaches over and lifts Mira up from the lying position to the sitting position so that they are facing each other; starts the Knock at the Door game) (See Appendix) (Singing) Knock at the door. (Tapping her forehead) Peek in. (Touching her eyelashes). Lift the latch. (Touching the tip of her nose) And walk in. (Touching her mouth).
Mira: (Mouth remains closed)
Vi: Oh, she isn't home. (Sounding disappointed)

Mira: Do it again.
  Vi: (Repeats the game)
Mira: (Mouth remains closed) Do it again.
  Vi: (Repeats again)
Mira: (Mouth opens)
  Vi: (Hugging her) Oh, I'm glad you're home!

Much of this session was spent in quiet time. Vi cradled Mira a couple of times, singing "Rock-A-Bye Mira" and later Brahms "Lullaby." During the latter, she lay in Vi's arms in a trance, with eyes half open and with her finger in her mouth. At another time, Mira said, "I want to lay down." She laid on the mat, and Vi chanted parts of her body as she touched them—"Here's your little head; here's your blond hair," and so on. To do her whole body, leaving nothing out, takes several minutes.

When Vi picked Mira up and put her in her lap, saying "It's time to get ready to go," Mira said, *"I don't want to go."* She reached for the lotion bottle and handed it to Vi, saying, *"You do it."* Then, after having had the lotion, she said, *"That's not nearly enough. I need a lot."* When Vi again said that it's time to go, Mira said loudly, "No, no" and held up her feet. Vi looked at her feet and said, "And I suppose you want lotion on them, too," to which Mira nodded in the affirmative. As soon as Vi began the lotion, Mira just lay back in Vi's lap and re-laxed, letting Vi do whatever she does. She only said something when Vi didn't do something right, such as when she put her socks on incorrectly. After she showed Vi how to do it, she again leaned back and relaxed.

Finally, Mira accepted and participated in saying the Goodbye. When Vi waved Goodbye by bending her fingers on one hand, Mira imitated Vi and did the same while saying, "Da-Da." Then she took the other hand and did the same thing, talking baby-talk and smiling. She looked like a baby.

Comments

Mira certainly was a very different child in this session. The most noticeable change was in the quality of her energy. She had a feeling of contentment about her as she got acquainted with her body, and she took delight in experiencing her bodily self. For example, after being touched, she would touch herself, feeling her hands and holding them up to look at them as babies do. She engaged in baby-talk. She looked like she was about two years old.

At the same time that she was more babyish, she was also more grown up. She expressed this both in the quality of her language and speech and in her ability to state clearly what she needed: *"I* don't want to go." "That's not nearly enough." "*I* need a lot." These statements show that she definitely has an "I" part of her now—the Observer part of her, her core self.

When Mira said to Vi, "You do it"—that is, take the lotion out of the bottle (something *she* always had to do before)—she was experiencing Vi as a "You" for her. With someone being a "You" for her, she could find her "I." These statements of hers demonstrate that Mira not only feels attached to Vi, but that she is also beginning to experience Vi as separate from her.

These remarkable changes are the result of the work Mira did before, especially sessions 2 and 3. After session 3, she was a changed child. From the very beginning, Mira allowed the cradling offered in Circle Time and some touching and cradling in the one-to-one period. But after session 3, she could not get enough touching and cradling. All of session 6 was devoted to cradling her or chanting her body parts as she lay on the mat or putting lotion on her hands and feet. She verbalized her need for touch ("I need a lot"). In session 6, Mira and Vi had a touching-verbal-dialogue. She could give herself permission to have this need now (to be touched). She has entered the stage of trust (Erikson, 1965).

The cradling, along with the vibrations from Vi's singing, provided the boundaries that gave Mira an inner world, a core self. The cradling experience protected her inner world from the outer world. Since the outer world has become separate from her, she can also relate to it now.

As the DP therapist, I experienced a new quality in Mira—a presence, a quiet solidness. She had the quality of knowing where she is going though neither she nor I know where that is yet. She was definitely in the attachment phase.

The growth that Mira accomplished in six weeks speaks for the potency of touch when done in a caring and sensitive way. The dialogue of touch begins the growth process.

Mira's changed behavior in session 6 also helped me to understand the meaning of Mira's resistant hyper behavior in session 3. Her behavior in session 6 shows that Mira lacked the experiences she needed to even be a two-year-old. No wonder she didn't know how to behave as a four-year-old! When I provided her with the experiences of a two-year-old, she both wanted it and didn't know what to do with it. It felt foreign to her. She couldn't handle it, so she screamed. That did not mean, however, that she didn't want it. She was a two-year-old trying to behave as a four-year-old. In session 6, she allowed herself to be the two-year-old that she was. From that place she relaxed. She enjoyed herself. She related and got acquainted with her inner self, probably for the first time. Now she was on track!

THE SEPARATION PHASE

The Separation Phase is a very exciting stage for both child and adult. Using her core self gained in the Hello part, the child asks for what she wants and guides the adult in the role she is to play. Each session is like a play, but neither the child nor the adult knows the script until the end of the session.

Session 7

During the session that followed her baby behavior, Mira began to assume a new role—that of a co-player. She wanted to contribute to the relationship—to do her part. She demonstrated this new role by bringing rice cakes to the session. (Rice cakes are the snacks Mary, the Leader, serves at the end of Circle Time.) To do this, Mira had to carry out a series of connected actions: She had to plan to do it; she had to ask her mother to buy the cakes and go with her to buy them; she had to find a store that carried them; and she had to remember to bring them on that Monday. That behavior showed a lot of emotional investment in her relationship with me, the therapist.

Unfortunately, my response to all her endeavor was to thank her for bringing the snacks and to lay them aside, saying we would have them later for Circle Time. Mira's response was to keep reaching over and picking up the crackers. When I kept putting them away, Mira finally gave up and followed my lead.

I was not seeing Mira at all at that moment. I was not present for her. I was not getting her message that this relationship meant so much to her that she wanted to make her contribution to it. I was thinking that snacks belong to Circle Time, that having snacks during our one-to-one time would disrupt the other pairs. The other children in the group would want some, too.

If I had not been so rigid and rule-oriented, I would have suggested that she and I have the cakes right then. Just she and I have a party! It would have been a wonderful thing to have done, and I would have acknowledged Mira's dedication to the relationship. If the other children had also wanted some (and they might not have even noticed us), I could have worked something out. This is an example of how children can help us become less rigid and of how I learned something about me from Mira. Mira gave up her autonomy to be with me.

In Circle Time, however, Mira did get seen by Mary, the Leader. Mary said that since Mira had brought rice cakes, we would have snacks first today instead of last. Mary was able to break the rules! Mary saved the day for Mira. Mira has entered the "domain of intersubjective relatedness" (Stern, 1985, p. 125).

Session 8

Mira hadn't learned the name of the Knock at the Door game, which she asked for by saying, "Do what you did yesterday. Peek." Mira said, "Do it again" four times. She is learning the game through this repetition as well as getting touched.

Session 11

This was the last session before the break over the holidays. Mira began this session by leaning over close to me and whispering, "Let's do Knock on the Door." The way she said it conveyed a quality of intimacy that had not been there before. This was our private, secret game. Before playing the game, I told her we would miss three meetings due to the holidays, but that I would see her after Christmas.

Mira first responded to this announcement with a startled and wide-eyed look. Then she asked if she would be staying with Mary and if the others would be gone. When I played her game, she said, "Do all the way around" (walking my fingers around her face). She offered her "kissable places," but then said they were all gone. She wanted to know if I lived with Mary. She said, "I don't like you," and that her toy (which she had brought with her) needed her to hold it because "It's too scared to be alone."

Session 12

Session 12 followed the three-week break over the holidays. This session shows (1) how Mira and I, as her therapist, reconnected after that break; (2) how Mira used her body for communication; (3) Mira's attachment to Vi; (4) Mira's separation from Vi; and (5) Mira's new verbal-dialogue.

Mira: (Greets Vi by holding up her fists and starting to hit her)
   Vi: (Grabs her hands) No hitting.
Mira: I'll get you. That's enough of that. (Not clear)
   Vi: (Taking Mira on her lap) My goodness. Well, Hello.
Mira: (Holding up her feet) Take off my "dooty" shoes.
   Vi: (Taking off a shoe) So, I haven't seen you for a long time.
Mira: I stayed home all day.
   Vi: Were you upset because I didn't see you?
Mira: (Grabs her shoe and throws it across the room)
   Vi: (Taking her other shoe) No, we don't throw shoes.
Mira: (Tries to throw her socks)

Vi: (Stops her) Are you upset with me because I didn't see you for a while? You haven't said Hello to me yet.

Mira: (Pulling away from Vi)

Vi: (Holding her)

Mira: (Yelling) I want that lotion.

Vi: All right. (Handing her the small plastic bottle)

Mira: (Throws the bottle right into Vi's face. Looks at Vi with eyes wide open, with a startled look and her mouth open)

Vi: ([For a moment, I was furious] taking bottle) We don't throw things.

Mira: (Squeals and points to band-aid on her finger) I got a boo-boo.

Vi: You have? Shall I kiss it?

Mira: Yeah. Take if off to kiss it.

Vi: (Turning Mira around to face her) I haven't said Hello to you yet.

Mira: Get away.

Vi: Well, tell me you're mad that I didn't see you for a while.

Mira: (Turns her head away and makes spitting sounds)

Vi: So that's the way you feel, huh? Remember I said I would be back, and here I am.

Mira: I want to sing a song.

Vi: Okay.

Mira: I want to do it with that. (The microphone)

Vi: Okay. I'll hold it for you.

Mira: (Moves her lips, but makes no sound) Now you talk. You sing a song.

Vi: You want me to sing?

Mira: Mhm-mhm. (Affirmative)

Vi: (Sings her usual Brahms "Lullaby")

Mira: (Smiling)

Vi: You're smiling.

Mira: (Half-way through, joins Vi in singing the song)

Vi: Great! You know that song. That's wonderful that you know that song.

Mira: You want me to sing it again?

Vi: Okay.

Mira: (Turning her back to Vi so that she is facing the room and can see everything going on with the other pairs) I want to sing it this way. I won't run away.

Vi: (Catching on to her and not believing her) But I can't see you that way. (Turning Mira so that she is facing Vi)

Mira: (Sings the whole verse with correct tune and words except one place. Instead of "bright angels around my child" she sings, "angels standing around.")

Vi: That's wonderful the way you sang that! You know that song. Did you sing that song when you were home?

Mira: Mhm-mhm. (Affirmative)

Vi: Did you sing it to your mother?

Mira: Mhm-mhm. (Affirmative) (Showing band-aid on finger) A boo-boo.

Vi: Shall I kiss it?

Mira: No. (Points to tiny part of band-aid)

Vi: Oh, right here. (Kissing that part)

Mira: (Pulls away) Fart.

Vi: Shall I say Hello to your nose?

Mira: No. Do Knock at the Door.

Vi: Knock at the door, peek in, lift the latch, and walk in.

Mira: (Mouth closed)

Vi: Oh, you're not home. (Disappointed tone)

Mira: (Moving her hand around her face) Go round. (Something Vi always did)

Vi: (Outlining Mira's face with her hand) So I walk around your face. I walk all the way around, and I see you looking at me. Let's see. I wonder if she's home. I wonder what she is doing.

Mira: Do it again.

Vi: Oh, do it again. (Repeats game, Mira's mouth is closed) What am I going to do? She's not home. Shall I look in the windows? (Putting her face close to Mira's, looking into her eyes as if they were windows)

Mira: (Giggles) Knock at the door.

Vi: (Repeats game) Oh, she isn't home.

Mira: (Giggles)

Vi: I got to walk around *again*? I climb the tree (Mira's head) and then I slide down. (Moving her hand over the front of Mira's face) I wonder what she is doing? Is she sitting in the house by the door?

Mira: No. The door's just locked.

Vi: Do I have the key?

Mira: You have to push the button, and it opens by itself.

Later in the session:

Mira: (Whiny voice) I didn't go to bed until midnight.

Vi: Let's rock, then. (Putting Mira in her lap and cradling her [in cradling, the child lies in the adult's lap, head on the adult's left arm. In this position, there is close eye contact between them], singing a lullaby)

Mira: (Lies quietly in Vi's arms with eyes open. Seems to be thinking about something. At the end of Vi's singing, still cradled, she looks up at Vi) You

165

know what? The other foot is the stuck one today. (Points to her foot, which she holds up)

Vi: (Ignoring Mira's foot but looking at her face) Did you bring any kissable places today?

Mira: (Still cradled, looks up at Vi's face) No, I didn't. (Pauses, thinks, still looking up at Vi) Do *you* see one?

Vi: (Laughing) Do I see one? Yes. I see one right here. (Kissing her on the cheek)

Mira: (Looking at Vi) That's not it.

Vi: Is it here? (Kissing her on the other cheek)

Mira: No. (Holds up her foot, looks at Vi, smiles)

Vi: (Taking her foot in her hand) Is it this foot?

Mira: Try. (looks at Vi—she is smiling and has an impish look)

Vi: (Kissing the held foot)

Mira: No. (Smiling—she is enjoying herself immensely)

Vi: Is it this foot? (Touching her other foot)

Mira: (Smiles—she is being playful)

Vi: (Kissing her other foot)

Mira: Ouch! (Sits up, examines her foot) A sore toe.

Vi: (Holding her, joins Mira in looking at her toe; Vi did not see any sore on her toe)

Mira: (Lies down facing Vi)

Vi: Here's your head, and here's your eyebrow.

Mira: You're not to sing songs, and you're not to say *words*!

Vi: Oh well, here is your head.

Mira: Stop doing that.

Vi: You're ordering me around today, and here's your nose.

Mira: Stop it. (Starts to kick Vi) Fart.

Vi: Are you still mad? There's your nose, and there's your mouth.

Mira: (Very softly) Stop that.

Vi: You have a dimple right there, and you've got teeth.

Mira: (Opens her mouth) Do you see my cavities in there?

Vi: No, I don't see any. (Counts her teeth)

Later in the session:

Mira: (Is restless, hears another child crying)

Vi: Turn around and look.

Mira: I got to go to the bathroom.

Vi: You can go at the end. (She never has to go and didn't go at the end) (Holds Mira facing her, with hand behind her head, rocks her up and down) Up and down . . . up and down . . .

Mira: I took a bath. Did you take a bath?

Vi: Yes.

Mira: Then why is your skin so rumbally? (Referring to wrinkles)

Vi: (Laughing) That's the way your skin gets when you get old. When you're young, like you, your skin is smooth. (Touching Mira's face)

Mira: When you're young. (Leans against Vi and tucks head into Vi's neck and closes her eyes; makes little humming sounds)

Vi: (Joins her in humming)

Mira: (Loudly) It's so dark.

Vi: Well, you can open your eyes. See, it's light now. If you close your eyes, it's dark.

Mira: There's a little light. I want some lotion on my feets.

Vi: Tell me which foot wants it. (Another child, Mona, yells, "Mary")

Mira: (Yells) Mary.

Vi: You said that because you just heard Mona say that.

Mira: Shut up.

Vi: How about putting some lotion on your face this time? (Putting it on Mira's face) Isn't that nice?

Mira: (Starts to put some on her own face) *It's so soft.*

Vi: (Ends the session with the usual cradling before going to Circle Time)

Comments

Reconnection. After a period of absence, nearly everyone experiences a period of awkwardness when meeting a close friend again. What shall I say to her? Will she be the same? Will she like being with me?

Mira and I, as her therapist, both experienced this awkwardness. How do we get reacquainted after missing three sessions? Mira, being a very active and take-charge child, initiated the contact by greeting me with held-up fists and by throwing things. After she threw the bottle of lotion right at my face, she connected by asking me to look at her band-aid finger. Then Mira contacted me in a very organized and focused way by saying that she wanted to sing a song (new behavior), followed by asking me to sing. I joined her, then Mira sang the whole song by herself. The song she sang was Brahms "Lullaby"—the song I had sung many times to her while cradling her. That song represented about as close and intimate a contact as she could get. Mira had learned that song and sung it at home over the holidays, possibly as a way to maintain contact.

167

Mira's behavior following her out-of-control bottle-throwing seemed to represent an attempt to make amends to me or reconnect with me.

Play Disruptions. When Mira doesn't know what to do, for example, after an absence or to begin a session, she tends to be very active, loud, energetic, and combative. After that initial introduction of herself, she relates well. In this session, the absence seems to have activated more of that behavior. Throughout, she engaged in what Erikson (1940) calls "play disruptions." These are behaviors that stop an ongoing interaction. They occur when the child is anxious, when the child doesn't know what to do or is trying to make up her mind, when the child is testing the therapist, when the child wants to be more in control, or when the child is practicing saying something because she knows the words.

Mira's "play disruptions" consisted of hitting, throwing things, calling the therapist names (fart, shut-up, fat lady), ordering the therapist not to do things ("You're not to sing songs and you're not to say *words*; stop doing that."). The play disruptions Mira used most often, however, were body hurts, and she used them a lot ("a sore toe; you're hurting my neck; you hurt my leg"). She never gave any evidence of feeling physically hurt. These sayings seemed to be just words, but they did serve to stop whatever she and the therapist were doing, at least for the moment. Once she had said she had a "sore toe," she paid no attention to her toe.

Mira also showed a more complex disruptive behavior in the form of moving or turning away from the therapist and saying things like, "I won't run away." Yet that is exactly what she'll end up doing if the therapist does not interrupt that urge in some way.

Mira's Use of Her Body as an Avenue for Communication. This session is replete with examples of how Mira used body language either to make contact or to disrupt contact. She began the session by hitting the therapist and throwing things—signs that Mira didn't know what to do or how to begin after a long absence. She pointed to a sore finger to make contact with the therapist after she had thrown the lotion bottle at her—a response to experiencing some anxiety. She made spitting sounds while her head was turned away. She communicated the pleasure of being touched by asking the therapist to repeat the Knock at the Door game six times, by initiating the stuck-foot game, and by asking directly, "I want some lotion on my feets." She used a "sore toe" (which was not sore) to disrupt or end a play. Finally, Mira expressed an awareness of the pleasure in touching her own face ("It is so soft").

Mira's Attachment to the Therapist. Since session 6, Mira has been building an attachment relationship to the therapist, because she trusts her now not to leave her no matter what she does. Mira showed this trust in the way she sometimes acted out using her body and using words. She feels free to do what she does. For example, she speaks perfect, grammatically correct English. Yet when she feels free or is in a baby place, she changes her speech to that of a much younger child ("I want some lotion on my feets. Me lay down").

It is the feeling of trust that allows Mira to feel close to the therapist: She asked the therapist, "Why is your skin so rumbally?" She learned Brahms "Lullaby." She remembers what they did from one session to the next.

Mira's Separation from the Therapist. Mira's separation process began in session 6, when she acknowledged the therapist's presence in asking her to put the lotion on (*"You* do it"). In session 12, she clearly expressed the separation in the following dialogues:

Mira: (Holding up her foot) You know what? The other foot is the stuck one
     today.
  Vi: (Ignoring her cue) Did you bring any kissable places today?
Mira: No, I didn't. (Pauses, looks at Vi) Do *you* see one?
  Vi: (Laughing) Do I see one? Yes. I see one right here. (Kissing her cheek)

In this dialogue, Mira stated her view ("No, I didn't"), and she asked the therapist for her view ("Do you see one?"). For the first time, Mira showed awareness of experiencing the therapist as separate from her. From this place, Mira not only sees the therapist as separate, but also as a person from whom she can learn.

Mira's ability to momentarily let go of her own need to be attended to and to respond to the therapist's focus also speaks for her ability to experience the therapist as separate.

Verbal Dialogue. Because Mira can experience the therapist as separate, she is able to engage in a truly two-way verbal communication. Up to now, Mira's verbal behavior was connected to touch and her body in the form of asking to be touched ("Do it again"). In session 12, she began using verbal language not connected directly to touch to express her desire to contribute to their relationship. For example, she said, "I want to sing a song." When the therapist said, "Great! You know that song," Mira asked, "You want me to sing it again?" And she sang it again, very beautifully and almost word-perfect. Here, instead of asking the therapist to do something for her, she is interested in doing something *with* the therapist, something together. Mira also wanted to show the therapist what she could do. She loved being acknowledged by the therapist. She accepted it. This level of verbal dialogue is very new.

Mira can engage in verbal dialogue because her words call up visual images and are less tied to her body. They are more abstract. She can imagine and create an event not present. She demonstrated this new ability in the following excerpt:

The therapist is touching her face in the Knock at the Door game, while Mira sits with her eyes closed.

Vi: (Walking with her fingers around her face) I wonder what she is doing. Is she sitting in the house by the door?
Mira: No. The door's just locked.
Vi: Do I have the key?
Mira: You have to push the button, and it opens by itself.

In that interaction, Mira used the imagery the therapist provided—imagining herself sitting by the door. She responded to the question, then added other images of her own, with directions to the therapist on how to get in ("You push the button, and it opens by itself").

In this example, two levels of behavior are going on at the same time—the body experience of being touched and the cognitive experience of creating images. This time, Mira's verbal instruction was based on a visual image, and in that sense, it represents abstract thinking. Mira can now carry on a verbal dialogue that deals with events not present.

This is all new behavior for Mira. In the past, if the therapist offered an image, Mira wouldn't say anything or would say one word—yes or no. This time, she responded to the image the therapist provided, but she also enlarged on it and added one of her own. She did this *twice* in that brief interaction. In addition, Mira's last response has the quality of a metaphor ("You have to push the button, and it opens by itself"). That is, you don't have to work that hard to enter Mira's world to play with her. Mira and the therapist are engaged in a truly verbal dialogue.

Thus, the body experience starts the growth process and is always present—a presence to which the child can return. It's home. Yet, the body is more than physical, sensual experiences. These experiences themselves contain images that are metaphors for guides for living. These experiences can be verbalized as well as experienced. One is an experience, and one is a thought.

Mira has now reached the stage where she not only can dialogue with touch (direct experience), but can also dialogue with words (abstractions that stand for those experiences). Mira's ability to create metaphors first showed itself in this session (session 12).

The Role of the Therapist. As Mira's therapist, I made some mistakes in the beginning part of this session. The first mistake was responding to Mira's request for the lotion bottle when she was already in an out-of-control place. Her bottle-throwing was predictable. It would have made more sense for me to have picked up the bottle and start one of the contact games or said Hello to her with a touch.

After the bottle-throwing, I could have said, "That made me very angry when you did that, and that hurt." I did not do it (although I certainly felt like doing it at the time), because I didn't think it would be useful for her at her stage.

Because the therapist said nothing, Mira reacted to her own behavior and did something about it by reconnecting in her own way with the therapist—singing the therapist's song.

I also discovered that interpreting Mira's disruptive acting-out behavior (hitting, throwing things, name-calling) as an expression of anger was not meaningful to her for two reasons: (1) Mira was not ready for verbal interpretations, and (2) she was not angry (her behavior showed that). Her name-calling was said softly while looking at the therapist, but never with any anger or much energy. After she said them, she went back to playing as if she had never said them. It was more like she said them to see what the therapist would do. After a while I simply ignored her words, and we continued our play.

When Mira turned her back to me saying, "I won't run away," I was ready. Holding on to Mira and turning her around to face me, I said, "But I can't see you that way." That time I got the cue.

I stimulated Mira's move toward experiencing me as separate by not responding to her request to kiss the stuck foot, but instead by offering her a new focus. Instead of doing something Mira wanted, I did something I wanted to do— offer Mira the opportunity to say what she brings to the relationship ("Did you bring any kissable places?").

Mira's response showed that she was ready for this stage. She not only answered me but also asked my viewpoint.

I also provided stimulation for the creation of images in the Knock at the Door game. Getting bored at so many requests to "do it again," I added, "I wonder what she is doing. Is she sitting in the house by the door?" To my surprise, this time Mira answered and added an image of her own ("No. The door's just locked"). When I responded to her image with, "Do I have the key?" she added another image ("You have to push the button and it opens by itself").

The role of the DP therapist is to keep up with the growth of the child and to change as she changes, to offer the child opportunities to experience herself in new and more mature ways. In the attachment process, children learn through imitation, identification, assimilation, and accommodation. This means that adults have to do something for the children to imitate, identify with, assimilate, and accommodate. In the above two examples, I provided Mira with new behaviors she could use in one or all of those ways.

As the therapist, I experienced session 12 as very rich, challenging, and exciting. I had fun with her in this session.

Session 13

Mira: (Taking off shoes) Take off my poo-poo shoes.

  Vi: You're taking your shoes and socks off; you're looking at me, and you're smiling.

Mira: (Giggles and smiles)

  Vi: (Touching noses) Hello.

Mira: (Gets the giggles) I want to get a drink. I'm thirsty.

  Vi: You can get one afterwards.

Mira: (Shaking her finger at Vi in her face, pretending to be very assertive) I want to get a drink.

  Vi: (Imitating her tone and gesture) You do. There's your nose. (Touching it)

Mira: There's your eyes. (Looking at Vi) Open your eyes wide. Your eyes are green.

  Vi: That's right. Open your eyes wide. You have blue eyes. (Holding Mira facing her and supporting the back of her head with her hands, lifts her up and down and rocks her in this position, chanting) Up and down . . . up and down . . . up and down.

Mira: (Rests her head in Vi's neck)

  Vi: (Chanting in sing-song way) Oh, you're snuggling your face into my shoulder . . . up and down. We can sing (la la la). Your face is so warm. [Mary, the Leader, said Mira looked like a nursing baby.]

Mira: Oh, my feet cold.

  Vi: (Warms her feet) You look real happy today. Are you happy?

Mira: Yes. Let me get a drink first. I'm sad. If you won't let me get a drink, I won't be happy.

  Vi: Oh, is that so. Where are you sad?

Mira: (Points to her chest and makes a little hum)

  Vi: Oh, do that again. (Patting her chest as she hums; Vi hums with her)

Mira: I want to lie on my stomach. (Turns over and puts her feet in Vi's lap)

  Vi: Shall I kiss this foot?

Mira: No. I can spell No. N-O.

  Vi: Can you spell Yes?

Mira: Yes. Y-E-S. Do Knock at the Door.

  Vi: (Plays game; Mira's mouth closed) Oh, she's not home.

Mira: I'm at the K-Mart, shopping. Just knock at the door and see if the door opens.

  Vi: (Repeats game; this time Mira's mouth opens)

Mira: (Leans over to Vi, puts her arm around her spontaneously and hugs her)

  Vi: Oh, it's so nice to see you again. What a tight squeeze you gave me.

Mira: Can I get a drink now?
  Vi: You can get one at the end.

Later in session:

Mira: (Pointing to her shirt) I have a T-shirt on, but I can't take it off.
  Vi: No. It's too cold.
Mira: No cold. I got some boobies. (Lifting shirt and showing Vi)
  Vi: That's nice. You are a girl.
Mira: And my daddy has boobies . . . big fat ones.

Later in session:

Mira: (Whispers in Vi's ear) Today is Jane's birthday.
  Vi: When is your birthday?
Mira: March December 29.
  Vi: (Laughs) How old will you be?
Mira: Five. (Holding up her fingers) I'm already four . . . not supposed to count
    this one (thumb) yet. Then I'll be five.

Later in session:

  Vi: (Rocking her up and down, facing Vi)
Mira: When I'm asleep, you're supposed to stop doing that. You do it, but when
    my eyes close, you just stop doing it.
  Vi: Oh, I see. When you go to bed at night, do you imagine I'm rocking you
    like this?
Mira: Mhm mhm. (Yes)
  Vi: You do.
Mira: No. I'm not touching no one right now.
  Vi: You're pretending you're asleep?
Mira: No. (Wants Vi not to touch her, so Vi removes her hands)

Very quiet; Mira not saying anything and Vi not saying anything.

  Vi: What are you doing right now?
Mira: Nothing.
  Vi: Time to wake up. It's morning.

Mira: You're not supposed to wake me until my eyes open like this. (Demonstrates) You just have to wake me up when my eyes are shut.

Vi: Okay. I'm coming to wake you up. It's time to wake up. (Picking her up) You put your arm around me, and we'll just rock a minute. Your cheek is so soft and you just snuggled into my neck . . . so nice. (She is totally limp)

Mira: (Hums with Vi; later raises up) Can you open just one eye?

Vi: Yes. (Does it)

Mira: (With some help, does it) It's bedtime!

Vi: (Starts to repeat the rocking, but Mira wants to do something else)

Mira: (Sitting in front of Vi) Now let me put my feet right here. (Sitting sideways across Vi's legs) Now you pull me up.

Vi: (Pulls her up close on to her lap) I'll show you a new game. (Putting her face close to Mira's face) Close your eyes . . . Open them . . . Boo!

Mira: (Giggles) That's a game. And now it's my game. It's really my game. Now you take these two feet (which are resting on Vi's shoulders) and now pull me up.

Vi: (Pulls her up into her lap; then plays the Close Your Eyes-Boo game)

Mira: That's *not* my game. (Said loudly)

Vi: So you have a game, and I have a game.

Mira: No. It's my game 'cause you already had your game. We go turns. It's my turn 'cause 'member you had your turn.

Vi: All right. So it's your turn.

Mira: (Sitting in front of Vi, trying to imagine herself in a pose . . . she talks it out) One arm goes like this, the other arm goes like this. I put my leg right here. (Yells) Pull me up.

Vi: (Pulls her up)

Mira: Can I have a drink now?

Vi: You can when we're through.

Mira: This is my game . . . one more time. (Putting her hand on her forehead)

Vi: You're thinking about it. You're tapping your forehead.

Mira: I know. I know.

Vi: You know how you're going to do it?

Mira: I'm thinking . . . I got it!

Vi: What are you going to do?

Mira: I'm going to hold your two pinkies . . . your two thumbs. Now pull me up.

Vi: (Groaning, pretending to pull her up) I can't get you up. (Vi then puts her hands around Mira's waist and lifts her into her lap)

Mira: (Laughs) Can I get a drink?

Vi: You can at the end.

Mira: (Gets more and more excited as she continues to improvise)
   Vi: It's time for Circle Time, so let's cradle.
Mira: (Sings the lullaby with Vi)

Mira In Circle Time

At the end of Circle Time, when the Leader asked the children what they liked best, Mira raised her hand and said it was the games she played with the therapist. Then she and the therapist demonstrated one of her creations in Circle Time. At the end of Circle Time, Mira stood up and hugged the therapist and gave her a quick kiss on the mouth (this was new).

After Circle Time, Mira reminded the therapist that she had said she could get a drink of water. She went to get it. When it was time to put shoes and socks on to leave, Mira got high and acted out by standing on a table. The therapist said to her in a calm voice, "Which do you want to be in the lineup (at the door), number four or number five?" She said number four, became calm, got off the table, sat down and put her shoes and socks on, and left calmly with the others.

Comments

In this session, Mira moved on to another level. To the touching dialogue, she superimposed and added a verbal dialogue based on images that she has created. Mira can now imagine being touched instead of always having to be actually touched. She is no longer bound to the concrete.

Mira demonstrated in this session that she is ready for the therapist to provide her with images that she can incorporate and use to create her own images. For example, Mira responded to the therapist's rocking her "up and down" with, "When I'm asleep, you're supposed to stop doing that. You do it, but when my eyes close, you just stop doing it." Here, Mira enriches the simple rocking with the meaning for her in this implied scene of a mother putting her child to bed. The therapist picked up on this with, "When you go to bed at night, do you imagine I'm rocking you like this?" She said yes. Mira then followed this unwritten script and was very quiet and still, as if she were in bed sleeping. The therapist played the mother role and woke her up when it was morning, and Mira gave the therapist instructions on how to do it. Later, Mira continued this play, saying, "It's bedtime." Mira was both the director of this play and a character in it (the baby). This was like "playing house" except real people were players instead of dolls.

This interplay, based on images created by the therapist and child, is new. The role of the therapist is to give meaning to the touching dialogue by supplying the images that accompany it. These images were useful to Mira, who incorporated them into her own life experience.

In this session, Mira showed a strong need to do, and be, like the therapist. In the role of a peer, she competed with the therapist, keeping track of the number of "turns" each had. She copied the therapist. For example, when the therapist showed her a "new game," Mira got very excited and she, too, had to create one right on the spot. She was intrigued by the sound of the word "game" and kept repeating it: "That's a game. And now it's my game. It's really my game." Then she proceeded to create a game. She had no idea ahead of time what she was going to do. She simply began by moving parts of her body (arms and legs), and that became the game. She was trying to understand the word "game."

In the role of a learner, Mira used the therapist as a teacher to help her create her game.

Mira: This is my game, one more time. (Putting her hand on her forehead)
Therapist: You're thinking about it. You're tapping your forehead.
Mira: I know. I know.
Therapist: You know how you're going to do it?
Mira: I'm thinking . . . I got it!
Therapist: What are you going to do?
Mira: I'm going to hold your two pinkies, your two thumbs. Now pull me up!
Therapist: (Groaning and pretending to pull her up) I can't get you up.
Mira: (Laughs)

What is important here for Mira was her investment and excitement in trying to create something and be on an equal basis with the therapist. The second point is that the therapist took the weak position and allowed Mira to be the successful one, and Mira always laughed. (Mira gave the therapist an impossible task, but the therapist left it as Mira had constructed it. The therapist did not teach her the "right" way to do it.)

For the first time, Mira defined herself in this session: as to age (four, about to be five); female (showing her "boobies"); a feeling person ("I'm sad. If you don't let me get a drink, I won't be happy").

These remarkable changes reflect Mira's total commitment to, and acceptance of, her relationship with the therapist. Up to now, most of the therapeutic work had been devoted to providing the conditions needed to create this attachmentseparation relationship. Mira put the finishing touches on it in this session. She initiated hugging the therapist for the first time (at the end of the Knock at the Door game) and kissing her at the end of Circle Time. Now she can give love as well as receive it. She accepted the limits set by the therapist (not leaving to get a drink), and her repeated testing indicated that she seemed relieved when the limits held. Her objections had a light, playful quality ("If you don't let me get a drink of water, I won't be happy"). She welcomed the therapist's input and help in creating her mother-child play and her new game. A child can use limit setting when she has a relationship. She sang the lullaby with the therapist at the close of the one-to-one session.

Now that Mira doesn't have to be so concerned about the relationship, she feels freer to focus her attention on herself, to do what she needs to do to define herself. She did that in this session when she defined herself, for the first time, as to age and sex. She also defined herself, through her games, as creative and powerful. She defined herself as a feeling person.

Unlike most of the previous sessions, which contained considerable play disruptions, physical aggression, and negative and chaotic behavior, session 13 was smooth, even, warm, playful, relaxed, focused, and organized. It depicted two people, a child and an adult, accepting of and being present to each other. Theirs was a two-way, I-Thou dialogue—both being givers and both being receivers.

Mira's organized behavior and sense of power carried over into Circle Time. She took the risk of sharing and showing off her new accomplishment— her new game—to a group of people (her peers). It was her idea. It didn't come from the therapist. She involved the whole group in what she did.

It took Mira thirteen sessions to complete this attachment-separation stage. These first thirteen sessions provide an opportunity for students to study how a young child learns to become attached, the effect of the attachment on the child, and the different roles the attached adult or parent must play.

The Role of the Therapist

This session illustrates the shift the therapist had to make to keep up with the child. The therapist not only responded to Mira's cues (noticing, touching, doing what she wants), but she responded in a different way by providing images and new possibilities for her. For example, she gave Mira an image that enabled Mira to create her mother-child play. She used a feeling word ("happy"), and Mira copied it. She offered Mira "a new game" which stimulated Mira to create her own new game. She coached Mira on her game by reflecting back to her what she was doing. The therapist used more verbal communication. Most of all, the therapist showed real enjoyment and delight in playing the roles in which she was placed by Mira. Because the therapist had fun, Mira experienced herself as a fun person and creating something new as fun and exciting.

Mira's response to the therapist setting limits (not letting her leave the room) had the quality of the children's game of "Mother May I." It felt like "playing house" where someone is the "mother" who tells them when they can do something and when they can't. It had a play acting quality.

THE TERMINATION

The Goodbye part of the Developmental Play group program is given special attention. First of all, it is an integral part of creating a relationship—first you say hello (form an attachment relationship), and then you say goodbye (separate yourself from what is not you). You have to say hello first; otherwise, there is nothing to say goodbye to. Growing up is a process of saying hello and saying goodbye.

In the Developmental Play group program, the Goodbye part is announced three sessions before the final one. Both the adults and the children were told in the first session that they would play together a stated number of times. A three-week reminder is about right for four-year-olds. ("We play today and two more times, and then we have to say Goodbye.")

The children use these three sessions perfectly. Most children in a DP group run by experienced trainers go through three steps: 1) experiencing pain and expressing negative feelings; 2) experiencing closeness and often showing it through presents to the therapist; and 3) experiencing both sadness and joy, a celebration of the new self.

GOODBYE PROCESS, PART 1: PAINFUL FEELINGS

Session 14

Mira: (Screaming)
  Vi: Stop that screaming right now. (Said firmly) You don't need to do that anymore.
Mira: You big fart! (Said softly)
  Vi: You haven't even said Hello to me yet. Is that dress new?
Mira: (Nods yes) [She had on a beautiful red dress, longer than her others]
  Vi: (Placing her hand behind Mira's head, starts the Rocking game as she sits facing Vi)
Mira: (Screams)
  Vi: (Ignores scream) Up and down. (Rocking her up and down)
Mira: Do that game "Close Your Eyes!" (The new game Vi taught her last week)
  Vi: Oh, you remember that one. Okay, close your eyes. (Placing her hands on the sides of Mira's head, touching her face with her face) Open . . . Boo!
Mira: (Smiles and giggles)

Vi: Oh, you liked that.

Mira: Pat my chest.

Vi: (Pats her chest gently)

Mira: (Makes sounds)

Vi: Can you make your voice go up . . . and then down?

Mira: (As Mira moves her voice down, Vi joins her, chanting and moving her
hand from the top of Mira's head to her feet)

Vi: See how the sound goes clear down to your feet?

Mira: Do that again. (Mira is lying down facing Vi)

Vi: (Repeats)

Mira: Do it again.

Vi: (Repeats)

Mira: (Grabs Vi's hand)

Vi: You're here (pulling her up), and I can see your teeth, and they are all
there.

Mira: (Giggles)

Vi: And there's a tongue.

Mira: (Sticks out her tongue) Do Knock at the Door game.

Vi: (Does the Knock at the Door game) Oh, the door is shut. I'll have to walk
around the yard. (Disappointed tone)

Mira: (Giggles) Knock on the Door again.

Vi: (Repeats game; Mira opens mouth) Oh, there she is. (Hugging her)

Mira: Knock at the Door.

Vi: (Repeats) Oh, she isn't home. I'll have to walk around the yard, and then
I'll slide down her tree. (Outlining Mira's face and sliding her finger down
the top of Mira's nose)

Mira: She went to the K-Mart, and she won't be back until vacation.

Vi: That's a long time.

Mira: Do it again. (Opens her mouth)

Vi: Here you are. I'm glad you're back. (Hugging her)

Mira: (Yelling) It's my turn to do my trick. I didn't get to do my trick.

Vi: *I have to tell you something first. I'm going to play with you today and* . . .

Mira: (Interrupting) Oh . . . Oh . . . I have to . . . I stayed up until midnight last
night.

Vi: You don't want to hear what I have to say.

Mira: I'm going to stand up, and I won't run away. (With a smile on her face)

Vi: (Still holding her hand) Well, stand up and let's see how you look in your
new dress.

Mira: Don't touch me anymore. I won't run away. (As she moves away)

Vi: (Stops her)

Mira: (Screams)

Vi: *I'm going to play with you today and then two more times and then the play program is over.*

Mira: (Closes eyes and is quiet for a second; then screams)

Vi: (Ignoring scream) Can you count?

Mira: Shut up. (Said softly)

Vi: I'm going to play with you today and two more times—one, two. (Counting her own fingers) Can you hold up your two fingers?

Mira: (Holds up two fingers)

Vi: Oh, you can. That's wonderful. There are two fingers right there—two times.

Mira: I can hold up three. (Demonstrating)

Vi: All right. (Taking Mira's hand and pointing to each finger in turn) Here's today, and here's next Monday, and here's the next Monday.

Mira: Now it's my turn to do a trick. (Yelling) You already did your trick.

Vi: Okay, what's your trick? (What she called her game last week)

Mira: My arms are here (Counting), one, two, three. Now pull me up.

Vi: (Pulls her up onto her lap, putting Mira's face close to hers) Close your eyes.

Mira: (Interrupts) You do that all the time.

Vi: Isn't that nice?

Mira: No. That isn't nice. (Said very quietly)

Vi: Are you thinking about us playing only two more times?

Mira: No.

Vi: Are you thinking about what you're going to do?

Mira: Yes. Okay. Here we are. (Phrase Vi uses a lot) My two arms . . . Hold your arms up right here . . . Now pull me up.

Vi: (Pulls her up; groans) That's a hard one. (Taking Mira's face in her hands) Now close your eyes . . . Open them . . . Boo!

Mira: Did I cheat? [Sometimes she opens her eyes before Vi says "Open"]

Vi: (Laughing) Did you cheat? No, you didn't cheat that time.

Mira: Now it's my turn. Hold my hands. Come on.

Vi: Okay. I got them.

Mira: (Counting to twelve) Pull me up.

Vi: Okay. (Groaning; pretending that it's very hard) This is so hard just from your hands. (Laughing)

Mira: (Laughing)

Vi: Okay, that was your trick, and now it's my trick.

Mira: I got my eyes closed.

Vi: Oh, you got your eyes closed already. (Talking very slowly) C-L-O-S-E your eyes . . . and ready . . . open them . . . Boo! (Kisses her eyes)

Mira: (Sitting on Vi's lap, starts to look down the neck of Vi's dress) I want to see . . . boobies. Can I see them?

Vi: (Stopping her) You can see them from right here.

Mira: Can I pinch them?

Vi: No, but you can rest your head against them, like this. They are like little pillows. Do you know what boobies are for?

Mira: Can I get a drink?

Vi: At the end you can.

Mira: I'm not happy. I wish I could stay in Blanche's room. (That is, not come) I don't want to rock anymore.

Vi: Where are you sad?

Mira: (Lies down)

Vi: You're going to lie down. After two more times, you *will* be staying in Blanche's room. (Touching her hair) Here's your hair. Are you dreaming?

Mira: Shut up. (Whiny voice). I want to sing.

Vi: I'll hold it (the microphone), and you can sing.

Mira: (Quiet)

Vi: Well, it's nice just to be quiet.

Mira: You sing it.

Vi: (Sings the usual Brahms "Lullaby" while holding her) It's just nice to be quiet like this. I can see your face. What color are your eyes?

Mira: Blue. (Loudly) I don't want to do this all the time. Let me go. (Pulls away; lies on floor)

Vi: (Touching her foot) Is this foot here today? Oh, she's asleep. (Lifting her up into her lap; Mira is like a rag doll; she lays her head on Vi's shoulder)

Mira: (Moving the microphone out of the way) That's in my way . . . (Sits up and makes a noise)

Vi: How about my doing my trick and then you doing your trick? You want to do that?

Mira: Uh, uh. (Yes)

Vi: Shall I start with my trick first?

Mira: No. Okay.

Vi: Okay if I am first. (Does the Owl game)

Mira: (Sitting quietly)

Vi: You look like you're thinking about something.

Mira: (With hand up ready to hit) I'll smack you!

Vi: (Stopping her) We don't hit in here, but you can tell me you don't like it
that we're going to stop in two more times.

Mira: (Almost under her breath) *I hate you, and I don't want to be your partner
anymore.* Let me go. I have to go to the bathroom.

Vi: Remember you do that at the end. [Mira never has to go to the bathroom]

Mira: (Lies down facing Vi; covers her eyes with her hands)

Vi: Mira's gone away . . . like she will be doing one day when we say Goodbye.
Can you see me when you got your eyes covered?

Mira: Mhm-mhm. (Yes)

Vi: I see you peeking out. What's it like in there behind your hands?

Mira: A little dark. (Raises up and puts her hands over Vi's eyes) Vi, is it dark in
there?

Vi: Yes, but I can see you even with your hands over my eyes.

Mira in Circle Time

Mira started to sob almost immediately. She sat in the therapist's lap and
cried the first half of Circle Time. Mary, the Leader, initiated singing, "It's All
Right to Cry." Mira didn't respond when Mary asked her if she was sad. One five-
year-old boy said Mira was crying because we were going to stop in two weeks.
Mira said, "That's not it." The other children were unusually quiet. Mira's crying
and pain got out into the larger world (the Circle), and it saw and heard her pain.
Mira expressed pain for the others. "Crying is the experience of the care-taking
self" (Levin, 1988, p. 173).

Comments

Several things stand out in this session. First, Mira's behavior is organized,
focused, and goal-directed. Once the agenda (the termination) was defined, Mira
organized the whole session in the service of dealing with that issue. She did her
own work in her own time, and needed little help from the therapist.

Mira responded to the announcement of the time of ending, first with
shock (closed her eyes and then screamed) and then by returning to her previous
focus on their games ("tricks"). At the same time, there was a change in her energy pattern and in the way she played these games. She took care that the therapist had her "turn." In being the receiver for the therapist's new game, she asked,
"Did I cheat?" She wanted to be on good terms with the therapist. She wanted to
do it right.

During a quiet period, the therapist, by asking "Are you thinking about us
playing only two more times?" moved the focus back to the subject of the termination. Mira replied, "No" quietly, without name-calling. She answered "Yes" to

"Are you thinking about what you're going to do?" What she meant, however, was how was she going to arrange her body in her new game which she had started last week. The interest in these games eventually gave out.

It was during her silences that Mira began to be aware of her inner feelings. She didn't want to continue the games, and she didn't want the therapist to rock her "up and down." She made wailing sounds as she sat in the therapist's lap, looking directly at her while trying to decide if she should do what she is thinking of doing. First, Mira expressed her feelings with her body—lifting her hand to hit the therapist in the face ("I'll smack you!"). Then, at the suggestion of the therapist, Mira expressed her feelings in words: I hate you, and I don't want to be your partner anymore" (said very softly while looking directly at the therapist).

Mira was then left with other feelings, which she wanted to get rid of by running away (to the bathroom). When this was not allowed, her energy pattern again changed. She became quiet and soft. She laid down facing the therapist and covered her eyes. She accepted the therapist's interpretation that she had gone away, as she will one day soon. She said, "Yes" when the therapist asked her if she could see the therapist with her eyes closed (although she was peeking). Then she sat up and put her hands over the therapist's eyes, asking, "Vi, is it dark in there?" (what Mira had said when her eyes were covered). The therapist told her that she, the therapist, could see her with her eyes closed. There was a feeling of intimacy between Mira and the therapist in these moments. Mira was very soft and close to tears.

Mira's tears came as soon as the other children and adults came together for Circle Time. Sitting in the therapist's lap, she began to sob—the deep, choking kind of crying that comes from the abdominal muscles, with tears running down her face. Asking her if she was sad didn't seem to be meaningful to her. One boy tried to help her by telling her she was crying because DP was going to end in two weeks. Mira was okay at the end of Circle Time. (Mira's mother reported that week that Mira told her that she had cried that day in DP because Vi hurt her leg. This is another example of Mira's use of her body to express feelings.)

What especially stands out in this session is Mira's ability to experience feelings toward the therapist, to define and verbally express those feelings directly to her, and to show these feelings with real crying (as opposed to her earlier whiny pseudo-crying). Her deep sobbing told her that something new and important was going on inside of her. Her tears were telling her that this relationship with the therapist was important to her. She took an immense risk to say "I hate you" to the therapist, adding a verbal dialogue to her dialogue of touch. In this session,

Mira experienced pain expressed physically, emotionally, verbally, and cognitively (with awareness).

The goal of Developmental Play is to build a relationship. To experience pain, a child must have had a solid attachment relationship in which the child trusted the adult and experienced a great deal of pleasure interacting with that adult. Mira's ability to experience pain speaks for the presence of a very close, intimate relationship, a true I-Thou relationship.

The fact that Mira said, "I don't want to be your partner anymore," rather than, "I don't want you to be my partner anymore" speaks for the strength of her core self. She speaks from her "I" position.

Along with the deep work Mira did on the termination issue, other behaviors stand out, the most obvious of which is her ever-increasing love for and longing for touch. She wanted to be touched from head to toe (which the therapist did in the beginning of this session when Mira asked her to "Pat my chest" while Mira made sounds). She had such a hunger for it, and she seemed to thrive on it. The touch was also stimulating her cognitive development and helping her to use more verbal dialogue.

The verbal dialogue shifted in two ways: first, Mira began using more words that referred to her behavior, her wants and thoughts; second, the talking had a two-way conversational quality. Examples: Mira: "Did I cheat?" Therapist: "No, not that time"(laughing); Therapist: "Are you thinking of what you're going to do?" Mira: "Yes. Okay. Here we are . . ." and so on. Mira's ability to share herself changed the flow of energy from a one-way direction (adult ———→ child) to a two-directional flow (adult ⇌ child).

Another behavior that stands out is Mira's increasing ability to use fantasy and imagination as the basis of her verbal dialogue. For example, in the Knock at the Door game, she used "she" instead of "I," showing that she could imagine herself in a different place, while at the same time being present in the here and now with the therapist. In that process, Mira was widening her world and experiencing it as a world larger than the small space containing her and the therapist.

The Role of the Therapist

Mira did much of her own work, and the therapist just needed to be present and supportive. The therapist, however, did three things that provided Mira with the conditions she needed to start the Goodbye process.

1. **The therapist stated the agenda.** Unlike the other sessions, session 14 did have a specific goal: to start the Termination process. The therapist did remind Mira once after her initial statement of the goal, and that was it. The therapist, however, did not push Mira to respond to the

Goodbye theme. Because the therapist did not pressure her, Mira's behavior shows the process she created in coming to terms with it on her
own, guided by her own inner self. She didn't need anyone to tell her
what to do. Her behavior showed a gradual awareness of a feeling
emerging that could not be ignored. And she expressed this feeling with
her whole self through her sobbing.

2. **The therapist set limits twice.** She stopped Mira from slapping her face
   and did not allow Mira to leave to go to the bathroom (and she didn't
   go at the end, either). Not allowing Mira to leave gave Mira the opportunity to stay present with the therapist along with whatever feelings
   she had. Mira wanted to leave immediately after saying, "I hate you . . ."
   because she feared some punishment (not verbalized by her). She was
   not sent to her room. That was when Mira became very soft, quiet, and
   later cried.

3. **The therapist provided a container for Mira's feelings.** The therapist
   held Mira's painful feelings. The therapist made it safe for Mira to allow
   these feelings because they were accepted and there was a place for
   them.

4. **The therapist helped Mira create images** that she could use after the
   termination; namely, she could imagine being with the therapist. She
   could pretend. She could fantasize. It was a very intimate scene when
   the therapist asked Mira if she could see the therapist with her eyes
   closed; Mira replied that it was a "little dark" with her eyes closed, and
   Mira covered the therapist's eyes, asking her if it was dark in there.
   Through that limit setting—keeping Mira there—Mira experienced a
   closer connection with the therapist.

Contrary to what some might think, it is this very experience of closeness
that enables the child to separate and say Goodbye at the end. It is this sense of
closeness that the child takes with her when she leaves. She does not go away
empty-handed.

The Circle Time also provided the conditions needed to be able to deal
with termination. It gave her the opportunity to share with others, and for them
to share with her this whole Goodbye process. The Circle Time experiences
helped the children bond with each other, especially since they came from the
same day care center. The Circle Time gave Mira the time and space to share her
tears. Her tears came in Circle Time. The Leader, Mary, allowed her to cry as
long as she needed to while she sang, "It's All Right to Cry."

Session 14 illustrates how one four-year-old child dealt with the beginning stage of the Goodbye process. It shows that Mira's ability to deal with the initial stage of experiencing the pain of saying Goodbye stimulated a lot of new growth in her. It showed what the therapist did to support this growth.

As the therapist, I was moved by Mira's ability to experience and express verbally very deep feelings. I was also struck, for the first time, with her physical beauty. In these three and a half months, she had changed physically as well as behaviorally.

GOODBYE PROCESS, PART 2: FEELINGS OF CLOSENESS AND EMPOWERMENT

Session 15

Mira entered the room in a happy mood, sat in my lap, and snuggled up close to me, face to face. She initiated contact by giving me a task that only she, Mira, could do. Holding up a tightly closed hand, she pointed to her first finger and said, "See if you can get that one up." I groaned as I tried, and finally said, "I can't get it up." Mira then said with great confidence, "Watch. I can do it." She repeated this with all her fingers with the same results. Mira enjoyed her success each time.

Then Mira got some paper off a shelf. I suggested she draw a girl. Sitting in my lap with her back against me, Mira put the paper on the floor and drew. After finishing one part, Mira would lean back against me and look pleased. After drawing a lot of hair on her figure, Mira said, "She's a lady."

Then I did a drawing of myself holding Mira, and under it I printed, "I love you, Mira." I read it to Mira, who had been watching intently. Mira then quickly snatched up another paper and said, "I'm going to write something you'll know how to read." She then printed some letters.

Vi: What does it say?
Mira: (In a tone that said, "I can't believe you're asking me this") You know what it says.
Vi: I think it says, I love you, too.
Mira: (Looking at Vi out of the corner of her eye, smiles) I love you very much. (Said very softly)

Turning toward me, Mira said, "I want to sing my song." I said, "Okay," and handed her the microphone that goes to the tape recorder. She loved holding that microphone (which had been there throughout her sessions). Then she got shy and self-conscious and told me to sing first. I sang her usual lullaby and handed the microphone back to her. This session was being videotaped, and Mira kept looking at the camera person (whom she knew), not wanting him to hear it. (Unfortunately, I was not getting her message.) Finally, Mira decided to do it. She made it as private as possible by putting her face under my chin and covering both our mouths with her hand. She made this song up as she went along and whispered it to me (I later got all of it by playing it back on my tape recorder).

Mira's Song

The trees and the apple seeds
and the bananas grow all the time
even the oranges.
Trees grow
because some trees are small
and then some animals come
and then every animal comes and plays
and then all the animals come
and they're all in bed in rosy time
for them to start to sing a song
for you and me.

I thanked her for the song (only part of which I heard). Mira wanted to sing another "song." At that point I took charge and said, "It's time for us to be together now before we have to stop." Mira lay on the floor in front of me and closed her eyes, turning her head from side to side at times as if she were asleep. I was quiet. She finally said, "You're suppose to rock me up and down." As I had done many times before, I put my hands behind Mira's head and back and lifted her, held her close, and gently let her down, repeating it as I chanted hypnotically, "Up and down." Mira was like a rag doll, totally limp. Her body was very heavy.

When I sang the lullaby at the close, I inadvertently changed one word (they will guard *thee* instead of they will guard *you*). Mira corrected me, then sang it with me to be sure I got it right.

When it was time to go to Circle, Mira said, "Pick me up and carry me *like* a baby." As heavy as she was, I did it. Mira's request is an example of a transitional phenomenon—creating a memory she will take with her (Winnicott, 1953).

187

Mira's Drawing

"She's a Lady"

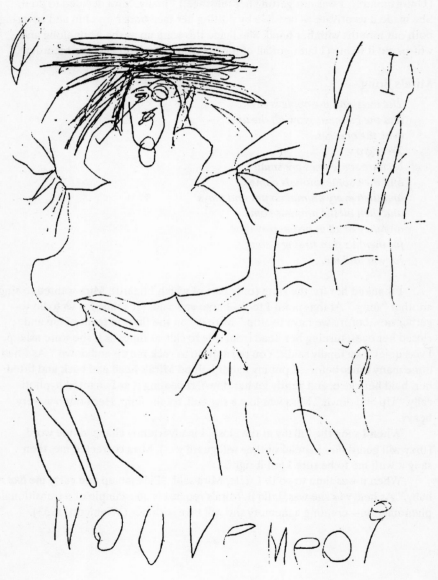

Comments

In this session, Mira was very much in charge of herself and in charge of what went on in the session—from the beginning (where she gave the therapist a task that only she could do) to the middle (where she gave the therapist a gift in the form of a very beautiful poem—her song), to the end (where she asked to be carried *like* a baby). In doing these things, she was happy and had a sense of quiet confidence as well as patience when the therapist wasn't getting her message.

Although termination was still the focus, neither Mira nor the therapist brought up the subject. Yet everything Mira did was guided by her awareness of the impending ending. Not that she had made plans ahead of time to do what she did in the session, but she was so organized and confident that it almost felt as if she had. It was almost as if Mira had said to herself, "Today, Vi and I are just going to be together and have fun. I'm going to tell her how much she has meant to me and I'm going to show her what I can do—sing a song, like Vi does. I'm going to do things to remember because it will be the last time just to be by ourselves. Next week, it'll be the end."

Mira's crying last week got her in touch with the loving part of herself and an awareness of her love for the therapist. The crying freed her or moved her to the next step—giving form to those feelings. Her "song" was one of those forms. This "song" is a symbolic, metaphorical representation of how Mira experienced the relationship. Her poem included all life—plant, animal, and human. Her poem is about life, growth, play, caring, love, and intimacy. The whole world celebrated their relationship ("and they're all in bed in rosy time to start to *sing a song for you and me*").

This poem shows Mira's new ability to use the abstract, representational mode of thinking. She has added the abstract to her basic mode of touch. Mira's imitating the therapist by printing letters to represent words ("I'm going to write something that you'll know how to read") is another example of this shift. Still another example was her drawing, another was her request at the end to "Carry me *like* a baby." Imagining herself a baby is very different from being a baby (as she was in the earlier sessions). Since she has experienced herself as a baby, she can now relive or recreate that experience through fantasy—a big step.

In this session, Mira showed her ability to function on two levels in the same session: the abstract (her poem) and the concrete ("rock me up and down").

Nearly everything she did in this session was new. This session is the only one (since session 4) in which she didn't ask to do the Knock at the Door game. She was too busy expressing her new self—being creative, independent, pleased with herself—empowering herself. For Mira, the second stage of saying Goodbye is one of empowerment and sharing of love.

The Role of the Therapist

At the stage where the child is empowering herself, the therapist's job is to step back and just support the child doing what she does. The therapist does less initiating and more responding. The therapist supported Mira when she set up tasks for her to do by playing the weaker role so that Mira could experience her power and independence (Vi: "I can't get it up." Mira: "Watch. I can do it.").

When the therapist did initiate something, it was in the service of supporting Mira in her new place—to give her a sense of accomplishment (for example, suggesting that Mira draw a girl and printing the words "I love you, Mira" under her drawing). Both of these examples helped Mira to see that feelings can be expressed in a form. She responded with excitement.

The therapist took charge after Mira had sung her song. Instead of allowing Mira to sing more songs, the therapist took over and said, "It's time for us to be together now." Mira welcomed this when she said, "You're suppose to rock me up and down." She is saying to the therapist, "You're supposed to take charge." The therapist saw that Mira was getting tired of trying to think up something. She relieved Mira of that need by initiating the cradling which is always done at each closing.

Sometimes, for whatever reason, the therapist may not always get the child's message, and the child does what she needs to do anyway. For example, Mira was so organized and focused that even when the therapist didn't get her message, she didn't let that deter her from singing her "song." Even though the therapist didn't quite get it—how self-conscious she was and how much she wanted this song to be something special and private, just between her and the therapist—she found a way to make it private and went on and sang it. Amazing!

As the therapist, I had suddenly become aware of Mira's physical beauty. She was a beautiful child. She had grown and her face was so alive. Now she looked like a five-year-old, close to her true age.

I am always surprised at the change in the physical looks of children after a few weeks of participation in Developmental Play. Mira was no exception. In the beginning, her looks didn't affect me one way or the other. I don't remember how she looked. I do remember, however, being surprised at how light her body was when I picked her up to put her in my lap. She seemed weightless. In the sixth week she clearly had a baby face and a baby body. She looked and acted like a baby. About the twelfth week she began to look and act like a four or five-year-old. Her hair got darker and thicker. Her face got fuller and showed the excitement and confidence of a child who enjoys life. By the end of the sixteen weeks, she became so heavy that I could hardly lift her when she asked me to pick her up and carry her like a baby. She was truly in her body.

This session was an unbelievable experience for me. Mira was so giving, loving, and present. I experienced her being able to love as well as allow herself to be loved. When I finally heard all of her "song" on my tape recorder, I was amazed that a four-year-old could create something that coherent and beautiful. And I didn't hear it with her (because she whispered it so softly). It is only now, as I work on this book, that I am beginning to appreciate the depth of this child's work.

THE GOODBYE PROCESS, PART 3: CELEBRATION AND INTEGRATION

Session 16

Mira: (Runs into the room and jumps up into Vi's arms)
   Vi: You ran and jumped into my arms and you got that pretty red dress on.
Mira: (After she is let down, she takes off her shoe and throws it)
   Vi: (Grabbing her other foot) That's what you used to do. You don't need to do that now.

A few moments later:

Mira: Let's do tricks. (Sitting in front of Vi) Now you have to just touch this (one toe) without nothing else. (Her legs are spread out with her hands on each leg) Wait 'til I count to two. One, two—okay, pull me up. (An impossible task)
   Vi: (Groaning, pretending to be working very hard) I can't get you up. (Reaching over and lifting her into her lap)
   Vi: Well, today is the last time we play together.
Mira: (Hugs Vi tightly)
   Vi: That's nice. Your face feels so soft.
Mira: (Smiles) I'm going out to dinner tonight at the Burger King, and if you want, you could come.
   Vi: Thank you for thinking of me, but I can't come because we have to say goodbye today. (Reviews her time with Mira—how she met and chose Mira)
Mira: (Listens quietly, then laughs) And now it's *my* turn. (Grabbing the microphone; pointing to the two parts of the microphone) This is mine, and this is yours. (Repeating what Vi had said to her in Session 15)
Mira: (Singing)

> *The rainbows and the sheeps and the apples*
> *the rain and the clouds will be from not a sunny day*
> *And then the sun comes around;*
> *Then that will be a sunny day*
> *And then all the animals come out and have a party.*

       Vi: Thank you. Now it's my turn. (Continues her story about Mira, reviewing things Mira did)
   Leader: (Comes around to take polaroid pictures of us)
       Vi: (to Mira) How do you want us to be?
     Mira: *You make a sad face, and I'll make a happy face.* (After picture is taken) *NO. I told you to be sad!*
   Leader: Why do you want Vi to be sad?
     Mira: 'Cause.
   Leader: 'Cause why?
     Mira: 'Cause I want her to.
       Vi: Did you want me to be sad because I'll miss you?
     Mira: (Quickly) Yes.
       Vi: Well, I will miss you. Are you a little sad that we are going to stop?
     Mira: (Hides her face behind her hands)
       Vi: Mira's gone away. Are you crying?
     Mira: (Crying with tears)
       Vi: (Holding her) Mira is crying because we're not going to play anymore.
     Mira: (Loudly) I'm going to tell my Mommy on you, Vi.
       Vi: What are you going to tell your Mommy?
     Mira: (Crying) That you broke my leg.
     Mira: (Crying; sits up)
       Vi: You're going to sit this way.
     Mira: (Moves away from Vi; lies on mat face down; looks angry; not crying)
       Vi: Are you a little mad right now?
     Mira: (Stands up)
       Vi: (Measures her to see how tall she is by having her stand close to her) Where does your head come?
     Mira: (Aggressively) My head is where it is. Can you feel it?
       Vi: Yes, I can feel it. (Touching it)
   Mira: Okay, now would you pick me up, please?

Mira jumps into Vi's arms and puts her legs around Vi's waist. She orders Vi to do impossible things—put Mira on Vi's head; let Mira fall backward without holding on to her.

Mira: Let's play Knock at the Door. That was fun!
    Vi: You like that game. (Plays the game; Mira's mouth is closed) She's not at home. (Running her fingers around Mira's face) I'll walk around the yard.
Mira: (Moving her hand from her chest down to her stomach) You're supposed to walk down here, too. Do it again. I love that game!
    Vi: (Repeats this game many times, each time covering more of her body as she walks around waiting for Mira to come home)
Mira: (Finally opens her mouth)
    Vi: Oh, she's home! (Said with delight)
Mira: (Giggles with delight)
    Vi: (Hugs her) I'm glad you're home.

Mira then puts her hands over Vi's eyes and says, "It's my game." She takes over and plays with Vi the "Owl" game that Vi usually plays with her. (Faces touching and eyes closed until the Leader says, "Open . . . Boo!")

Mira: You're not supposed to open your eyes until I tell you. (Said firmly)
    Vi: You have to tell me, then.
Mira: Okay. Close your eyes. Open them . . . Boo!
    Vi: You do know how to do it. That's nice. You could show your mother how to play these games.
Mira: She never knows what to do.
    Vi: Who?
Mira: She never knows what I want.
    Vi: Your mother?
Mira: (Covers her face)
    Vi: (Ends the session with cradling Mira and singing a lullaby)
Mira: (Reaches up and touches Vi's hair; turns and sits sideways on Vi's lap, quietly looking out and thinking)
      [Circle Time called] Carry me like a baby.
    Vi: (Picks her up and starts walking)
Mira: Pretend I'm your tiny baby.

Mira in Circle Time

Mira provided the focus for the whole Circle Time by putting herself into the center and acting out her fantasy of being a new baby in the family. With eyes closed, she tipped her face up in front of each person to be seen and to be touched. Children and adults both enjoyed touching her face. At the end, when the Leader asked, "Of all the things you did, what did you like best?", Mira, the first child to respond, raised her hand and said, "What I liked best was when we did our trick, Vi couldn't get me up." She laughed (See Circle Time).

Comments

Beginning with the announcement of the termination in session 14, Mira has been preparing herself for the Goodbye. In this, the final session, Mira brought together a sample of everything she had done before that was meaningful to her, together with something new (a new game) to take home with her. By the end of the one-to-one and the Circle Time, Mira's behavior showed that she experienced a sense of celebration of her new self.

First of all, from the moment Mira entered the room, she invited, asked for, and demanded a great deal of touching. In the Knock at the Door game, she wanted her whole body touched, not just her face. She asked the therapist to carry her several times and do baby-like things, such as put her on the therapist's head. This was new. And the therapist did respond and give her the touching contact that was possible. These touching contacts helped Mira center herself, feel her own body, and create memories that she can call forth when she needs to feel her core self.

Mira reviewed all the games she had played. She continued to work on her own creation, her game which she had started back in session 13. In this act, Mira showed an ability to create an interest, to keep it on hold, and to develop it.

Mira expressed feelings physically and verbally. She cried and said, "I'm going to tell my Mommy on you, Vi . . . that you broke my leg." (This is another example of how she uses her body to express feeling.) In the same hour, she also expressed feelings verbally when she said to the therapist in the picture-taking, "*I told you to be sad.*" (Mira wanted to feel that she was important to the therapist.) In asking for a last time play of the Knock at the Door game, she said, "*It was fun. I love that game.*"

Mira also prepared herself for the final Goodbye by learning the therapist's Owl game so that she could do it to others when she went home. She wanted to be the initiator of that game, not just the receiver. Mira needed some coaching from the therapist because she was leaving out the instructions ("Close your eyes"). Both she and the therapist were pleased that she "got it." To be the initiator of that game requires that a child have a core self and have boundaries that enable her to distinguish herself from the one to whom she is teaching the game. Mira's ability to do this indicated that through these games she is defining her boundaries.

Mira also showed her ability to create her own inner world of quiet and peace through the simple act of imagining herself being held and cradled. ("Pick me up and carry me like a baby. Pretend that I'm your tiny baby.") She knew the difference between the fantasy world and the real world. She could be in the real world and fantasize being cradled at the same time. She can now imagine herself being cradled by the therapist anytime she needs to. The therapist becomes an "evoked companion" (Stern, page 111).

Finally, in this last session, Mira offered another "song" that was a metaphor for her experience in therapy, in particular, and for life experiences, in general.

> *The rainbows and the sheeps and the apples*
> *the rain and the clouds will be from not a sunny day*
> *And then the sun comes around;*
> *Then that will be a sunny day*
> *And then all the animals come out and have a party.*

Her song has living things (sheeps and apples), happy times (rainbows), sad times (clouds), time for nurturing and renewal (rain), and times when people are not happy (not a sunny day), then "the sun comes around" and people celebrate (have a party). In other words, life has its ups and downs, but in the end "the sun comes around" and everything's all right.

Mira's ability to give form to her experiences in this symbolic way is very unusual for a four-year-old. She was motivated to do it because the therapist sang songs to her, and she wanted to give something back to her therapist. She identified with her therapist. First of all, she had a form in mind—a song ("my song"). From then on, she just made it up on the spur of the moment. What she made up, she doesn't really understand. A child at this age can create concepts that she won't understand until later. Thus, a child, even at this age, has a higher self that knows more than what she can express in the moment. Yet, at the same time, her "song" did express the ups and downs, the ins and outs, and the resistance and acceptance she experienced in these sixteen sessions.

Mira continued her organized behavior right into the Circle Time. She provided the structure around which the whole Circle Time activity was organized. Through her new baby fantasy, she got both the adults and children in touch with

her and with each other in a quiet, loving family-like way to celebrate their to-
getherness and the birth of something new—another metaphor—an image and
memory for all of them to take home.

As the DP therapist, I was moved by all the hard work she did. I felt a wave
of deep sadness come over me when she said her mother doesn't know what she
wants. I was immensely pleased with her creative role-playing in the Circle and
the enjoyment both she and the other children got out of her little play. I was
happy with her when she laughed at the end when the Leader asked what they
liked best and Mira said, "What I liked best was when we did our trick, Vi
couldn't get me up."

Postscript

In talking to Mira's mother a short time after this session, I asked her, "Do
you ever play those games with Mira?" She said, "No. I don't know how. But
would you show me?" I showed her by playing the Knock at the Door game on
her. Later, she said that her two girls ask her to do that game with each of them
every night before bedtime.

THE THERAPEUTIC PROCESS AND THE ROLE OF THE THERAPIST

Let's look at these sixteen sessions one more time. This time the focus will
be on the therapist and her role as an active participant in this dialogue of touch
in an attempt to understand the effect of her participation on Mira's behavior.

For me, as the therapist, Mira's therapy was like watching a baby get born
and go through infancy, early childhood, and late childhood up to age five. Once
Mira could allow the touching, she used me as a mother to provide her with the
basic experience of body awareness through touch. The intensity of Mira's longing for this touch indicated that she had been deprived of this basic touch. For
about the first ten sessions, Mira related to me as a mother. In session 11, Mira
began experiencing me as separate from her and started relating to me as a playmate. As a play partner, Mira kept track of everything I did, seeing to it that I
played fair and took turns. To experience her independence, Mira created for me
tasks that only Mira could do. In the last three sessions (14-16), Mira saw me
more as a friend from whom she could learn and with whom she could share feelings, images, and thoughts in a verbal dialogue. At the end, Mira composed a
poem ("My Song") that expressed the intimacy of our relationship.

WHAT THE THERAPIST DOES

DP therapy sees the changes in the child in terms of what the therapist did to provide the conditions the child needed to make those changes—in other words, defining the "facilitating environment" needed for each stage. Children learn through imitation and identification with the adult. What is the adult doing and what is the child imitating?

In Developmental Play therapy, the child's growth takes place within and through her relationship with the therapist. The Developmental Play therapist uses touch to create relationship. This is not a simple therapeutic approach, nor is it easy to do. It is not adequately described as any physical contact with a child. The therapeutic efficacy of touch lies in the *how* of it, in its qualitative aspects.

One form of touch I chose to use in Mira's therapy was cradling while singing to her. Singing is, in itself, a kind of touch, as the singing voice sets up vibrations in the listener. When I sang to Mira, I could feel my singing reverberate in her body and quickly help her to relax. Sometimes I sang a lullaby; sometimes I chanted the names of parts of her body as I lightly touched them; sometimes I sang about what I saw her doing; and sometimes I just softly hummed. Sometimes I was quiet. Whenever I sang, I felt a flow of energy from Mira to me. I felt connected to her, and I knew that my voice helped her feel connected to me. The singing helped me stay present.

Cradling and singing was the avenue through which we first communicated with each other. The communication was at the body level—through touch, sound, and vibration—the dialogue of touch. It took Mira three sessions to learn to become a participant in this dialogue of touch.

SESSIONS 1 AND 2

In session 1, Mira allowed the touching (her hands, the Knock at the Door game, and the cradling), but she wasn't experiencing the touch. She just sort of let me do it. She did, however, say, "Do it again" to the Knock at the Door game. As for Circle Time, none of the five children could handle themselves in a group. They screamed and yelled, Mira included. During the cradling that closed the Circle Time, however, Mira totally relaxed in my arms and reached up and touched my hair, as babies do with their mothers.

In session 2, Mira definitely began to react to the touching. She disrupted the touching activity periodically, saying "Shut up" to me, calling attention to other people in the room or saying I was "hurting" her. Then she would return to the touch, which she controlled—for example, picking up the lotion bottle saying, "*I* want to put it on." (She wouldn't allow me to put it on her.) This behavior showed that Mira was being more present. She was feeling something, and it was new and unfamiliar. She didn't know if she wanted this experience, but she was trying it out.

In the end, however, Mira did let me in. She did this through her "stuck-knee" game—a game *she* created. That game was her way of saying, "Touch me. I need love." That game was her way of opening the door to me and saying, "Come in." She also used this game in many later sessions as an avenue for making contact.

What the Therapist Did

The therapist gave Mira something to respond to. I noticed her, I introduced Knock at the Door, a touching game, and I cradled her. To feel seen through being touched was new for Mira. Her approach had been to get seen through yelling and telling others what to do. Here, she didn't have to do anything except to allow herself to be touched.

The Effect on Mira

First of all, Mira came alive. She *felt* something, and that feeling mobilized her to respond. Her mildly disruptive behavior (name-calling, hitting, kicking) showed that Mira was trying to figure out what to do about this new feeling. Her behavior showed that she both liked this new experience and that she resisted it. Through experiencing herself touched by the therapist, she experienced herself, her body self (her inner self).

SESSION 3

Mira pulled out all the stops in this session to resist being touched or noticed. She fought the contact with her whole body—hitting, screaming, throwing shoes, and trying to run away. Even so, she showed she had moments of enjoyment, but as soon as she became aware of this feeling of enjoyment, she fought even harder to wipe it out. Nevertheless, in spite of all the resistance, by the end of the session, Mira was allowing herself to be cradled by the therapist. She looked like a little baby as she lay in the therapist's arms. She reached up and touched the therapist's hair.

What the Therapist Did

First of all, I was in charge. I didn't allow her to control me. Yet she was free to do whatever she needed to do. Outside of not allowing her to hit me, throw things, or runaway, I wasn't controlling her, either. I wasn't making her do anything, but I did give her something to respond to by noticing her, saying what

I saw, and touching her. I carried out her requests even though that didn't seem to help. I stopped the cradling when she complained. I didn't punish her or abandon her no matter what she did. She couldn't get rid of me. I was always present in very physical, concrete ways.

The DP Therapist Sets Limits

In session 3, the therapist set limits in two ways: (1) I did not allow her to leave the scene, hit me, or throw shoes; and (2) I refocused or "reframed" her negative behavior by turning it into something positive and fun. For example, when she spit, instead of saying, "That's not allowed," I held up the palm of my hand toward her and said, "Do it here." Then I pointed to my cheek, "Do it here," also a way to get her to experience me through touch. I kept varying the way I held her. For example, I changed the cradling into rocking her in a boat. Pretending we were in choppy waters, I said, "I have to hold you tightly so that you won't fall out." Soon she began to enjoy this, saying, "Do it again."

The Therapist's Experience

Without a doubt, this session was the most difficult one for me, both physically and emotionally. The intensity of Mira's resistance made me be present with her every second. It was this intensity, without letup, that made it hard even for me, an experienced therapist. I certainly felt her energy and her aliveness. And *she certainly felt me touching her.* She was certainly present.

It wasn't until later that I understood her behavior. I realized that the experiences I enabled her to have were very new for her. She wanted them, yet at the same time she could not allow herself to have them. I also realized that I had provided her with the conditions she needed in order to experience her inner self, her core self. This core self was born through this interaction with the therapist. Now she can relate. At the end, I realized that she and I had begun a relationship.

SESSIONS 4 THROUGH 10

From session 4 on, Mira became a very different child. She could not seem to get enough touching ("That's not nearly enough. I need a lot.") These sessions revolved around two touching dialogues: (1) Mira being cradled in the therapist's arms or lying on the floor in front of the therapist, while the therapist sang and gently touched and named the parts of her body; and (2) playing the Knock at the Door game. She asked for this game to be played over and over. Mira and the therapist were relating on the body level.

Mira was clearly in the attachment phase. She took in everything the therapist did—her words, the sound of her voice, her expressions. She learned the lullaby the therapist always sang to her. She remembered from one session to the next what she and the therapist had done.

What the Therapist Did

At this stage, the therapist responded to Mira's need to be mothered. This was not a role I played. I was a mother. I did what mothers do, and I felt like a mother. I responded to her cues to be touched in certain ways and to have the touch be repeated ("Do it again"—the Knock at the Door, which is a touching-the-face game). I didn't require her to do anything. I supported her to lie quietly in my arms while she was in her trance. I allowed her to be in her baby place with her baby talk as long as she needed to be.

The Therapist Initiates Touching Games

The DP therapist not only responds to the child's cues, but she also gives the child something to respond to. I initiated the Knock at the Door, a touching-the-face game that says Hello, Are you home, Can you come out and play? It is a more complicated peek-a-boo game. I knew I was in tune with her when I saw how much she loved this game.

SESSIONS 11 AND 12

Through the attachment process—allowing herself to be seen, touched, and cradled—Mira developed a core self. To be complete, however, the core self has to be shared with another who is experienced as separate from her. Mira first experienced the therapist as not her, as separate from her, in sessions 11 and 12. By separating the therapist from her, Mira created a person with whom she could share her core self and make herself complete. Now there are two people (the therapist and Mira), each with her own "I." Now sharing is possible.

At this period, Mira has shifted from her self-experience being regulated by the therapist to sharing her subjective experience with the therapist and experiencing how each influences the subjective experience of the other. In Stern's terms, Mira has added to her "core-related self" an "intersubjective-related self" (Stern, 1985, p. 125). To the experience of physical intimacy, Mira has added the experience of "psychic intimacy," the ability to experience empathy. She has a feel for where the other person (the therapist) is coming from.

Mira first showed this psychic intimacy in session 7, when she brought the rice cakes to share. From then on, she watched the therapist and assimilated and incorporated everything the therapist did. Nothing escaped her. She was like a sponge.

This psychic intimacy was reflected in Mira's addition of a verbal dialogue to her dialogue of touch. Up to now, she had used words to invite touch: "Do it again"—a one-way conversation. Now she could engage in a two-way conversation, and her words contained images and feelings not directly connected to the body, as demonstrated in sessions 11 and 12.

SESSION 11

Mira moved close to the therapist and whispered, "Let's do Knock on the Door." What was new was the feeling she communicated through her action and her voice, namely, that this is a very special, private, intimate activity not to be shared with anyone else. That act demonstrated a commitment to the relationship that had not been there before and a commitment that she would do her part. At that crucial moment, the therapist had to tell her they would not see each other for three times because of the holidays.

The intensity of Mira's reaction made her aware of how much this relationship meant to her. In the process of dealing with this separation, Mira moved into a verbal dialogue that defined psychological states or relationship feelings. First, she experienced shock (shown physically), then fear of abandonment (who is she going to stay with), withdrawal (her kissable places offered have "gone"), anger (hitting the therapist and saying, "I don't like you"), and saying she wanted to hold the toy that she had brought with her because *"It's too scared to be alone."* Her projection of the fear to be alone onto her toy speaks for her ability to empathize and to experience feelings.

In session 11, Mira looked as if she were thinking for the first time. She really concentrated and explored her thoughts. She spent many moments just being quiet while she did her thinking. (The other children were extremely noisy, but she didn't even seem to hear them—very new.) For the first time, her face was that of a thinking child.

SESSION 12

During the return after the holiday break, Mira showed her awkwardness about reconnecting after the break by her old acting-out behavior: hitting, name-calling, and hitting the therapist in the face with the lotion bottle.

Some therapists might interpret this behavior as anger that could not be expressed in session 11 because of the parting, like children expressing anger to their parents when they return from a trip because now it's safe to do so.

As the therapist, however, I saw it more as out-of-control behavior because she didn't know what to do. She needed to feel safe, and she needed limits instead of interpretations. I rarely offered interpretations; when I did, they made her behavior more out of control. In fact, what I needed to have done was *not* to have given her the lotion bottle.

Interestingly, Mira got scared at her own behavior and started controlling herself on her own by her usual method—asking for touch. She showed the therapist a "boo-boo" on her finger. Then she offered to "sing a song." The therapist held the microphone for her. She moved her lips, but no sound came out. Mira then suggested that the therapist sing, and Mira joined her singing the lullaby.

Therapist: Great! You know that song! That's wonderful!
    Mira: You want me to sing it again? (With eager tone)
Therapist: Okay.
    Mira: (Sings the lullaby correctly except for one place. Instead of "bright angels around my child," she sings, "angels standing around.")
Therapist: That's wonderful the way you sang that! You know that song. Did you sing that when you were home?
    Mira: Mhm-mhm. (Yes)

What is new here is Mira's ability to take charge of her own behavior. She could react to her own behavior and do something about it. She felt relieved that the therapist liked her singing (especially after she had just hit the therapist) and offered to do it again when the therapist said she liked it. She really enjoyed being liked.

What the Therapist Did

The therapist set limits. She stopped Mira from hitting her. Later, when Mira said she wanted to sing her song "this way" (with her back to the therapist), saying, "I won't run away," the therapist turned her around, saying, "I can't see you that way." The therapist did not believe her when she said, "I won't run away."

Two-Way Conversations

Mira's experiencing the therapist as separate is reflected in her two-way conversations:

Therapist: Did you bring any kissable places today?
    Mira: No. I didn't. (Thinking) Do *you* see one?

Mira: Do it again. (Touch her face in Knock at the Door game; request re-
peated several times)
Therapist: (Getting bored; with impatient tone) I wonder what she is doing. Is
she sitting in the house by the door?
Mira: No. The door's just locked.
Therapist: Do I have the key?
Mira: You have to push the button, and it opens by itself.

What the Therapist Did

In the first example, the therapist had ignored Mira's cue to kiss her foot
and had asked this question instead. Mira's response showed that she could let go
of her need (temporarily) and respond to the therapist. In addition, for the first
time, Mira asked the therapist for her view on something. (Her "thinking" behavior in session 11 stimulated by her anxiety over the holiday break had continued.)

The therapist was no longer responding to Mira's every request. Instead,
the therapist did something she wanted to do and that she felt was needed. In
other words, the therapist made herself more separate.

In the second example, Mira was able to let go of her dialogue of touch and
enter a dialogue of words, words that contained images not directly connected to
touch or the body. She is discovering that language is another way to be in relation to the therapist. The therapist's contribution was to give Mira an image
(Mira sitting in her house by the door). Mira had to experience herself being
present, and at the same time, she had to imagine herself in another place.

"Play Disruptions" (Erikson, 1940)

Erik Erikson used this term for disturbance in play that is due to repressed
material becoming conscious. In the beginning, Mira exhibited a number of play
disruptions in the form of yelling, screaming, hitting, name-calling, and trying to
leave the scene. Her play disruptions, however, were not set off by a break in the
defenses, because she had not yet reached the stage of having defenses. She
didn't have a core self when she began, which is a requirement for defenses. Mira
used play disruptions when she didn't know what to do or when she wanted to
test me. Sometimes she just seemed to enjoy saying certain words ("fart"), to
hear herself say them, and to see the effect on me.

What the Therapist Did

The few times the therapist tried to interpret ("You're mad because we
didn't see each other for three weeks."), she got no response at all, not even an

answer. That was because that wasn't what was going on with Mira. Mira simply did not know how to reconnect after the holidays, and she felt safe enough to try those words. After that, the therapist just ignored her play disruptions and refocused her on relating through touch. That nearly always worked.

Children this age, or with this developmental lag, are not ready for verbal dialogues. They don't have a thinking process going yet. It wasn't until session 11 that Mira showed signs of being able to introspect.

SESSION 13

So many lovely, exciting things happened in this session that it's hard to know where to start. First, Mira's commitment to this relationship became complete and total in this session. This commitment was sealed when she hugged the therapist for the first time in the one-to-one and kissed her at the end of Circle Time. She had accepted hugs before but had never initiated them.

Second, the quality of her energy and essence had changed. Throughout, Mira had such an air of presence, confidence, security, and most of all, sheer joy in everything that she did. She felt so happy with herself. (As Brazelton says, when a child feels good about himself, you know that child is going to make it.)

This *joie de vivre* may be the result of her having dealt with the three-week break over the holidays (session 11) and having to reconnect again (session 12). Now she can get back together with the therapist and do her thing freed from having to deal with an outside event that intrudes upon their privacy.

In session 13, Mira added a new role for the therapist—that of a playmate. At the same time, she didn't give up seeing the therapist as a mother, but the mother-child interaction changed—it got more intimate. The verbatim sessions show that in nearly every session, Mira functioned on two levels at the same time: a very early level and a very advanced level. She never leaves the infant stage while she's doing something very advanced; in fact, she goes deeper into that early period. In that same session, she will be showing very advanced behavior. Session 13 is an example of this duality.

The Cradling

In the later sessions, I changed the way I did the cradling. I held Mira facing me, and with my hands supporting her head and back, I lifted her up and down, chanting "Up . . . and down . . ." In this session, Mira just let her head fall into my neck, as a tiny baby does. She trusted her body totally to me, even more than she had before. Mary, the Leader, commented that she looked like a nursing baby. This was her body saying she is committed to this relationship.

Whenever Mira's behavior showed she didn't know what to do or she started taking care of the therapist, the therapist initiated the rocking.

The Effect on Mira

In the later sessions (11-16), the rocking had the centering and quieting effect needed to bring forth memories and images that moved Mira into more advanced verbal dialogues. For example, in session 13 Mira created a mother-child play that incorporated this rocking experience. Mira started this play during the rocking when she said, "When I'm asleep, you're supposed to stop doing that." The therapist then supported this mother-child image when she said, "When you go to bed at night, do you imagine I'm rocking you like this?" Mira said, "Yes." From that place, Mira took off and developed this mother-child play in which she was both the director and the child.

What stands out here is Mira's ability to connect the past to the present, to bring something from the past into the present and, above all, her awareness that she can create this play. To create this play, Mira had to have an image of herself at bedtime (a memory of her mother putting her to bed) and being awakened in the morning (by her mother) and an image of her being rocked (by the therapist). She had to have experienced both the mother and the child in order to direct the therapist in the mother role. Her play gave form and meaning to past experiences through reliving these experiences in the present with the therapist—through the dialogue of touch.

Mira's play is an excellent example of how children return to an earlier period in their lives to bring it forward to make their lives more complete, not as they experienced that period then (Mira does not remember herself as a baby), but as they experience it in the present (Levin, 1985). Mira's play gave her a new self-awareness. She also enjoyed creating this play. Mira experienced herself as the creator of her experience.

Mira's play is also an example of how the basic touching experience furnishes the foundation for the next stage of development. Out of the presymbolic concrete stage develops the symbolic and abstract stage. Psychological awareness is added to the body awareness.

What the Therapist Did

The therapist's contribution to Mira's play was to be a player—the mother. This time, however, the therapist was playing a role—a "pretend" mother. And Mira also knew she was playing a "pretend" child. This is very different from session 6, in which Mira was experiencing herself as a baby and the therapist was doing what real mothers do. It is out of that experience that Mira was able to create her play. The therapist helped Mira see what she was really doing when the therapist gave her another image ("When you go to bed at night, do you imagine I'm rocking you like this?").

Playmates

When Mira needed a playmate, the therapist moved into that role. In that role, the therapist and Mira took turns showing each other games they had created. For example, after Mira had created her game, the therapist said, as she finished doing what Mira had asked her to do ("Pull me up"), "I'll show you a new game" (the Owl game). Mira reacted as if the therapist had upstaged her, and she accused the therapist of not taking turns ("We go turns"). Then she said, *That's not my game.*

Mira was not quite ready to share as an equal partner. She felt deserted when the therapist offered her a game instead of paying attention to Mira's production. Mira was also in the process of defining what was hers and what was the therapist's. She needed to feel seen and validated before she could respond to the therapist. Above all, Mira needed to feel her own power and to validate herself before she could attend to another. Mira's awareness of this need to be seen and acknowledged was new.

What the Therapist Did

The therapist got Mira's message. Mira was delighted when the therapist turned her attention toward her, as in the following response:

Mira: This is my game . . . one more time. (Putting her hand to her forehead in a dramatic gesture)
Therapist: You're thinking about it. You're tapping your forehead.
Mira: I know . . . I know. (In dramatic tone)

The therapist did not help Mira with her game or do anything unless Mira asked for it. Mira was trying to imagine her body in a certain position, and she was trying to create something when she had no idea what she was trying to create, but she was struggling with it, sort of talking it out as she moved an arm or a leg. The therapist didn't interpret or suggest anything. She just observed Mira and said what she saw Mira doing. Mira liked that and responded verbally and emotionally. Being noticed did not destroy her feeling that she was doing something on her own.

When Mira asked the therapist to do something that was impossible to do, the therapist didn't tell her it was impossible or suggest something else that would be possible. The therapist played the role of a weak person, groaning and pretending to work hard, saying, "I can't get you up." Mira felt very empowered because she had created something the therapist couldn't do. In other words, the therapist played her game and Mira felt seen, understood, and empowered. Her feeling of empowerment was so important to her that her very last words at the end of the program were, "What I liked best was when we did our tricks, Vi couldn't get me up."

This interaction is an example of the therapist backing off to allow the child to experience her success as hers and not the therapist's.

The Dialogue of Words

The two-way verbal dialogue that started in session 12 increased in Session 13: the mother-child play, Mira's work on creating her game, Mira's verbal response in the Knock at the Door game, and Mira's defining herself as to age and sex.

What the Therapist Did

In the Knock at the Door game, the therapist provided images for Mira starting with session 12. Up to that point, Mira's responses to the game consisted of "Do it again," "Do all the way around." In session 12, the therapist required more. When the therapist said, "I wonder what she is doing," Mira responded with, "The door's just locked." In session 13, Mira's response showed that she had learned from session 12 that she can use her imagination without needing to be stimulated to do so by the therapist. For example, she gave an entirely new response: "I'm at the K-Mart, shopping. Just knock at the door and see if the door opens."

This example illustrates two things about children's needs and their growth. First, at a certain stage in the touching dialogue, the therapist needs to provide the child with images that grow out of the touching but may not be connected to it or the body directly. Second, if the therapist is in tune with the child, the child will take in the image she provides and use it to learn that she, too, can create events through imagining them. In addition, the child, in order to share her images, learns to use words, learns that language is another way to be in relation to others. The fact that sometimes Mira's words didn't fit the action shows that she is just learning to use words.

Limit Setting

Children experience limit setting as the attachment-person's caring about them when it is done sensitively and at the right time. For example, Mira actually seemed relieved when she wanted to go get a drink, and I said she could do that at the end. She asked four times, but after each response from me, Mira returned to what she was doing without any name-calling or acting-out. She seemed to be testing me, but in a playful way ("I'm sad. If you won't let me get a drink of water, I won't be happy."). After enjoying being rocked, she said, "Now can I get a drink of water?" She didn't show any feeling one way or another when I said, "At the end." She actually seemed to enjoy obeying a rule. This acceptance of limits seemed to be part of her commitment to this relationship, a commitment she expressed in everything she did.

Another way of setting limits is illustrated in my response to Mira's acting-out behavior at the end of the session (putting shoes and socks on to leave). Mira had demonstrated her new game in Circle Time, kissed me goodbye at the end of Circle Time, got her drink, and then she lost her composure. She got on top of a table and began to dance around in a wild way. She could have fallen and hurt herself. I knew that if I reached for her, Mira would have jumped or fallen. I first quieted myself, and then said in a quiet voice, "Which do you want to be in the line-up at the door, number four or number five?" She immediately said, "Number four," got down by herself, put her shoes and socks on, and got in line, ready to leave.

TERMINATION

In the Developmental Play group program, the beginning and the end are set. It is like school in that sense.

The goal set in the beginning—to create an attachment separation relationship through touch—was met in session 13. The basic work is complete. Mira now has the basic tools for relating to others, both through a touching dialogue and through a verbal dialogue. She has a core self that enables her to assess herself. She has an intersubjective-related self that enables her to relate to others. She has what she needs to say goodbye.

SESSION 14

Mira responded to the announcement of the ending with a moment of panic followed by asking to play the Owl game, the game that upset her in session 13 when the therapist presented it. First, she was unusually cooperative, asking once in playing this game, "Did I cheat?" Finally, she could no longer hold back her feelings about ending this relationship. She started to hit the therapist and said, "I hate you, and I don't want to be your partner anymore."

What the Therapist Did

The therapist provided a holding environment for all her feelings. First, the therapist did not allow Mira to leave the scene after expressing her anger. From that, Mira learned that it was safe to stay. The therapist wasn't angry with her. Second, through their interactions, the therapist demonstrated to Mira that while she will not be with the therapist anymore, she can imagine being with her. The therapist had her practice, with her eyes closed, seeing the therapist. When Mira sat up and put her hands over the therapist's eyes, the therapist said, "I can see you even with my eyes closed. I can see you right inside my head." The therapist was saying, "I'm remembering you, too. I won't forget you."

In the Circle Time that immediately followed, Mira began to sob while the therapist held her. She allowed the other children and adults to see her in tears and pain. She experienced herself having permission to cry. No one told her to stop crying.

Mira's crying, while being held by the therapist in Circle Time, represented another moment of intimacy for her. Feeling herself cry with her whole body got her in touch with the caring and loving part of herself (Levin, 1988).

To experience pain and share it openly while crying is one of the most healing things a child (or adult) can do. Many children never cry because they don't have an attachment relationship that allows it.

SESSION 15

This session was not like any session before or after it. From the opening gambit, Mira took charge. It was her show. From the moment she walked in, she seemed to know exactly what she was going to do, as if she had planned it beforehand. This taking-charge behavior, however, was very different from her old taking-charge behavior of yelling and telling others what to do. In this session, she shared herself, her feelings for me, and asked for what she needed quietly and appropriately. Except for the rocking at the end, everything she did was new. This is the only session in which she did not ask for a touching game (although throughout the whole session, she was sitting in my lap).

The second difference was the quality of her energy and affect. She did what she did with so much joy, light, and love. From beginning to end, it was a love feast—quite a contrast from the pain experienced the previous week in her crying.

Yet, it was Mira's ability to experience the pain that made her aware of the importance of this relationship to her and the awareness of the love inside her. Mira had learned to love as well as to be loved. In this session, Mira experienced both: she gave love (her "song") to me, and she could ask for love from me ("carry me like a baby").

Session 15 was new in still another way. All of the interaction was carried out in a verbal dialogue. To the dialogue of touch, a presymbolic concrete mode, Mira added a symbolic verbal mode. For example, she expressed her experience in therapy in a metaphor (her "song") that described her experience in terms of seeds and plants growing and animals playing and being close at the end of the day with Mira and me ("They're all in bed in rosy time for them to start to sing a song for you and me"). Mira's request at the end ("carry me *like* a baby") had both abstract and concrete elements.

In the beginning of the session, Mira took charge by asking me to do something that only Mira could do (lift the fingers on her hand). In that interaction, Mira experienced her power and felt acknowledged by me for her strength. At the end of the session, Mira took charge by asking to be "rocked" and "carried like a baby." In that interaction, Mira felt accepted and acknowledged as a child with a need to be held. She can be strong and have needs at the same time. It is also okay to be close and intimate.

The force that stimulated all this new behavior was the awareness (although not verbalized) that next week would be the last session.

What the Therapist Did

Since Mira was doing extremely well providing most of the structure, the therapist just responded to her cues. Mira was the initiator, and the therapist was the responder. To Mira's initial challenge (pull up her fingers), the therapist again took the role of the weaker one. The effect on her was one of delight and sense of power.

In the figure-drawing time, the therapist presented the idea that feelings can be expressed in writing when she wrote on her drawing, "I love you, Mira." The effect on Mira was to immediately write something on her drawing and ask the therapist to read what she had written with her ABCs ("I love you, too.").

What the Therapist Missed

Because the therapist was distracted by the videotaping and wanted the words to Mira's song to be heard, she was not in tune with Mira, who was very self-conscious and shy about singing her song. Mira wanted the song to be private, for the therapist's ears only. The therapist was telling her to sing it louder, and Mira wanted to sing it very softly.

Mira was very aware that she was not reaching the therapist and said, looking frustrated, "I'm tired of this." She was very patient, however, and worked it out so that she did her song her way (privately). She mastered her shyness. Her "song" was very beautiful (although the therapist didn't hear all of it; she had to play it on her tape recorder later). And Mira really enjoyed creating it, which she did in a very quiet, confident, undramatic way. This behavior speaks for Mira's empathic ability and her emotional maturity.

SESSION 16

When a child has what it takes to say goodbye, the Goodbye process is a very integrating and empowering experience. What it takes is a core-related self and an intersubjective-related self. That means that she is aware of her own inner experience (her core-related self), and she is aware of how her subjective experiences influence others and how their subjective experiences influence her (her intersubjective-related self). The latter has to do with the ability to experience empathy and mutuality. Mira's behavior showed that she had what it takes (Stern, 1985).

Mira took charge of herself in session 16. She did everything she needed to do to say Goodbye. She worked on *her* game again. She tied up all the loose ends. She said how she felt. She cried a little. She mentioned her mother. She asked for a tremendous amount of touching. She played her favorite game one more time ("That was fun. I love that game."). She created another "song" that said it all.

> *The rainbows and the sheeps and the apples*
> *The rain and the clouds will be from not a sunny day*
> *And then the sun comes around*
> *Then that will be a sunny day*
> *And then all the animals come out and have a party.*

Finally, Mira showed that she is learning how to recreate or relive an earlier experience through fantasy ("Pick me up and carry me *like* a baby. *Pretend* I'm your tiny baby."). In this request, Mira is still experiencing herself being really cradled and held, but she is also building a memory in her body so that she can recapture this experience at a later time when she isn't being held by me. Not only did Mira end the session by getting held by me, she also brought her fantasy into the Circle Time and created an atmosphere where everyone reached out and touched her. In so doing, she was also providing a model for the other children:

they, too, can recreate this loving touching feeling by "pretending" they are here again—in their imagination. It was very beautiful and loving. Instead of competing with the other children, she invited them to participate in her fantasy-play.

What the Therapist Did

Again, as Mira organized the whole session, the therapist simply responded to what she put out. Sometimes this meant giving feedback on what she was doing. For example, when Mira was learning to be the initiator of the Owl game, she accused the therapist (as the receiver) of not doing it right. The therapist told Mira that she had left out the instructions. Then Mira did it correctly.

Mira worked out several issues in the process of learning the therapist's game. First, there is the issue of boundaries that depend on whether she is the receiver of the game—that is, being the one done to or whether she is the initiator who has to tell the receiver what to do. That is what Mira was dealing with when she left out the instructions. She was learning to switch roles from being the receiver to being the initiator or giver.

Another issue that got resolved had to do with Mira's negative reaction to the therapist when she first presented this game in session 13. In session 14, Mira asked for the "Owl game" (perhaps indicating some undoing or making-up behavior). In session 16, Mira handled her competitiveness by learning how to do the game herself. She identified with the competitor.

This is an example of the child's learning through identification with the adult. Identifying with the therapist, Mira can show this game to someone at home by doing it to them.

The therapist responded to Mira's demonstration that she could do the Owl game by acknowledging her success and connecting her to her mother: "You do know how to do it! That's nice (with excited tone). You could show your mother how to play these games." The therapist felt sad when Mira said, in a sad voice, "She doesn't know what I want."

This statement of Mira's shows a lot of awareness of the subjective experience of herself and of others (her mother, her therapist) and the effect each has on the other. She would like her mother to do with her what the therapist does. She sees that is not where her mother is (see the Postscript, page 247).

The therapist's suggestion gave Mira the opportunity to express feelings about her mother. The therapist, in doing this, is providing Mira with conditions to help her reconnect with her mother.

Most of the time, the therapist did not offer interpretations of Mira's behavior. For example, in the Goodbye session, Mira said she was going to tell her mother that the therapist "broke her leg." The therapist just let Mira say it her own way without adding anything. At another time, however, in this same session, when Mira said she wanted the therapist to be "sad" ("I told you to be sad."), the therapist said, "Did you want me to be sad because I'll miss you?" Mira said, "Yes."

In this interaction, Mira wanted some indication from the therapist that the therapist valued this relationship, that the therapist had a good time, too, and that there'll never be another quite like this one.

One way the therapist tried to help Mira develop her core self was to show her how she can recreate and relive experiences through imagining them ("When you go to bed at night, do you imagine me rocking you like this?"). The work of the therapist seemed to have paid off when Mira expressed this concept verbally by using the word "pretend" for the first time. In the final Goodbye session (16), Mira started practicing imagining being with the therapist when she said at the very end, "Pick me up and carry me like a baby. *Pretend* that I'm *your* tiny baby" (Winnicott, 1953).

In this act, Mira created her own experience of closeness. It will stay with her as a memory for a long time because she created it and because the memory is one of being touched. Mira is internalizing the therapist, who becomes her inside therapist, or what Stern (1985) calls an "evoked companion." The "companion's" job is to assess ongoing interactions by comparing them with the memory of the earlier experiences.

The therapist allowed the extra amount of touching that Mira initiated in the last session: for example, jumping up onto the therapist, wrapping her legs around the therapist's waist and asking to be carried. This was a spontaneous act and the first time she ever did it. (Note: Both Jason and Kenny did the same thing in their Goodbye session—see Chapters 3 and 4.)

In addition to playing all the games one more time (which Mira did) as part of the termination process, it is also very important for both child and therapist to talk—what did they do, what they liked or didn't like, and how are they going to say goodbye. The therapist initiated this conversation. With Mira sitting on her lap facing her, the therapist told the story of how they came together, how she chose Mira as her special friend, the games they played, what Mira said and did. In telling her story, the therapist conveyed to Mira how much she valued their relationship.

Then Mira responded by telling her version. She wanted a crayon to take home (one she found in the room). The therapist told her she was going to get a picture of her and the therapist to take home. At the end, Mira was quiet. Then she looked at the therapist and reached up and touched her hair (something Mira did in the very first session). Then, sitting sideways on the therapist's lap, Mira sat there quietly thinking until Circle Time was called. She asked to be "carried like a baby" to Circle Time (Winnicott, 1953).

THE ROLE OF TOUCH IN MIRA'S THERAPY

Mira's therapy was based on touch. Touching and cradling provided the foundation for everything she did in the sixteen sessions. Touch was an integral part of every therapy session. However, it played a different role and served different functions for each stage in her therapy. The quality of the touching and the way Mira used it changed as she progressed.

At first Mira looked like a passive receiver of the touching, lying quietly in my arms or on the floor while I touched her and sang to her. Once she could allow herself to be touched, she could not get enough of it. She was like a hungry child who is getting nourishing food for the first time. Although she was quiet, often lying in a trance with her finger in her mouth, she was not passive. In the cradling she was allowing her body to absorb the touch and herself to enjoy total relaxation without any intrusion from the outside. She felt her own body—its energy and its aliveness. She felt her own presence and her own existence. She felt the pleasure in this new awareness. She felt seen and touched. These are focused inner experiences. She is experiencing her Beingness. That is not a passive act.

Touch at this stage served the purpose of providing the conditions needed for Mira to become attached to the therapist. It was the immense pleasure and sense of joy, when touched, that moved Mira to relate to and want to be with me, the therapist. She didn't want to lose this new-found reality, the sense of aliveness and being she got when touched. It was her awareness of the pleasure and aliveness that she experienced through the touching that moved her to the next stage.

The pleasure and aliveness she experienced from being touched moved Mira to the next stage; namely, asking for the touch. First, she did this nonverbally through body language. For example, if one hand was touched, she held up the other hand to be touched. When cradled, she reached up and touched my hair. Then she used verbal language: "Do it again." "I need a lot." At this stage she could take some responsibility for getting her needs met, now that she knew what some of her needs were.

Knowing what her needs were and communicating these needs to the therapist organized Mira from the inside out. She wanted to be with the therapist because that is where she felt her Beingness. The touching dialogue initiated the attachment process.

The touching experience enables the child to use her body as an instrument of communication. Mira used body language to communicate what she wanted just as all young children do. In Mira's case, however, that language was not easy to decipher because the same body words meant different things at different times. For example, calling my attention to "a sore toe" was her way of initiating contact with me, and it was also her way of disrupting or ending contact. She never actually had a sore on her toe. She used the word "hurt" in the same way. When she said I hurt her neck or her back, sometimes it meant she wanted me to stop; at other times it meant she wanted me to make it better. She never gave any evidence that she was hurting in any physical way. Rather, she used this body language to express her degree of comfort or discomfort in her relationship with me. When Mira cried in dealing with the termination, she said she was going to tell her mother that I "broke her leg." Mira was using words, but her words referred to body parts.

These examples show how the experience and awareness of the body provide the child with the basic language of communication—the dialogue of touch. Body awareness furnishes the bridge from the dialogue of touch to the dialogue of words.

The touching experience also furnishes the child with images and memories needed to relate through language. The skin doesn't forget. The memory of the touch remains in the skin, and that touch can be retrieved any time the child focuses her attention on that experience or relives that experience. At this stage, the child discovers the word "pretend." In the last session Mira said to me, "Pick me up and carry me like a baby. *Pretend* that I'm your tiny baby." In this request, Mira is making use of her memory of being cradled by the therapist. She is visualizing herself being held by me one more time so that she can take that memory with her. Touch then leads to seeing and visualizing. "Seeing is touching at a distance."

As an example of this visualizing process, Mira used her body to try to create an image of something she had never done; namely, a body game to play with me to compete with her. She sat in front of me and tried to imagine ahead of time what she would do. The only way she could do it was to move a leg or arm first, and then an idea came to her—how to involve me. What she asked me to do was impossible to do. Out of that experience she got a sense of power because she had thought up something for me to do that I could not do. That activity demonstrated the creative process because she didn't know how it was going to turn out, and neither did I. That was the excitement of it.

In sessions 12 through 16, Mira used the touching as a base to create images that enabled her to relate through language, the dialogue of words. For example, she shifted from body-connected words to words not directly connected to her body; from "Do it again and go all the way round" in her favorite game, Knock at the Door, to "She went to the K-Mart and she won't be back until vacation." The last statement has no connection with the body, yet it came out of the experience of being touched in the game and from sitting on my lap. Again, this example illustrates the primordial function of touch for human development. Mira could both experience herself as present and imagine herself being some-place else so long as she was in touch with me.

Lastly, the touching experience made Mira aware of the therapist as a sepa-rate person and aware of how much she wanted to be with her. To give form to her feelings, she began to relate through language. Her verbal communication contained feeling words ("hate, sad, love, happy"). In sharing these feelings with the therapist, she became even more aware of these feelings. She could hear her-self say them, and she could see the effect of saying them on the therapist. For ex-ample, Mira showed great joy in playing her favorite game, but in session 16 she put her feelings into words: "Let's play Knock at the Door. It was fun. I love that game." Mira's ability to create two poems (her songs) to represent her feelings moved her into another realm—the realm of an intimate I-Thou relationship. They were abstract expressions of the relationship. *The touching dialogue has be-come a verbal dialogue. The physical connection has become a psychological con-nection.*

This shift, however, does not mean that Mira doesn't need touching any more. The touching and body awareness is embedded in, and is a part of, the higher functions. For example, when Mira was expressing abstract thinking in her two poems, she was sitting on the therapist's lap. The more Mira used verbal dia-logue and abstract expressions, the more she wanted to be touched, the more she demanded it. For example, after Mira had created her abstract poem in session 15, she said to me, "You're supposed to rock me up and down now." At this stage, the touching serves as a stabilizing centering function—a place to which she can return any time. Mira seemed to know that. The touching then was like a friend that accompanied her through her stages of growth. The memory of it will always be there, and she can ask for it whenever she needs it now. She can create her own world from the inside out—very different from trying to create it from the outside by ordering other people around. The role of the touch was to help Mira experience her own body as a friend and guide.

SUMMARY OF THE THERAPIST'S WORK

The DP therapist is always guided by the belief that touch is the basic form of communication, that the child's awareness of her bodily self through being touched by a caring person is the experience needed for the emergence of the inner or core self. To implement this principle, the therapist touches and cradles. The cradling helps the child turn inward and focus on her own inner rhythms. The cradling helps the child experience her own presence and the presence of the therapist. It is the beginning of the dialogue of touch. It is the beginning of a relationship.

Although I knew that I would be touching and cradling Mira sometime when I began seeing her, I had no pre-session plan as to how I would do it for any one session. I began by looking at her, noticing her, telling her my name, asking her to say her name, and saying briefly why we were together. In doing this, I noticed her and touched her. Her response to being noticed and touched started the communication, the dialogue of touch. In other words, I take charge, initiate the contact, and select the activity that we will be doing together. That leaves Mira free to do what she needs to do. She doesn't have to wonder what to do, or to take care of me. Because I am not telling her what to do (as many people do), I am not giving her anything to oppose. Her opposition, when it does come, will not be to me. Rather, it will be an expression of her discomfort at being seen and touched.

The Struggle—Period 1

When I cradled and touched Mira in session 1, she gave me very little to respond to. By session 3, she did respond—in the form of earsplitting screams, hitting, biting, name-calling, and pushing me away. Even when she did ask for the touching, which she did do sometimes, she began her screaming almost as soon as I started the touching.

I responded to this behavior, not by forcibly holding her for some length of time as some therapists do, but by varying the way I held and touched her. I cradled her for short periods of time. When she objected, I changed the way I touched her, or asked her to show me the part that she said I hurt. I just kept trying different kinds of holding. For example, I discovered she liked the touching when it was done in a game or while moving. She liked my Row, Row Your Boat game which required me to hold her tightly so she wouldn't fall out of the boat. She liked being held tightly. By the end of that session, Mira was allowing me to cradle her for a longer period. She totally relaxed.

The Meaning of the Struggle

The cradling brought out into the open two contradictory parts of Mira: one part that said she needed and liked the cradling, and the other part that said she was too big for this. In fact, Mira said in session 1, "I don't need a hug." Mother also said, in hearing her baby-talk, "She knows better than that." Mira was not conscious of this contradiction, but her body certainly expressed it. She was experiencing the tension of being trapped between the two parts and the terror of not knowing what to do.

What the Therapist Did

I stayed with it and with her, not giving up, but adjusting the touch to her. I was consistent and present. She could not get rid of me no matter what she did. The effect on me was total exhaustion, yet something in me made me hang in there with her. It wasn't a case of me deciding to do it or to not do it. There wasn't time. She needed what I did, and I did it. The effect on Mira was to give her a feeling of trust and safety, to be whatever she needed to be—a baby.

Infancy—Period 2

This period could be described as a mother with a new baby. Mira invited the touching and the cradling. I rocked her and sang to her. It was as if Mira and I were the only ones in the world. She asked for the Knock at the Door game over and over. Although we did the same things each session, Mira always added something new each time so that the touching game became more complex, and I never knew what she was going to do. I was never bored with her. This period was as easy as Period 1 was hard and difficult. It was relaxed and enjoyable for both of us. I provided the touching and the cradling, and she took it. She was the receiver and I was the giver. Much of this period was spent just being quiet, she lying still as I chanted or sang while holding her.

Playmates—Period 3

In this period Mira organized her own world. She put out where she was and what she wanted. She created games to show me her power and that she could do things on her own. I responded by respecting this stage in her. I backed off and gave her space to do her thing, to struggle in defining what she was doing. I simply observed more and waited for her to tell me what she wanted (she never had any trouble doing that). She was the initiator and I was the responder. She was both a giver and a receiver. She began using more verbal language.

This shift in her also freed me to be more separate from her and to introduce something new instead of limiting myself to just responding to her. When I did this, she let me know she didn't like it. Sometimes the interactions had the quality of two playmates trying to defend their turf. My focus was helping her define hers.

Friends—Period 4

This period included the last three sessions and the termination process. As Mira expressed her feelings about the termination, she did most of the initiating.

218

She did a wonderful job of organizing her goodbye. I served her in several ways. I was a container for her feelings. I listened to her. I held her when she cried. I helped her prepare for the parting and her future in two ways: first, by showing her how she could imagine herself seeing me with her eyes closed; and second, by printing the words "I love you" on my drawing to show her feelings can be expressed in writing. I set limits by not allowing her to leave the room after she had expressed her anger toward me. Doing that enabled her to experience some close feelings that led to her deep crying.

In this period, Mira treated me more like a friend, a person from whom she could learn. As an example, she wanted me to show her how to do my Owl game so she could do it at home. I did that. At the same time, she felt safe enough to ask me to carry her like a baby and pretend that she was my tiny baby. I cradled her at the end, as always.

Review

Mira turned out to be quite a disturbed child. When a child makes the kind of gains Mira made in a little more than four months, one tends either to forget what she was like in the beginning or say that she couldn't have been that disturbed in the first place.

In the beginning (especially session 3—both the one-to-one and the Circle Time), Mira was a very controlling, demanding, loud-mouthed child who got attention through disruptive behavior such as screaming and yelling and telling others what to do. At this period, she was not a very pleasant or giving child, nor was she a very happy child. In the beginning of the program when the adults had to choose one of the children, no one wanted her except Vi.

Mira was lacking at the basic attachment relationship level. Her hyperactivity and inability to stay focused came from her trying to be a four-year-old when developmentally she was only two. Because she had such excellent speech and because she was so active, she may not have seemed that disturbed. However, as soon as she was required to relate to a person—child or adult—she showed it. Although she had a high level of speech, she did not use it for relating. Instead, she used it to say she didn't need a relationship ("I don't want to give her a hug. I don't need a hug").

However, in spite of all this, Mira showed phenomenal growth in a short time when given what she needed. What was she given?

In reviewing what I did with Mira, I chose four things that seemed to me to be the most crucial: (1) the touching and cradling throughout, but especially in Stages 1 and 2; (2) my backing off in Stages 3 and 4 to give space and support to her newly discovered core self; (3) setting limits by not allowing her to dilute her feelings by leaving the scene when she felt deeply about something; and (4) being present in all of her stages (most of the time). Mira felt my presence and also my enjoyment of her.

At the end, I was very moved by this child and the depth of her work. I was amazed at her creative ability and what she said in her poems. She helped me understand how this creative process comes about in a young child. She helped me become aware of my own rigidities. I enjoyed her as much as she enjoyed me. I wish that all mothers could have this experience with their four year-old girls. It is the child's first experience of loving and being loved. It reminds the mother of her first experience of love with her mother.

Mira's drawings of a girl. The day care center was asked to collect drawings periodically from the children in the DP program. They were asked to draw a "girl" or a "boy," as the case may be. The children did the drawings with crayons; colors could not be duplicated here.

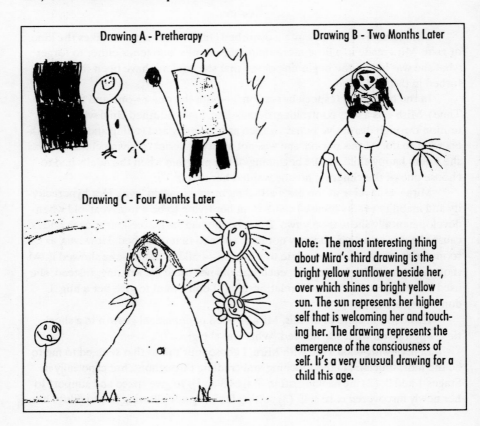

Drawing A - Pretherapy

Drawing B - Two Months Later

Drawing C - Four Months Later

Note: The most interesting thing about Mira's third drawing is the bright yellow sunflower beside her, over which shines a bright yellow sun. The sun represents her higher self that is welcoming her and touching her. The drawing represents the emergence of the consciousness of self. It's a very unusual drawing for a child this age.

SUMMARY OF THE THERAPEUTIC PROCESS

The course of therapy describes the evolution of the core self in a young child, Mira. The core self begins with the experience of the body being touched by a caring person. To receive touch, the child has to allow the touch. Mira could not allow the touch because she had no core self to receive or hold the touch, and she needed the touch to find her core self. Without a core self, Mira tried to get a sense of who she was by controlling others.

The first three sessions were devoted to learning to allow the touch. At the end of session 3, Mira decided to let herself have it. From then on she could not get enough touching.

Sessions 4 to 10 were Mira's infancy period. When the therapist held her and sang to her, she relaxed into another world (her trance). She looked and acted like a baby. Feeling herself touched provided Mira with an inner self, a self that sought the touching because the self got born through the touch. Through the dialogue of touch, Mira discovered her core self.

To be complete, the core self needs to share itself with another. Through asking for the touch ("Do it again"), Mira experienced the therapist as separate from her ("Do you see one [a kissable place]?") From then on, Mira had someone to whom she could talk and she also had something to share—her core self. Since the therapist was also separate, the therapist also had something to share: her responses to Mira and her views.

In sessions 11-13, Mira experienced the therapist more as a playmate with whom she actively shared and also competed. Through this playmate interaction, Mira began to be in relation through words as well as through touch. Through the dialogue of words, Mira discovered her intersubjective-related self. By the end of the 13th session, Mira had what she needed to be in a relationship with another—the goal of this therapy. She had a core-related self (an awareness of what she is experiencing) and an intersubjective-related self (an awareness of what the other person is experiencing).

The last three sessions (14-16) could be described as Mira's grown-up period, grown-up in the sense of being a mature four-year-old. Our relationship was more like two people having a conversation, sharing experiences. Mira experienced her relationship with the therapist as very special, personal, and private. It had the qualities of preciousness, innocence, and intimacy. She gave form to these qualities in her two poems. It was an I-Thou relationship.

Mira demonstrated that she could empathize with the therapist. For example, when Vi didn't get her message, Mira told her so. Then she went on and figured out a way to do what she wanted to do anyway, but in a very gentle way. She had the ability to allow herself to feel deeply, including crying, and to give form to those feelings by sharing them with Vi. She had this exquisite ability to feel deeply and to come out of it with a sense of joy and empowerment. Mira could take charge now—this time from the inside out. It was herself that she took charge of, not others. Through being touched by Vi, she got in touch with herself.

Developmentally, Mira moved from a young two-year-old to an advanced five-year-old in the sixteen sessions.

In review, Mira's growth followed four stages of development:

1. Resisting the touch.
2. Infancy: asking for the touching. The dialogue of touch: a receiver.
3. Playmates: interactive and confrontal state. The dialogue of words. A giver.
4. Joining the collective: a giver and a receiver. The I-Thou dialogue of intimacy.

Mira's growth took place within a Developmental Play group program that included both a one-to-one relationship with her therapist and a group or family relationship involving four other children, four adults, and the Leader, Mary, during Circle Time each week. In the next section, we'll look at Mira's behavior in the Circle Time sessions. We will look at the role of the Leader in a DP Circle Time.

PART 2: CIRCLE TIME

Circle Time gives the child the opportunity to practice with peers what she has learned in the one-to-one segment. This interaction with peers also helps the child separate from her adult partner. Circle Time is designed to help the children learn to relate to each other through the dialogue of touch. The child has the opportunity to be the center of attention, to be touched and seen by peers. Circle Time is also designed to give the child a feeling for boundaries. She learns that certain activities belong to the beginning, or Hello part, certain activities belong to the play part, and certain activities belong to the ending, or Goodbye part.

As with the one-to-one, the adult—here, the Leader—takes charge to provide the conditions needed for the children to engage in a touching dialogue with each other. She does this in two ways: first, she leads the children in an activity; and then, as they are ready, she invites individual children to lead or show what they can do. Much of what the Leader does in Circle Time comes from observing the children and making what they do into something for all to do.

The Leader lets the adult partners know when it's time to stop the one-to-one play and bring their children to the circle. She may do this by walking around and telling them they have to get ready to come to the circle, or she may put some music on as a signal for all to come. The adults sit in a circle holding the children in their laps.

HELLO CIRCLE TIME

The following are examples of some of the activities used in a first Circle Time, or in the Hello part of every Circle Time.

1. **Follow-the-Leader Hello song.** The Leader begins by looking at one child and sings (to the tune of "Frere Jacques") "Hello, Billy" (children repeat). Leader: "I see your blue eyes" (children repeat). "I see you look-ing at me" (children repeat). "I see you moving your hand" (children repeat).

   As the children are ready, the Leader asks one child to be the Leader and say Hello to another child (or adult). Then that child chooses another child to be the Leader, until all have had a turn.

2. **Follow-the-Leader with hand movements to music.** The Leader moves her hands to music and asks the children to follow: "Follow my hands." After the children get into the rhythm, the Leader may invite a child to touch another's hands as she moves to the music. Or the Leader may in-vite different children to be the Leader and to choose someone else when they have finished. Moving her hands, the Leader says to the child, "And now, can you put an ending to your hand dance?"

   These hand movements to music help the children become aware of many qualities of their bodies, including their beauty: "Notice how beautiful your hands are when they move." Children learn about form when they are asked to put an ending to their movements. They learn to use their body to make an ending statement. Some children stop their movement by crossing their hands, by laying them in their lap, by putting their hands together as if in prayer. In this way, they learn to experience the difference between moving and not moving, being quiet. They can observe the feeling of the body moving and observe the feeling of the body being still.

3. **Saying "Hello" with your feet.** The Leader moves her feet toward the center and invites the children to touch feet. (Many children will take their shoes and socks off, although this is not required.) The Leader no-tices different size feet and toes. Hearing this, one child may wiggle her

toe. The Leader might make this child feel noticed by saying, "Oh, look what Amy can do. Let's all do that."

This foot-touching "Hello" often leads to the children saying "Hello" to other children with their feet, or to making a bridge with all their feet, with some feet under the bridge and some on top of the bridge. Sometimes this leads to singing "London Bridge is falling down," which is a way to end this foot play.

As much as possible, the Leader should allow these feet interactions to come naturally from the children. She should not be putting out organized games for the children to play.

4. **Saying "Hello" with your hands**. The Leader might start by putting her hand out to one child and saying "Hello," followed by other children saying "Hello" to each other with their hands. With less organized children, the Leader might say, "Let's all say 'Hello' with our hands" as she moves toward the center and holds out her hand. Again, how these games develop will depend on the children and on the ability of the Leader to make something out of what she sees the children doing.

5. **Pass-it-on**. The Leader might start by gently touching the hand or a knee of the child next to her, looking at her and saying, "Would you pass this on?" That child passes the hand-touch or knee-touch on to the next child, and so on around the circle, until the touch comes back to the Leader. Then, if it feels right to the Leader, she could ask a child to be the Leader and pass something on. That child chooses someone else to be the Leader, and so on until all the children have had a turn.

A CIRCLE TIME SESSION: SESSION 3

The following transcribed Circle Time session illustrates what a Circle Time looks like and feels like. The five child-adult pairs, of which Mira and the author are one pair, is the same group presented earlier. As you read this dialogue, you will get a feel for what these children, including Mira, were like in the beginning of the program, and you will also get a feel of what it's like to be the Leader of this group in its beginning stages.

This Circle Time (session 3) was the one that followed Mira's one-to-one session 3. To get the whole picture of Mira's behavior at this stage, review her one-to-one session 3 (pages 153-157), and then look at the transcribed Circle Time session 3.

A Transcribed Hello Circle Time

Setting: The Leader, sitting in her place on the floor, has put on some soft music and called, "Circle Time." The adults finish what they are doing and bring their child to the Circle area, sit down, and hold their child on their lap. The Leader takes charge.

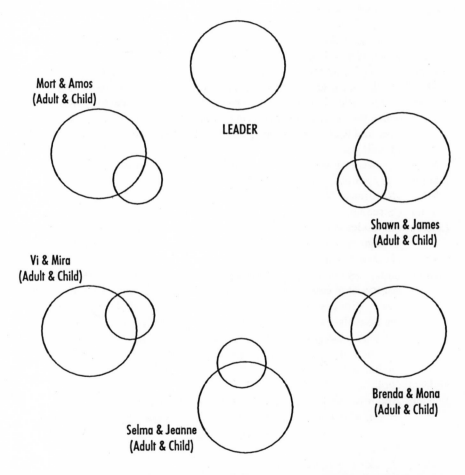

Mort & Amos
(Adult & Child)

LEADER

Shawn & James
(Adult & Child)

Vi & Mira
(Adult & Child)

Brenda & Mona
(Adult & Child)

Selma & Jeanne
(Adult & Child)

Leader: (Looking around as adults bring their children to the circle) Everybody is here. Follow my hand. Listen to the music. (She moves her hands to the music, observing children)

Children: (Imitate Leader and move their hands to the music)
  Leader: That's right, Jeanne. (Touches the palms of a child across from her)
          Anyone across the circle you'd like to touch their hands?
   Amos: (Touching Leader's hand)
  Leader: That's right, Amos.
   Mira: (Yells) Mona!
  Leader: Here's Mira and Mona. Here's Mona saying Hello to Amos. That's
          very nice. There you are.
 Jeanne: (Reaches toward Amos)
  Leader: Here, Amos. Jeanne wants to touch you.
 Jeanne: (Crawls on all fours to reach Amos and touches his hand)
   Mira: (With loud voice) I want to touch James. (Moves toward James)
  Leader: Very gently. Well, let's ask James if it's okay. (To James) James, Mira
          wants to touch hands with you. Is that okay with you? Can she come
          over and touch your hand (Touching him) like this? (To Mira) I think
          he said yes.
   Mira: (Crawls over on all fours to reach Amos, and touches his hand)
  Leader: Very gently . . . very gently, Mira.
   Mira: (Returns to Vi's lap and screams)
   Mona: (Screams)
  Leader: (In louder voice) Everybody follow me. (Moves her hand to the music
          in large movements) Move your hands up. Both hands straight up.
Children: (Follow her and screaming stops)
  Leader: Here they come down. (Moving her hands toward the floor) You've
          got to watch closely. Here they go. (In sing-song tone) That's the way,
          Amos. (Smiling at him) That's the way, Jeanne. (Smiling at her) Let's
          see how high we can stretch. (Moving her hands up) Oh, Amos is re-
          ally high. (Laughing at him) Now let's see how far we can go forward
          and then up again (Moving hands up) and then fall down again. (Mov-
          ing hands to floor)
Children: (Follow)
  Leader: And now, while the music is very quiet, we're going to take turns.
          Mona, who would you like to touch? . . . very gently . . . reach across.
   Mona: (Crawls over and touches Mira)
  Leader: Mira, okay?
   Mira: (Looking at James) Hi, James.
   Mona: (Continues touching others, guided by her adult partner)
  Leader: (Names them as she touches them)
   Mira: (Making noises)

Leader: (Continues naming) And Mary, and Vi, and here's somebody else
    ready. (Looking at Amos)

Mira: Me.

Mona: (Touches Amos)

Leader: That was very nice, Mona. And you said Hello to everybody. Okay,
    Jeanne, it's your turn. Listen to the music and see who you'd like to
    touch.

Jeanne: (Touches all of them in turn)

Mira: (Pulls her hand back when touched by Jeanne) Eh!

Leader: That was very nice, Jeanne. And now it's James' turn. Who would you
    like to touch with your hands, James? Listen to the music.

Amos: (Holds out his hand)

Leader: Oh, Amos, would you like him to touch you?

James: (Reaches over and touches Amos in the stomach)

Leader: (Laughs) Oh, right in the tummy, okay. Well, that was very nice,
    James. And now we'll move right around here and it's Amos' turn. Hi,
    Amos.

Amos: (Names the children he touches in a quiet, gentle way)

Mira: (Making noises and hitting Vi's knee)

Leader: And now there's one person left. And you know who that is?

Mira: (Points to Vi)

Leader: (Laughs, and so do the children) I think it belongs to Mira. Anybody
    you'd like to touch? Very gently. (Names them as she touches them)
    Very nice.

Mira: (Ends her touching with a little yell)

Leader: (In a louder voice) And everybody had a turn. Sometimes, it's hard to
    wait your turn, isn't it? But everybody got a turn, huh! I'll tell you what
    we're going to do now.

James: (Softly) I want a turn.

Leader: You'd like another turn.

Mira: (In a loud voice) I want a turn.

Leader: Hold on here a minute. We'll see how turns go. Your turn, James.

James: (Touches others)

Mira: (Loudly) My turn.

Leader: Just a minute. Let's see if there's anybody else he wants to touch.

Mira: (Softer voice) My turn.

Leader: We're going to go in a different order than we did before. And so it's
    Mira's turn. So who would you like to touch?

Mira: (Touches each child)

Mona: (Loud voice) My turn.

Leader: And now it's Amos' turn. Who would you like to touch?

Mira: I touched myself. (Touching her knee)

Vi: She said she touched herself.

Leader: Oh, okay. And now it's Jeanne's turn.

Jeanne: (Reaches over and touches each child)

James: (While touching going on) I'm hungry.

Leader: Okay, everybody. It's cradle time. Everybody in our Circle, we're going to have a cradle time. So big people, get in a comfortable place. (Shuts off the music) Here we go.

Vi: (Turns Mira around in the cradling position)

Mira: (Screams, stiffens her body, then relaxes)

Leader: (Sings Brahms "Lullaby")

Mira: (Lets herself be held. She turns her face toward Vi, reaches up, and touches Vi's hair. She closes her eyes and lies totally still during the singing)

James: (Sits up in Shawn's lap during the singing)

Jeanne: (In cradling position she is very tense and moves her body a lot)

Mona: (Stiffens her body, fights the cradling by moving her body in strange positions with her legs up in the air)

Amos: (Sits up, leaning against Mort)

Leader: (Continues singing, then chants) Just lean back right on your partner and see how warm it feels to rock. James and Shawn are rocking close, and Mona and Brenda are rocking, too. Jeanne and Selma are rocking, and Mira and Vi are rocking, too. Amos and Mort are rocking, la la la ... (to end the singing) Now everybody stay real still with your partner and the two of you remember what the trick is you're going to do. You want to be the first, Amos?

Amos: (Nods yes)

Leader: Let's make a little bit of room in the center of the circle. Now wait a minute, you guys, because we've got a lot of people in this group, and the first one to do a trick is gonna be right here. (Pointing to Amos and Mort) Does anybody know who they are?

Jeanne: Amos and Mort.

Leader: Right. Which one is Amos? And this one? Okay, everybody pay attention because in the center ring of our circus, we have Amos and Mort.

Amos: (With help from Mort, does a headstand)

Leader: Stand up and take a bow, Mort and Amos.

Amos
and
Mort: (Stand up and bow)
Others: (Applaud)
Leader: (Introduces Mira and Vi in the same way)
Vi: (Removes Mira from her lap and lays her down in the center; she has one knee bent) This knee won't work. How many kisses does it need to make it move?
Mira: (Holds up her two hands)
Vi: (Kisses her knee ten times and then the knee does move)
Mira: (Stops Vi from picking her up) The other knee.
Leader: This is a two-knee trick.
Vi: (Repeats the trick, asking the others to help her count)
Leader: It does work. (The other knee) That's a very nice trick. Now will you stand up and take a bow? You could do a curtsy. (Stands up and shows her)
Mira: I don't want anyone to see my underwear.
Leader: Oh, no. They won't see your underwear. Just hold your skirt.
Mira: (Giggles, gets silly, loses her balance, and then loses her composure)
Vi: (Reaches out and pulls her back into her lap)

Other children do their tricks, except Mona, who can't.

Leader: (Passes out rice cake snacks and asks each child to share with her partner)
Mira: No.
Others: (Share snacks)
Leader: (Sets up a game with the snacks) Let's see if we can make them crunch together. (Holding up her cracker) Everybody get it ready right in front of your mouth. Ready: One, two, three. (Bites into cracker)
Children: (Follow: Each child has a turn to be the leader and count)
Leader: (Offers Vi a bite of her cracker) That's all for turns today.
Mira: (Screams)
Leader: Wait a minute. I would like for you all not to yell in here because it hurts my ears.
Mira: (Screams)
Leader: Did anyone have a good time in here today? Did you, Jeanne?
Jeanne: (Nods yes)

Leader: Would you turn around and tell Selma?

Jeanne: (To Selma) I had a good time today.

Leader: Did anyone else have a good time?

Children: (Hands went up by all the children, including Mira)

Jeanne: I had a good time with Selma.

Leader: I'm glad to hear that. Okay, it's time to put your socks and shoes on. If you want to give your partner a hug, you can. Anyone who wants to give their partner a hug?

Mira: I don't want to give her a hug. I don't need one.

Other Children: (Hug their partners)

Leader: (Sings the Good-bye Song; says time to put on shoes and socks)

Mira: (At end of song, goes around and hugs each child)

What the Leader Did

These verbatim Circle Time excerpts demonstrate that the Leader was in touch with these children and really saw them. She showed this by providing them with the structure they needed to feel seen. She helped them feel seen through touch and helped them see other children through touch. This is the goal of Circle Time.

The Leader began by using soft music as a way to provide quiet energy that would help everyone to feel present. Then she involved the children in a Follow-the-Leader hand movement activity, all moving their hands in unison. Then she individualized the movement by inviting the children to take turns reaching across the circle to say Hello to another child with their hands. Here the children had a choice, and they had to take charge of themselves. First, they had to decide if they wanted to do it. Then they had to look and decide who they would want to touch. These children all needed guidance from their adult partners to do this. Eventually, they all lost control, as shown by the screaming.

The Leader responded by returning the children to a unison body movement—all moving their hands in unison, up and down, following her lead. She contained them through the music, through a unison body movement, and through the hypnotic quality of her voice. The Leader's actions demonstrated her ability to see and understand what these children needed. They needed to feel connected to her through her voice and common body movements without having to do anything else. The way the Leader responded to the children in their chaos is another example of seeing and touching children so that they feel seen and touched.

Another example of the Leader's connection with this group of children is illustrated by her choice to have the cradling part early in the Circle Time.

Usually, the cradling belongs to the closing and Goodbye part of circle activities. These children, however, needed it earlier. They needed a quiet time just to be with their partners without having to do anything but be there with them. The cradling provided Mira with just what she needed. More than any of the other children, she used the cradling to relax, to touch and look at her partner, and to shut out everything from the outside to be present with herself and her partner.

Following the cradling, the Leader introduced an activity where each child had the opportunity to be the center of attention and be seen by all (the Trick Time). Even when the adult partner helped the child plan her trick, as demonstrated by Mira, these children did not find doing "tricks" easy. They showed that they did not know how to be the center of attention in any organized way.

The Leader initiated the Goodbye part with passing out snacks. She gave each child one rice cake and asked them to share with her partner. They all did, except Mira. Then the Leader initiated a game using the crackers to bring the group together, each child taking turns counting before all take a bite.

The Leader ended the session by focusing the children's attention on their experience of the session: "Out of all the things we did, what did you like best?" In this early session, these children had a hard time answering this abstract question. The Leader helped them out by asking, "Who had a good time today?" and "Did you have a good time, Jeanne?" She also invited them to be a giver by giving their partners a hug. All the children did this except Mira. However, Mira did hug all the children.

The Children

The transcribed Circle Time 3 shows how difficult it was for all five children to relate to each other in a group setting. Yet these children all knew each other at some level because they attended the same class in the same day care center. This is also the third time they have met here in Circle Time. The behavior of these children shows that they were lacking in a core self. The Leader responded to this lack by having all the children do hand movements to music in unison, guided by her. Then the children felt their own bodies and their own presence as well as feeling the Leader's presence.

Although all these children could talk (with the exception of Mira, who talked constantly), they said almost nothing except, "I want a turn. My turn." Even though all the children had speech, they were not able to use verbal language as a way of being in relation to another. Verbal language emerges out of the body language of touch. These children needed to learn to relate to each other through the dialogue of touch as the first step.

The Leader recognized this need when she invited the children to take turns choosing and touching one person at a time. The children, however, had a hard time waiting their turn. It was as if they all needed the touch and the attention immediately ("I want a turn. My turn"). They needed to be seen through touch.

A study of the two parts of Mira's DP shows the connection between the work done in the one-to-one and the work done in Circle Time. For example, Mira's knee trick was created in the one-to-one when Mira said one leg "don't work." When Mira didn't know what to do for a trick in Circle Time, the therapist suggested the "knee trick." Thus the Circle Time provides the children the opportunity to practice what they have learned in the individual session in a larger arena with a larger audience. The Circle Time helps the children to transfer what they have learned with their therapist to the other children.

The cradling experience in Circle Time is another example of the carry-over from the individual time. The only time in the whole Circle Time that Mira experienced herself relaxed, with no need to demand attention, was during the cradling. Again, the cradling was something she finally allowed herself to have at the end of the one-to-one. In Circle Time, Mira began the cradling by screaming and stiffening her body. Then she realized she knew how to do this, for she had just let herself be cradled in the one-to-one a few minutes earlier. Then she relaxed. She looked at the therapist, reached up and touched her face, then closed her eyes and just let herself be. She looked and felt like a baby. The cradling was probably the most meaningful thing for Mira in the Circle Time. None of the other four children did the cradling. The two boys just sat up in their partners' laps with eyes open. Mona fought being held, and Jeanne was constantly moving.

For Leaders

The interaction between Mary, the Leader, and the children in this Circle Time shows that what the Leader chooses to do is not a question of what game or activity to do that day. Rather, it is a question of providing the conditions that enable the children to relate to each other where they are that day. To meet the needs of this DP group, the Leader selected activities that were body-focused and concrete, such as moving hands, touching another, cradling, eating, counting, Follow-the-Leader, and taking turns.

Two activities were more verbal and abstract: the "tricks," and the question at the end, "What did you like best?" All the children had a hard time doing their "trick" because they didn't know what to do and it was new. The children needed an immense amount of help from their adult partners (therapists). Mona couldn't do it at all. Yet, at the same time, Trick Time added something new and exciting.

Because none of the children could say what they liked best, the Leader changed the question to, "Did anyone have a good time in here today?" This could be answered verbally or nonverbally. Mira raised her hand with the rest of the children to indicate she had a good time.

The Leader reconnected the children to their therapists when she asked the children to share the cracker with their therapists (all did, except Mira). At the end, the Leader invited the children to give their partners a hug (all did, except Mira).

This Circle Time illustrates how you begin the DP process and what DP looks like in its early stages. This Circle Time also illustrates the three parts of a Circle Time: the Hello part, the middle or play part, and the Goodbye part. For the Hello part, the Leader had the children follow her doing hand movements to music. She invited each child to say "Hello" to another child through touching. The middle part consisted of something new created by the children—the Trick Time. In the Goodbye part, the Leader passed out snacks and asked the children to say what they liked best. She invited them to hug their partners. There is no one specific thing the Leader has to do in each of these parts of Circle Time. Whatever the Leader chooses to do, she needs to base that choice on providing the children with what they need in order to relate to each other, which is the goal of Circle Time.

The behavior of the children in this Circle Time showed that they were at a preverbal stage of relating, even though they all had speech. That is, these children needed to relate to each other first through nonverbal avenues such as touch, seeing each other, moving their bodies, and making sounds. These experiences furnish the foundation for the development of the verbal dialogue.

Leading a Developmental Play Circle Time looks easy, but it is difficult to do. The Leader has to respond to the cues of all the children and create an activity that speaks to these cues.

THE GOODBYE PROCESS IN CIRCLE TIME

Each Circle Time has a Goodbye part, and the last Circle Time is a Goodbye Circle Time.

In contrast to the middle part of the Circle Time session—the part in which the children create and try out new experiences with the help of the Leader—the Goodbye part is more set or fixed. The Goodbye part is a ritual that is more or less the same for each session. This ritual helps the children to integrate and give form to the things they did, and it helps to center them so that they can return to their class, or wherever they go, feeling good about themselves.

Each Circle Time ends with some or all of the following: (1) the adult partners cradling their children while the Leader sings a lullaby; (2) snacks; (3) the children and adults saying what they liked best that day; (4) the Leader singing a Goodbye song (to the tune of "Good Night Ladies"); (5) the Leader inviting the children to give their partners a Goodbye hug. In the Goodbye song, the Leader names both the child and her adult partner, and the group sings it back ("Goodbye James and Shawn," group repeats) until all have been sung to. The Leader may do this while sitting in the circle, or she may sing it while walking around the circle, placing her hand on the head of each child and adult as she names them.

The Termination

Goodbye Circle Time differs from all others for two reasons: (1) the children and the adults know that this will be their last time to be together like this, and (2) the Leader provides the children with specific experiences that they can take with them to serve as a bridge to relating to others when they leave.

Preparing the Children for Termination

Many children never have the opportunity to experience and deal with a separation or a goodbye such as school ending, parents getting a divorce, family moving to another area. Children see and know these events are happening, but no space is provided for them to share in these events. It is as if the children weren't there and didn't matter.

In Developmental Play, children do get the opportunity to experience and deal with goodbyes. In the very beginning of the program, the children and adults are told that they will be in this play program for so many weeks (young children count the weeks on their fingers and are also reminded of the ending three sessions before the end ("We play today and two more times and then we have to say goodbye, and we won't be playing with you anymore"). This gives the children, the adults, and the Leader three sessions to bring this program to a close.

A transcribed Circle Time of Mira's DP group illustrates what one Leader did and what one group of children did in their last Circle Time. By comparing the children's behavior in the first and last Circle Time, you will notice how the children, especially Mira, have become more related to each other—the goal of Circle Time.

THE GOODBYE CIRCLE TIME: SESSION 16

Setting: Leader is sitting on floor, with music playing, as adults walk in with their children.

Selma: (Walks in with Jeanne)

Vi: (Walks in carrying Mira)

Mira: (To Vi) Pretend I'm your tiny little baby.

Leader: Vi has a little tiny baby. Don't wake the baby. (Looking at Jeanne) Oh, my goodness. Looks like Jeanne is asleep, too. There are two sleeping girls with their partners, and we've got one boy watching the girls sleeping. And we've got one lap empty. And here comes another partner with a little one. (Brenda enters, carrying Mona) (Amos was absent)

Mira: (Sits up and starts rubbing her eyes, which are closed)

Leader: Mira is starting to wake up a little bit. Everybody just be quiet with your partner just a minute. Lean back on your partner.

Mira: (Rubbing eyes and yawning, eyes still closed, moves into center)

Leader: I think Mira is starting to wake up.

Mira: (With eyes still closed, lifts her face up toward the Leader)

Leader: And there's her little face. (Reaches out and touches her face) Okay, everybody, big folks, let's rock.

Mira: (Leans her face out toward James)

Leader: I think Mira would like James to touch her face.

James: (Reaches out and touches her face)

Leader: How about Shawn?

Shawn: (Reaches over and gently touches her face)

Mort: I'd like to touch her face.

Leader: Right over here, Mira.

Mira: (Leans her face toward Mort, with her eyes still closed)

Mort: (Touches her upturned face)

Brenda: I want to say "Hello" to her face. (Touches her face)

Mira: (Sitting in center of circle; eyes closed, yawns, then moves over toward the Leader with her face upturned)

Leader: You want some more. Big yawn here. (Cups Mira's face in her hands)

Group: (Laughs a little)

Leader: Would anyone else like to have their face Helloed to?

Jeanne: (Touches Mira's face)

Leader: And Mira's trying to say Hello to Jeanne and they've both got their eyes closed, and now she's patting her. And now let's see—I want to say "Hello" to Jeanne's foot, too. (Touches her foot) And Mira's saying "Hello" to Mona. And Mona's saying "Hello" to Jeanne's foot over here. And Jeanne is looking to see who's saying "Hello" to her.

Jeanne: I got my foot on Mort's sock.

Leader: You've got your foot on Mort's sock. And you've got Mort and Mary
and Selma. Vi, would you like to put your foot in and say "Hello" to
Jeanne's foot?

Vi: (Puts her foot in center with the rest of the feet)

Leader: She's (Jeanne) got Vi and Shawn at the same time.

Brenda: Oh, I'm going to put my foot in. Look at that.

Leader: And you've got Mort and Vi over here at the same time.

Mort: Oh, your feet are so nice and warm. (To Jeanne)

At this point Mira starts walking around. The Leader holds her a few minutes.
Then Jeanne wanted to be held by the Leader. The Leader offered that they
could sit with someone other than their partner. Jeanne and Mira did. James and
Mona wanted to stay with their partners. There was some restlessness at this
point.

Leader: And you know there's somebody who's not here today.

Jeanne: Amos.

Leader: Know where he is?

Mira: Home.

Leader: And there's one other person who hasn't been here, but he's here
today.

Children: James.

Leader: That's right. I'm glad you're here today, James. Okay, you guys. Today
is the very last time to play together. Anybody got anything you want
to say about that?

Jeanne: (Loud voice) No.

Leader: No. Okay.

Jeanne: I happy.

Leader: How come you're happy?

Jeanne: Because I like it.

Leader: You can look across the circle and see your friends. Well, I have a surprise. You may have noticed that I've been taking pictures, and Mort
has been taking pictures. Mira, will you go back and sit with Vi, because we're going to look at pictures. Mona is going to help me pass
them out. Each kid can look at the pictures with your partner. Each
kid can pick *one* picture to keep.

Pictures are passed out with help from the Leader.

Leader: Look at your pictures with your partner.

Talking going on as pairs look and decide which pictures they want.

Leader: Everybody hold up the picture you're going to keep.
   Mira: (Runs out of the circle)
Leader: Mira, I want you to stay in the circle. You can sit with Brenda, but you have to stay in the circle. (Mona is being held by the Leader)
Leader: (To Mona) No grabbing, Mona.
   Mira: (Sitting by Brenda, looks at her picture and throws it away)
Leader: (Picks it up and hands it to her) Let's see which one James chose.
Leader: (To Mona) Would you like to show your picture of you and Brenda?
   Mona: (Hides her picture)
Leader: Mona doesn't want to show her picture.
   Mira: (In her old baby-talk voice) I'm not going to let anybody see mine. (Imitating Mona)
Brenda: I'd like to see your picture, Mira.
Leader: Mira, may I see yours?
   Mira: (Holds it up for the Leader to see it) Don't show it to Mona.
Leader: Thank you.

Jeanne and Mira show each other their pictures.

   Mona: (Yelling at Mira, who was stealing a glance at her picture) Quit peeking, cheater!
Leader: Mona doesn't want to show hers right now. (In her take-charge voice) I'll tell you what we're going to do. For one last time, we're going to say "Goodbye" to our partners.
  James: (Interrupting) We going to have snacks?
Leader: We're going to have snacks. One of the things I remember, James, is your saying "I want snacks." You're my snack reminder. Everybody get out of your partner's lap. Everybody stand right up. Look around and you can sit on the floor in between anybody you want to.

Children move and sit in a new place away from their partners except James, who stays with Shawn.

Leader: (Passes out snacks; the children said they wanted a whole cracker) Here's a whole one for Jeanne. (And so on) Let's see if one more time we can all crunch at the same time. When I count three, we all go crunch. Ready? One, two, three. Crunch. Now, while you're eating your cracker, would anybody like to say the thing that you liked the best out of the whole time?

Mira: (Immediately raising her hand) Me!

Leader: Okay.

Mira: I liked it the best when we did our tricks (In the one-to-one) and then Vi couldn't get me up. (Smiles, looks tickled)

Group: (Laughs; Mira laughs)

Leader: You liked that. Who else wants to say what they really liked that happened in here?

James: I like my friends.

Leader: You like your friends. Are these all your friends? Can you say everybody's name?

James: Yes.

Leader: And you like them. How about Jeanne. What did you like the best?

Jeanne: I like snow.

Leader: You like snow (puzzled)? Where did you have snow in here?

Mort: (Offers explanation) On those postcards you sent us from Colorado.

Leader: Oh, I put those in the mailbox far away and they came to you.

Mira: (Leaves the circle, where she had been sitting next to Brenda)

Leader: Mira, I'd like you to stay in the circle.

Mort: (Carries her back)

Leader: (Asks adults to say what they liked best) Vi, what did you like the best?

Vi: Let me see.

Mira: (Pipes up) When we played Knock at the Door? (Looking at Vi)

Vi: Knock at the Door? Yeah! I liked that one. And when I played it, what would you say?

Mira: I said you have to knock on the door again and maybe somebody will be there.

Leader: You both liked the same thing. What did you like best, Shawn?

Shawn: I liked it where James crawled over and touched my nose. What I liked best was that James came back.

Leader: I think James liked that where he rolled over and touched your nose because that's the picture he chose.

James: I want another cracker.

Leader: I'll share this with you, James. Mira, you have so many crackers, would you like to share with someone?

Mira: Nope. (Said firmly)

Selma: What I liked best was when we touched noses.

Leader: Instead of the cradling, we're going to do this. All hold hands.

James: *I want to cradle* in the blanket.

Leader: That's okay. Before we do that, we're going to do this. We're going to hold hands like this. Take the hand of the person next to you and sing along with me: On Monday morning.

Group: On Monday morning.

Leader: We all came to play.

Group: We all came to play.

Leader: And each one of us had a partner (Group repeats)
And when I touch your nose (Group repeats)
Say what your partner's name is. (Group repeats)
(Touches Mira's nose)

Mira: Vi.

Leader: (Touches James' nose)

James: Shawn.

Leader: (Repeats with each adult)

Mona: (When her nose is touched) My mama comes here.

Leader: And after we all had partners. (Group repeats)
What a surprise. (Group repeats)
My partner picked me. (Group repeats) And this is the very last time (Group repeats) We're going to play together. (Group repeats)
But I'm going to remember (Group repeats)
James (Group repeats) and Shawn (Group repeats)
and Jeanne (Repeated) and Vi (Repeated) and Selma (Repeated)
and Mira, and Mort, and Mona, and Brenda, and Mary.
And sometimes when I'm quiet, I'm going to remember a lot of special things we did and somewhere I have lots of friends.
Before we go, James wanted to do something all you guys like to do.
So, we're going to swing James in the blanket and anyone else who wants a turn can have one.

Mira: I want a turn.

Leader: Okay. Put your pictures over here and you can get them later. Shawn, would you get on the other end of this (the blanket) and help me swing James?

Leader: Okay, everybody help me sing. Goodbye, James. (Group joins, sung to the tune of "Good Night, Ladies") Goodbye, James, Goodbye, James. We're glad you came to play. Shawn, would you like to pick up James and help him put his shoes on, ready to go? It looks like Mona is next.

Leader: Brenda, will you help me swing Mona? (Song repeated as they swing her) Would you take your little friend and help her put her shoes on? (Repeated with Jeanne)

James: I want to help.

Leader: Mira's turn. (Leader and Vi swing Mira)

Children leave with the Leader.

COMMENTS

The Children's Relationship to Each Other

A comparison of the two Circle Times shows the children's growth in relating to each other—the goal of Circle Time. In doing this relating, the children showed new ability to use the group to get their needs met. That is, more of the work of Circle Time was defined and created by the children and less by the Leader. For example, the Goodbye Circle was initiated by Mira when she placed herself, with eyes closed, into the center of the circle and invited others, without words, to see and touch her. The children and the adults responded by touching her. Mira and the group provided the structure. The Leader simply reflected what was already going on.

First, the children related to each other through the dialogue of touch as they reached out and touched Mira's face—quite a change from the screaming, yelling children who didn't know what to do or how to relate in the beginning. Then individual children began touching each other and touching feet.

Later, the dialogue of touch became a dialogue of words when the children shared their pictures with each other. Mona, for example, who never said anything in the beginning, said to Mira, "Quit peeking, cheater." The children who said almost nothing in the beginning talked more; and Mira, who talked constantly in the beginning, was much quieter. When she did say something, it was a statement of where she was rather than a demand for attention.

The Children's Relationship to the Leader

The last Circle Time also shows the children's growth in relating to the Leader. The Goodbye Circle shows that the children had a relationship with her. They also began to be in relation to her through language. For example, Jeanne, who never showed much affect, responded to the Leader's question, "Anybody got anything to say about this being our last time to play together?" with a very loud "No!" She clearly communicated that she didn't want to talk about the parting.

240

James came out of his shell first by relating to the Leader. First, he asked for food. He took the risk of opposing the Leader when he said he wanted to be "cradled in a blanket" right after she had just said they weren't doing cradling. He said, "I want to help" rock the others, and "I like my friends"—all in response to the Leader.

Mira, who was very negative in the beginning, also developed a relationship with the Leader. For example, when Mira threw her picture down, the Leader picked it up and handed it to her. She accepted it. When Mira said, in imitating Mona, "I'm not going to let anybody see mine," the Leader asked to see hers. Mira held her picture up for the Leader to see, saying, "Don't show it to Mona." Thus, she had learned to accept the Leader as a person with whom she can have a dialogue.

The Quality of the Energy

The quality of the energy in the last Circle was very different from the energy of the first one. In contrast to the yelling and screaming and demands for attention, the energy of the last Circle was quiet, flowing and smooth. There was a feeling of presence and acceptance. The children could hear and respond to the Leader. That is, the children felt seen and heard (because they could allow themselves to be seen and heard), and the Leader felt seen and heard (because the children responded to her).

This feeling of calmness and acceptance also came from the children's increased ability to allow themselves to be touched and to be cradled. In the first Circle, only Mira could allow the cradling. In the last Circle Time, three children had their partners carry them to the Circle (Mira, Mona and Jeanne). The two girls sat very quietly as they observed Mira being touched by James and adults. They were just present—no screaming or yelling or negative words. The cradling enabled the children to get in touch with their inner or core self, the quiet part of them that experiences what they do and feel as coming from inside them. They have become aware of their inner life. From that quiet place, they could observe both their own behavior and the behavior of others.

Mira

To understand how the one-to-one session and the Circle Time session each contribute to the integration of experiences in the process of saying Goodbye, turn back to pages 191-193 and reread Mira's Goodbye individual session and follow it with a rereading of the last Circle Time.

Everything Mira did in the one-to-one was in the service of dealing with the termination. She left nothing unfinished. She ended the session by acting out a fantasy (being a "tiny baby") that would provide her with a memory of being held and loved by the therapist, an experience she could relive any time she focused her attention on it. When the Leader called Circle Time, Mira did an interesting thing. She brought her tiny-baby fantasy to Circle Time. She shared her fantasy with the outer world, the group, and invited them to participate in it.

In doing this, Mira created not only a memory of being held by her therapist, but also a memory of being seen and touched by the whole group. Above all, she created a memory of how *she* had provided this experience for *herself*—evidence for the existence of a core-related self and an intersubjective-related self. This means that she can recreate this experience any time she has the need.

In the Goodbye Circle, however, Mira did have moments of being anxious, which she showed by twice walking out of the circle. (Mira always let you know when she was upset.) When she was brought back, however, she became involved again and was present. Because of her relationship to the Leader, she could accept the Leader's help.

Mira's behavior in the Goodbye Circle also reflects the security and trust she felt in her relationship with her therapist and how that relationship helped her to function in the larger world, the Circle group. For example, the two times she left the Circle were followed by making connections to her therapist: (1) in answering the question of what she liked best ("I liked it best when we did our tricks and then Vi couldn't get me up" and (2) when the Leader had asked her therapist what she like best, Mira answered for her, "When we played Knock at the Door?" It was very important to Mira that she and her therapist like the same thing.

Thus, Mira ended the DP group program feeling good about herself. This good feeling came from her ability to share herself and her experiences with the Circle family. It also came from her ability to utilize the Circle family to help her feel touched and seen and her ability to involve her peers in a goal-directed activity. She could ask them for something she needed, very different from her initial behavior of screaming for attention. The Circle Time experience enabled Mira to practice in a larger world what she had learned with her therapist.

What the Leader Did

The Goodbye Circle Time illustrates how the Leader provided the conditions needed for these children to integrate their experiences and say Goodbye in a way that enabled them to end the program feeling good about themselves.

First, the Leader responded to the children's cues when they provided the structure they needed to say Goodbye (Mira's tiny-baby play). The Leader reflected and supported what they were doing on their own. The Leader did not shut off this play (to provide their own structure is one of the goals of Circle Time). The Leader helped them to develop it further and stayed with it as long as something was developing.

Then the Leader gave the others the opportunity to sit in the center and be "helloed to," but no one responded. The Leader let that go and brought the group together by touching Jeanne's foot. This led to everyone touching feet in the center. The group said "Hello" to each other through foot-touching. Jeanne said, "I've got my foot on Mort's sock."

Following this, the Leader demonstrated limit setting by holding Mira when she started to walk around. Then Jeanne also wanted to be held by the Leader (she was developing a relationship to the Leader). The Leader then said they could sit with a different person other than their therapist.

At this point, the Leader brought up the issue of termination by asking if anybody had "anything to say about this being our last time to play together." Only one child responded. Jeanne said loudly, "No."

Note that the Leader did not invite the children to go into their feelings about parting at this stage. The approach at this stage is to help the children integrate what they have already experienced and to give their experiences some form—a ritual and a meaning that would provide them with an image that they will remember when they need it.

For example, the Leader passed out the Polaroid pictures of each child with her therapist and gave time for the children to walk around and share their pictures with each other. These pictures serve as a bridge to carry the experiences in DP into the child's life after DP. The good experience of DP can be recalled by looking at the picture. Winnicott (1953) called these objects "transitional objects."

The Leader's sensitivity to the differing needs of these children is illustrated in the different ways she responded to the negative behavior of two children, Mira and Mona. When Mira threw her picture down, the Leader quietly picked it up and handed it to her. She accepted it. When Mira said she wasn't going to show her picture to anyone, the Leader asked if she could see it, and Mira held it up for her to see. These were exactly the responses Mira needed. Mira's negative responses were imitations of Mona. The Leader's approach to Mira helped her to move out of her negativity (which was mostly a habit rather than an expression of anger) and to realize that's not who she is. In so doing, the Leader gave Mira a chance to experience herself in a new way—a related way—by ignoring her negative behavior and by presenting her with a new focus. Mira's response to the

Leader's invitation showed the Leader to be in tune with Mira; that is, seeing her as ready to share.

On the other hand, Mona's negative behavior (hiding her picture and saying to Mira "Quit peeking, cheater") came from a child who was just beginning to relate. In the beginning, she could not allow the touching and she said almost nothing. Mona was not in a place where she could share because she had not experienced herself owning anything, including a self. (A child cannot share until she feels she has something to share.) Mona is sharing that she doesn't want to be seen; that is a beginning. The Leader respected Mona's position when she said to Mira, "Mona doesn't want to show her picture." The Leader was also teaching Mira to respect Mona's position.

During snack time, the Leader gave each child and each adult the opportunity to say what they liked best in this program. Then all held hands while the Leader reviewed for them the story of how they came together, asking the group to repeat after her. She brought each child and therapist together one more time by asking each child to name her partner when she touched the child's nose. Finally, the Leader honored James' request to be "cradled in a blanket."

All the children wanted to be cradled this way. Each child was put into the blanket by her therapist, who then held one end of the blanket so that she and the Leader could swing it gently. The other children lined up on the sides and helped to rock it. At the end of the song, the therapist lifted her child and helped the child get ready to leave.

SUMMARY OF THE LEADER'S WORK

As you read the transcribed sessions of the two Circle Times (sessions 3 and 16), you feel the Leader's presence. The children also felt her presence. From the beginning session to the last session, the children never had to wonder what to do.

In the first Circle Time, when the children didn't know what to do or what to expect, the Leader provided them with the condition needed for them to feel her presence. She gave them something to respond to—her touch. Then she invited them to experience the presence and existence of each other through touch. Relation began with the dialogue of touch.

When the children did know what to do and were doing it—one of the goals of Circle Time—the Leader simply said what she saw them doing. She did not interpret. For example, the Leader responded to the group involvement in Mira's "tiny baby" play in the Goodbye Circle by reflecting what they were doing and by inviting other children to participate. Her response helped the children to become aware of what they were experiencing, and they felt seen, heard, touched, and validated by the Leader.

The Leader also gave the children the experience of learning to respond to her focus. For example, in the Goodbye Circle, the Leader directed the children's attention to the process of saying Goodbye. Through having them share their pictures, saying what they liked best, holding hands while listening to the story of how they came together, and the cradling in the blanket, she showed them how to say Goodbye—not by talking, but by doing things together and sharing.

In doing this, the Leader helped the children build sharing experiences that they could relive later and also use as a guide for making new relationships. The children will remember these experiences for a long time because they involve bodily felt experiences (touch: the skin never forgets), being seen (touch through the eyes), and feelings and emotions (sadness and joy). The children had both the experience of being touched, seen, and heard by the Leader and the experience of seeing, hearing, and touching the Leader—an interactive relationship.

To run a DP group in this way is not easy. It takes a tremendous amount of concentration and, above all, presence. It can, however, be very rewarding and exciting, different from the rewards of being a therapist for one child.

THE ROLE OF TOUCH IN THE GOODBYE PROCESS

Touch plays an important part in the Goodbye process as well as in the Hello process. Although one might think that the children would require less touch in the process of separation, these children demanded even more—both in the Circle Time and in the one-to-one (see Mira's session 16). This need seems to represent both a way to handle the anxiety over the ending of the program and to provide a way to create a memory or experience that they can take with them. In this Circle Time, this extra touching just before parting seemed to stabilize the children, to enable them to feel okay about saying "Goodbye."

Many parents provide this extra touch for their child when they are about to leave by kissing and hugging her. Unfortunately, some parents have a need to add, "Now you be good" or "You be good to your little sister" or "Stay out of the cookies." In doing that the parent loses her connection with the child. The child does not feel the parent's presence.

The last Circle Time *began* with a touching activity initiated by the children. Mira's "tiny-baby" play enabled the whole group to create a family atmosphere of warmth and acceptance where they all (children and adults) could be in touch with each other without having to do anything. The children could identify either with Mira, the one being touched, or with the loving parent, the one doing the touching. That was the way the Goodbye Circle Time began, initiated by the children.

The Goodbye Circle Time also *ended* with another family-like scene, again initiated by the children, this time by James. When James said, "I want to be cradled in a blanket," all the children wanted to be cradled this way. His request again enabled the group to become a family, a family in which every child got heard, seen, and touched. Every child had the opportunity to share her core self with the others as her therapist placed her in the blanket held at each end by the Leader and her therapist. The others participated in the gentle swinging of the blanket while singing the "Goodbye" song.

Looking up, the child could see all the faces of her family looking at her. At the end of the song, the therapist lifted her child out of the blanket and the next child had her turn. After James had his turn, he said, "I want to help"—evidence that he is feeling a part of this group.

James' request to be "cradled in the blanket" led to a perfect ending for the Goodbye Circle. The Leader had planned not to include the usual cradling by the therapists as a way of helping the children separate from their partners. Instead, she had the whole group hold hands. James, however, felt the need for cradling before saying Goodbye. The cradling in the blanket enabled the child to maintain contact with her therapist through her eyes (touch at a distance). (The ability to see comes out of the ability to be touched, which is the next step.)

The dialogue of touch provided the foundation for the emergence of the dialogue of words. Yet the ability to be in relation through language did not eliminate the dialogue of touch. Touch always remained as a kind of "Home" place for the child's core self. Thus, the demand for extra touching or cradling just before parting was a move on the part of the child to experience one more time this wonderful sense of self so that she won't forget it—so that she can remember who she is.

Cradling for the child is like meditation for the adult. This need for cradling is not a regression but rather a progression. The cradling experience enables the child to turn inward to experience her inner self—the *I* part of her that can quiet her fears or focus her attention on some creative activity.

OVERVIEW

These two Circle Time sessions illustrate the role of the dialogue of touch in helping young children relate to each other through touch and through words, especially children with no core self. The children in this group of four-yearolds had no core self: four were passive, withdrawn, and nonverbal (although all had speech); Mira was hyper, aggressive, controlling.

In the beginning, none of these children could relate even at the presymbolic, concrete, experiential level—through the dialogue of touch. Though they all had speech, they did not use it as a way to be in relation because they lacked the experiences that give content to speech. In other words, these children had no experiences to talk about. They literally had nothing to say. Psychologically, they were dead children, including Mira. Although she was very active, her activity was not person-related.

Once the children experienced the touch as pleasurable because it made them feel alive, they had something to talk about ("I want a turn"). Relating through language gives the child a vessel or form into which she can put her experiences. Through the dialogue of touch, the child gets a core self. Through the dialogue of words, the child becomes *aware* that she has a core self.

The Goodbye Circle shows the gains these developmentally delayed children made in learning to relate to each other both through touch and through words. They had just begun to really talk to each other when the program ended.

The change in these children seen in the Goodbye Circle is both the product of their work with their therapists in the one-to-one and with their work with the Leader of Circle Time. Providing both a one-to-one experience and a group experience in one program gives the child the experience of forming an attachment relationship to one adult and the experience of using that attachment experience to relate to others—another adult and peers. The Developmental Play group program is unique in that way.

POSTSCRIPT

Everyone who comes in contact with DP eventually asks this question: What happens to these children after they leave this program? Many who have seen videotapes of this work say that they don't think it's fair to drop these children in such a short time, especially after receiving such loving contact from the adults in this program.

In response, I always say that *these children are not the same children they were in the beginning*. At the end, if the program has been successful, they have become children who have a core self and who can relate. They talk to their parents more, and they reach out and touch their parents more. Most parents welcome this, and they, in turn, start touching and talking more to their children.

MIRA

Mira's mother reported that Mira began touching her more right away. She would push her body against her mother's body when they were sitting together. When she watched Mira on the videotape, her mother said she had never seen

Mira so quiet and calm as she was in session 6 (page 159), "except when she cuddles against me now."

Her mother recalled that Mira had colic as a baby. She said she carried her around a lot because she didn't know what to do. She said Mira had some kind of rash on her face, so "I never took any pictures of her because she was so ugly."

Her mother also reported that Mira took medication when she had asthma and when she was on that medication, she was high and couldn't calm down (she was not on medication all the time). When Mira was tense, she would take a piece of her mother's pants between her two fingers and make a sucking noise.

After she looked at the videotape, I asked Mira's mother if she ever played that Knock-at-the-Door game with Mira. Mother said, "I don't know how" (which is what Mira said about her mother). Then she said, "Would you show me how?" I then played this game with her in exactly the same way I played it with Mira. Later, her mother reported that her two girls asked her to play that game with them every night just before bedtime.

Mira's mother also reported that Mira is more emotional now. When she cries, she cries deeply, as if her heart will break. She keeps the Polaroid picture given to her at the end of Circle Time with her things, and no one is to touch them. When she goes to bed at night, she puts the picture on the stand next to her bed. When her mother told Mira that she loved Vi, too, Mira said, "You can't love Vi. She's just for kids."

Mira's Post-Therapy Contact with the Therapist

About six months after termination, Mira called and wanted to go out and eat with me. I made arrangements with her mother for me to go to breakfast with her and the two girls. In the restaurant, Mira moved over and got on my lap as she ate, and wrote her ABCs. The following year she called me and said, "I'm in the Brownies now," and then she didn't know what else to say. A few months later, she called me and had a lot more to say: "I have a friend, Lila, and she likes me, too."

The following year, when I went to her house to get her mother's signature, Mira, her sister, and the new baby were all present. This time Mira went over and sat on her mother's lap, and her mother very lovingly put her arms around her. She did not seek any touch from me, but came to me and said, "I'm seven now," and asked me to solve a little puzzle. As I was going out the door, Mira said, "Goodbye, Vi." That was Mira saying "Goodbye." I was very pleased with Mira, and a little sad. I was pleased with the whole family.

Mira's behavior here demonstrates that she has transferred her attachment from the therapist to her Mother. She did this by internalizing the therapist, who becomes an internal guide for creating other intimate relationships—this time, her mother. With this internal guide, Mira could touch her mother and let her mother know what she wanted. She could also accept contact from her mother, who began providing it. Her mother said Mira was very sensitive to her and knew when she was depressed, and she would ask her mother what was wrong. Mother and daughter became more present with each other, both giving and both receiving. I felt this loving energy flowing from one to the other when I was in their presence.

School Behavior

Mira's mother reported that she had some difficulty staying on task when she first entered first grade. She got distracted by the other children. The teacher, however, placed her where there was less activity, and then she seemed to do well. Her mother said she was not interested in reading, but she was interested in sports.

Mira is now ten and in the fifth grade. Her mother said that Mira has been free of asthma and has not been on medication since she left the Developmental Play program at age four.

APPLICATIONS

Settings

The Developmental Play group program has applications for many settings. It was originally created in 1970 as a school therapeutic program for teacher-referred children. In 1974, its effectiveness as a program to help first grade children with "social/emotional problems" was tested through a grant from the U.S. Office of Education. The IQ gains were not only statistically significant, but they were maintained over time (Brody, Fenderson, and Stevenson, 1976). The Developmental Play program is currently listed in the National Dissemination Network's "Educational Programs that Work."

Since 1970, children from the public schools, Head Start, and day care centers either are or have been benefiting from participating in Developmental Play group programs (Brody, 1976, 1978).

A current (1993) example of the application of Developmental Play is illustrated in its use in the public schools of Buffalo, New York. Here it is part of the regular school program and is carried out by members of its staff. The Special Education Department has been providing for a number of years a Developmental Play group program for the children in this department. This program is under the direction of Barbara Moran, the supervising school counselor. She runs

groups herself and trains and supervises school counselors and psychology graduate students from the University of Buffalo. She reports that the graduate students say that the DP training is the best clinical training they receive. She
reports that even with running eight or more groups, they are not able to meet
the referral demands. The children helped include those from all elementary
grades.

Other settings where the DP group program has been found to be effective
are in hospital settings, residential treatment facilities, therapeutic pre-schools,
and day treatment programs (I was in charge of a Day Treatment program within
a school for one and a half years for four to six-year-old psychotic children. It was
very effective, and our work was much appreciated by the principal of the school
in which it was housed.) (Brody, 1978).

The uniqueness of the Developmental Play group program lies in the nature and quality of the training of those to be child partners or Leaders. The
training is the focus of the next chapter.

6 TRAINING: THE SUPERVISORY MODEL

Chapter 6 focuses on the training part of the Developmental Play group program. The Leader is in charge of training.

Training of adults in Developmental Play therapy is organized around the conviction that experiences are indispensable for learning to be a skilled helper to children; experiences are also necessary for the thorough understanding of therapeutic principles and methods. To be caring touchers of children, adults themselves need to experience the effect of touching and being touched. The didactic material presented is always wedded to guided experiences.

The Schedule of the Training Sessions

Preprogram training: Two three-hour training sessions are held before the Developmental Play group program begins.

Presession training: A one-hour training session precedes each Developmental Play group meeting.

Ongoing supervision by the Leader during the one-to-one part of each Developmental Play group meeting.

Postsession training: A one-hour training session follows each Developmental Play group meeting.

Postprogram training: One (or two) three-hour training sessions are held after the Developmental Play group program with the children has ended.

To help you understand and experience what goes on in the training sessions, we will look at the process as it unfolds in one Developmental Play group program. The verbatim material excerpted from the training sessions is intended to give a sampling of what takes place in Developmental Play training. It is also intended to encourage a sense of what it feels like to be an adult partner to a child in a Developmental Play group and to share one's experiences of work with a child with other trainees under the guidance of a supervisor.

The Setting, the Children, and the Trainees

This Developmental Play program took place in a preschool sponsored by an agency for families on welfare. Six four-year-olds—three boys and three girls—participated. These children lived in public housing in a crime-infected, drug-involved community in which police arrests were common. One child had been a cocaine baby. Three of the six trainees are members of the staff, and the other three are experienced therapists. The Leader is the author.

THE FIRST PREPROGRAM SESSION

The purpose of the preprogram sessions is twofold: (1) to provide the trainees with the opportunity to learn how to be present; and (2) to build a community within which the trainees can learn to experience their own presence through meditation, touching and being touched, seeing and being seen. These are the experiences they will need to be able to touch, see, and understand the children with whom they will be working when the Developmental Play program begins.

MEDITATION

The Leader greets the new trainees and welcomes them. Each session always begins with a centering which may be long or short. The centering for the first meeting is a *touching-the-body meditation*—a long, centering exercise.

Leader: We are going to say Hello to the body. Make yourselves comfortable. Close your eyes. Focus your attention on your breathing. You have a little cradle inside of you that rocks you. Just feel that rhythm of your breathing as you breathe in . . . and out . . . in and out. See what part of your body starts to relax . . . just feel the in and out of your breathing. Now put your hands together and feel them touching each other. See what they feel like touching each other. Feel the temperature and the texture. Do your two hands like each other? See if you feel some pulsing between your two palms. If you put your attention on the tips of your fingers, you may feel some throbbing there. Just listen to your body.

Now put your hands on top of your head. Do you feel some heat there on top of your skull? Touch your hair and feel its texture. Move your hands up under your hair and touch your hair in a way it would like to be touched, as if it is saying, "Oh, that feels so good. Do it here." What's the quality of your hair? Feel the back of your head. Just let yourself enjoy this without having to do anything else or without judging yourself.

Now put your hands on your forehead and feel your hand touching your forehead. Does your forehead like it? If you start in the middle of your forehead with your two hands and move out to the temples on each side, you'll find a little sensitive place there where you can feel some throbbing. Sometimes it feels good to press a little on that place.

Now touch your eyebrows. Do they like it? If you take your two thumbs and place them in the corner of your eyes and then move them under the bony arch over your eyes, that feels good. Follow it around to do under the eyes. Stay off the eyeball. Now move to your nose, your cheek bones, your mouth, your lips, your chin.

Starting with the chin, move the hands up the jaw, and you'll find some ears. Move your fingers all around the curlicues in your ears, put your finger in your ears and plug them up and listen to the sound inside your body, take your thumb and forefinger and go around the rim of your ears, and then end by pinching the ear lobes. Now take a minute and just feel your face. Does it feel different?

This meditation continues until the whole body is done, including the torso, arms, hands and fingers, legs, ankles, feet, toes, back of the leg, buttocks, backbone, back of neck and to the top of the head, where it began.

Now say Hello to your voice by just making a little hum with your next breath. Put your hand on your voice box and feel the vibration. Touch your lips and feel the vibration. Just move the pitch or the sound around until it feels like your sound. Listen to just your own sound. Now listen to your sound and also the sound of the whole group. Now let your sound flow out the window into the cosmos until you can't hear it anymore.

Now just be still and feel where you are right now. Do you notice the change in the energy in this room? What would it be like for you to have more of this in your life—the feeling you have inside you right now?

When you get ready to come back, just open your eyes gently and just let them see what is in front of you without analyzing it. Just let your eyes see.

Sharing the Experience of the Meditation

Trainees: Relaxed, melted.
　　　　 Peace.
　　　　 Because of the noise outside, I had a hard time relaxing.
　　　　 Relaxed. I didn't want to come back. I feel sad.
　　　　 I could feel my sound empty me out, and I felt sad.
　Leader: In this approach, we will be touching children. So how was it for you touching yourself. Any part of your body you liked more?
Trainees: My feet.
　　　　 My neck.
　　　　 My head.
　　　　 My arms are kind of neat.
　　　　 My voice.
　　　　 I didn't like touching my face—gets my make-up all messed up.
　Leader: So when you look in the mirror to put on your make-up, enjoy the feel of it, the feel of saying Hello to yourself—Hello to yourself being present, and then you feel your aliveness.
　　Ida: I noticed one thing. When I came here, I said, "Have I bitten off more than I can chew because I thought of all the things I'm doing?" I felt I was racing (during the meditation), racing, racing. The more I said calm down, the more I realized I was racing. But now I find since we did that whole thing, I am at peace and I haven't had that for a long time. I used to have this and then I got started doing all these things. I have to ask myself, "Do I want peace or money?"
　Leader: How much time did that take? About ten minutes. Are you worth ten minutes? What was it like getting in touch with your voice?
Trainees: I liked the sound of all the voices together—very calming.
　　　　 We were united.
　　　　 It was like a cosmic chord.
　　　　 I couldn't get relaxed until we did the voice.
　　　　 When we made the sounds, I didn't hear all the noise outside.
　　　　 Energizing.
　Leader: What was it like when you plugged your ears?
Trainees: Like the ocean.
　　　　 Like a big storm.
　　　　 I had something. Like I was more contained. I can't escape anymore.
　Leader: Who created this feeling, this place?
Trainees: We did, ourselves,
　Leader: If you created it?

Trainees: We can do it again.
  Leader: It's getting in touch with the loving and alive part of you. How do you get in touch with it?
Trainees: Reach in and touch it.
  Leader: So when you are working with children, if you are in this quiet place, you can see the children. It's the quality of your energy that influences the children, not what you say. That's what they copy.
  Leader: What was the effect on you of using your eyes to look?
    Cora: Strange, because most of the time when you look at somebody, you're carrying on a conversation. When I was looking, I wasn't carrying on a conversation. It felt strange, like I was staring and I was trying not to think what the other person was thinking.
   Clara: I had the sense of settling into myself—surprise to me when I look at anybody, I get present—a "I know that kind of feeling."
    Paul: I was aware I wasn't present (because of the noise).
    Gill: It was okay for me to look. I was aware others were uncomfortable.
     Ned: I felt awkward. It felt like I was staring.
  Leader: Look at all the things that go on inside of us when we're not saying anything and just looking—how hard it is just to see and be without judging or analyzing.

  The goal here in this training is to create an environment in which you feel safe to say anything you need to say that's related to the work. If it's something I say or do that disturbs you, you can feel safe to tell me. You can feel safe to share wherever you are in this group.

  Now, close your eyes again. Focus on your breathing and notice what part of your body lets go. Just observe it. You don't have to do anything. Just feel your stomach muscles go in and out as you breathe. Hear the air come into your nostrils when you breathe in, and feel the air go out your nostrils when you breathe out. With eyes still closed, say a word that describes how your body is feeling right now.
Trainees: Calm.
Calmer.
Peace.
  Leader: So open to that feeling of peace, calm, calmer, comfortable, relaxed. Say to yourself, "I am (your name), and I am peace" (whatever it is).

  With your eyes still closed, I'd like you to get an image of a child you'd like to work or play with in this program. As you look at that child in your imagination, what does that child say it wants from you? What does it say it really needs?

(Passes out pencils and paper) Now, I'd like you to draw a picture of you with that child—how you'd be with that child.

On the back of your drawing, write a statement saying what you were saying to yourself as you drew, what you were trying to show, and the quality of the child.

CIRCLE TIME EXERCISE

Leader: Now, how about sitting on the floor. (Trainees sit on floor in a circle with the Leader) What I'm going to do with you are samples of what we're going to be doing with the children. (Pointing to their feet) Look at all these feet. Some have socks on, and some don't. Some are big, and some are small.

(Pointing to Clara's feet) Look at the way she moves her toes. (Others laugh and remove their shoes) This toe goes up, and that one goes down. Oh, look, Cora can do it, too. Let's all do what Cora does. (Others imitate her)

Gill's saying Hello to Ned with her big toe. I'm going to say Hello to Ida. (Reaching over and touching Ida with her foot)

Trainees: (All are reaching over and touching each other's feet and laughing. Their feet are all crossed over each other in a pile.)

Leader: Close your eyes and see if you know whose foot yours is touching. (Quiet moments) Now, let's start to say Goodbye. Begin with the feet on top. (One by one they separate their feet)

Leader: (Holding out her hand) We can also say Hello with our hands.

We are all going to be in this project together for 16 weeks. Those of you who are willing to be here and be present to the best of your ability, raise your hand.

Trainees: (All raise their hands)

Leader: So, now go inside and find a word that describes how you feel about starting this group.

Trainees: Anticipation.

Curious.

Open.

Rush and slow down.

Depressed.

Tense, more like excitement.

Introductions

The trainees introduce themselves by stating their names, what they do, what they want to get out of this group, and what they have to give to a child.

Responses: Several said to help them with their clients and with their own young children. Some said they had seen the value of this program with other children and wanted the children of this agency to have the benefit of it. Ned, the teacher, said, "To help me with the children, and myself, too."

The Hello Circle Time Song

Leader: Sing what I sing (to the tune of *Frere Jacques*). Hello, Clara (all repeat, Hello, Clara), I see your brown eyes (all repeat), and you have your hands crossed like this (all repeat), etc.

Leader: Now, Clara, will you pick out someone and sing what you see? (Game continues until everyone has had a turn)

Leader: In this song, you say just what you can see with your two eyes without any qualifications or judgment. That's hard to do because everyone always wants to add, "Your *beautiful* brown eyes," or *"nice* hair."

Clara: When you said that to me—seeing my brown eyes—I felt very special. (Others share their experiences of being seen)

Leader: Yes, I had to really look at you to see what color they were. We tend to use so many qualifiers that they lose their value. When you work with a child, you have to provide some structure. You don't expect the child to do all the work. Children need to be seen. When they feel seen, they respond. All you have to do is say what you see. For example, what happens if you say to a child, "I see you brought your hand there?"

Paul: She'll show you the other hand.

Leader: Yes. A healthy child is aware that when she is touched by a caring person, she feels her aliveness. She invites the touch to feel that aliveness. When you work with a child in a Developmental Play way, you help the child develop her inner self first through experiencing her bodily self when she feels touched and seen by you. That's what you will be doing— touching, seeing, noticing, listening to the child, and responding to her reactions to being touched and noticed.

DEMONSTRATION: HOW TO SAY HELLO

Leader: I am going to demonstrate how you say Hello to a child in your first meeting. I need a volunteer. (Ida volunteers and sits on floor facing Leader) All I'm going to do today is to say the Hello part. (To Ida) You just be who you are. (Looking at Ida) Hello, Ida.

Ida: Hello, how are you?

Leader: You are the one I chose for my play partner. My name is Vi.

Ida: Hello, how are you?

Leader: Can you say Vi?

Ida: Vi.

Leader: And your name is?

Ida: Ida.

Leader: Say your name again. I like the sound of it when you say it.

Ida: Ida.

Leader: Did you hear it when you said it?

Ida: Yes.

Leader: Well, I'm going to play with you every week for 13 weeks. (Taking Ida's hand) Can you count?

Ida: (Touching each finger, counts to 13)

Leader: Oh, your hand is so warm. And it's got knuckles, and I see you looking at them. I said Hello to this hand.

Ida: (Holds up her other hand)

Leader: Oh, this hand would like me to say Hello to it—Hello. (Touching it) (Taking both hands in hers) So I'll say Hello to both of them like this. You just did something very interesting. You put your fingers between mine. See that? You're looking at it. This finger is saying Hello to me, and I'm saying Hello back. (Moves her finger in return) I can hold your hands inside mine, like this. (Cupping both of Ida's hands inside hers)

Ida: I can do this. (Putting one hand on top)

Leader: You put your hand on top. It's so warm inside. I'm looking at you and saying Hello to your hair (gently touching it), your nose, your shoulders. Can I say Hello to your eyes?

Ida: (Nods Yes)

Leader: I'm going to say Goodbye to you now.

Ida: No.

Leader: You liked it. But I'll see you next week.

Ida: Why?

Leader: Goodbye for now. (Hugging her)

◆ ◆ ◆

Ida: Can I say something?

Leader: First I want you to go inside and see what this felt like.

Ida: Happy—a little racing, happy racing, emotion—emotion like reaching out—like somebody is a little scary because for a little child . . .

Leader: Just be yourself, where you are right now.

Ida: Racing, comfortable, neat to reach out because you were in charge, since you were calling the shots.

Leader: What was that like, that you didn't have to take charge?

Ida: It was all right—relaxed. I let you take it 'cause I was trying to take over.

Leader: *You were.*

Ida: I almost started to do it again.

Leader: What was it like when you realized that you didn't have to?

Ida: Safe, secure, structured.

Leader: I sensed that you were nervous and tense, and you didn't quite let me in. You kept wanting to give something back and to take charge as if you had to give something back.

Ida: That's a dynamic always present in me.

Leader: I felt that in you. I was trying to convey to you, through my touch, that you don't have to do anything. All you have to do is to experience me touching you. So what you experienced and what I experienced matched. It's great that you got that right at the beginning of the training because your job is to be present and help the child experience your touch. You don't have to do anything, and the child doesn't have to do anything. You saw what it would be like for a child not to have to take care of the adult when you tried to take care of me in the demonstration. When the child lets you in, that's giving to you in the sense that now you and the child have a dialogue.

Ida: I got it.

Leader: Just now, when I touched your hand, your hand let me in. Your energy is much quieter, shown in your voice and in your body. Do *you* feel it?

Ida: Yes.

Trainees Practice Saying Hello to Each Other

Leader: Now, I'd like you to look around and see who you would like to have as a partner and then go over and sit in front of them. (Members do this)

Now, I'd like you to make an honest statement to each other as to how the two of you got together; for example, saying, "I didn't know who I wanted so I just let someone choose me." Or, "I chose you because I really wanted you." (Time allowed for this)

Now, decide which one of you is an apple and which an orange.
(Time allowed; some giggling)

Who are the apples? The apples will be the adult partners, or the
Givers, and the oranges will be the child partner, or the Receivers. The
Givers are to practice saying Hello to your partner as if you were meet-
ing her for the first time. (Time allotted for this)

Sharing Time

Leader: Close your eyes and see what it was like to be the adult, or the Giver.
Hard or easy? What was it like to be the child, or the Receiver? How
did you experience your adult partner? When you are ready, come back.
Receiver—pick out one thing your partner did that you liked best and
one thing you wished she had done differently and share it with your
partner. (Time allotted for this)

Leader: What was it like to say Hello to this person?

Clara: I had a lot going for me. Part of me said, "How can I do this for a half-
hour?" (To Cora) I felt protective about saying anything about your
face. Instead, I went for your earrings. I wanted to touch your face.
When I noticed your feet, they really responded to me. I could feel it. I
felt like they wanted to be touched, too.

Leader: (To her partner, Cora) What was it like for you?

Cora: I don't like anybody to touch my face.

Leader: So you see, Clara, you got her message. That's the dialogue of touch.
What each of you experienced matched. Clara, you wanted to touch her
face, but you didn't, and Cora didn't want her face touched.

Gill: The most difficult time I had was slowing myself down. I got stuck on
hands. I guess I had to give myself permission to be stuck on hands. The
sense I had was what do I do next? And he (Paul) was comfortable with
the hands, but always this little voice back in my head, "Gill, you're not
doing enough. You got to do more."

Paul: I was surprised when she said that. I just felt so there. I was surprised
when you said "stuck" because it felt so natural. I felt like you knew
what you were doing.

Ida: I sensed in me anxiety. I was a little anxious and there you (Leader)
were above me, and I had a need to perform. My mind was spinning. I
do better with adults.

Leader: Was there a place where it got better?

Ida: When I noticed his shoulder.

Leader: You simply said what you saw.

Ned: (Her partner) I enjoyed it. I just sat back and took it all in. Although I had sweaty palms, it was neat.

Leader: Here are two examples in which the partners did not match: Paul and Ned felt given to by their partners, but Gill and Ida did not experience themselves as giving. (To Gill and Ida) Are you two aware of what stopped you from feeling this connection?

Ida: I was thinking I had to perform and I wouldn't be good.

Gill: I was in my head telling myself that I wasn't doing enough, so as a result, I wasn't present.

Leader: Right. As a result, there wasn't a dialogue of touch. Yet in another sense, there was one because your partners said they experienced a calmness from you even though you weren't aware of this because you weren't present. What would it be like for you to experience your own energy in tune with their energy? To accept that they felt given to by you?

THE CLOSING

Leader: Before we close, I'd like each of you to give a one-liner stating where you are right now.

Paul: I feel a whole lot calmer and present.

Cora: I'm looking forward to the next time.

Gill: I feel like I've got that center back again.

Clara: I'm amazed at what happened in here. (Pointing to her body) It feels real nice.

Ida: I'm looking to the next session to change some of the things I can do.

Ned: I'm real relaxed. I came in here all tense, real hyper, and I'm just real calm, real collected. (Others laugh)

Leader: Let's stand and hold hands. Just find your quiet place before you go so that you can take it with you.

COMMENTS

This first preprogram session accomplished the following:

1. The six trainees began the process of getting to know each other in intimate and touching, seeing ways.
2. They got in touch with their own bodies through touching themselves, being touched, and touching others in very simple, playful ways.

3. They experienced the presence of others through being touched and touching, through being seen and seeing.
4. They became aware of what they do to shut off their experience of being present.
5. They experienced, by practicing with each other, what it might be like to work with a child in a Developmental Play way.
6. They came away with a sense of calmness, excitement, and eagerness to start.

THE SECOND PREPROGRAM SESSION

Leader: Let's begin by taking a minute to go inside and see where you are right now.

Trainees: Anxious; excited; slowing down; tired; tense; tense.

Leader: What was it like to share that and let somebody see that?

Trainees: Indifferent; starting to relax; comfortable; sharing; didn't make any difference; I still feel anxious.

Leader: There are two parts to getting in touch with your inner self: first, you go inside and see what you are experiencing, what your body feels like. Second, you share that with someone you trust. Then notice how that sharing affects your experience.

Anyone have anything they want to report that happened during the week related to what we did last week?

Gill: Practicing over the week this sense of peace—it nourished me for the week.

Ida: She (Gill) got the peace from here. I got the feeling there *is* peace. (Laughs) I was anticipating coming here not to regret it, but it'll be a little time when I don't have to rush around. I can get in touch with myself. I don't have to be "on" all the time.

Leader: Would you be willing to turn to somebody and say, "I don't have to be on all the time"?

Ida: Now it comes scary to say that.

Leader: Would you be willing to say it to me?

Ida: (To Leader) I don't have to be on all the time.

Leader: How was that?

Ida: Okay.

Leader: What happened?

Ida: The scaries sort of went away. I realized more than ever before how guarded I am.

MEDITATION

Leader: It's a good idea, before doing anything, to close your eyes and go inside, and see where you are. Once you learn how, you can do it in five to ten minutes. Now we're going to do a longer one. We're going to do the one we did yesterday except this time without touching yourself. However, if you need to touch your body to feel it, touch it.

Close your eyes. Focus on your breathing. You don't have to do anything but feel what your body is doing. Notice how the energy changes when you focus on the in and out of your breathing. Put your two hands together and feel them touching each other. Feel the throbbing that goes on between them and at the ends of your fingertips. Just be there a minute without doing anything and see how nice that is. Now part your hands. Focus your attention on each hand. Can you feel the other hand touching it even though, right now, your hands aren't touching? The touch of the other hand is still there. You just have to focus your attention on it, and it's there for you.

Keep feeling your breathing, and put your attention on the top of your head. How does the top of your head feel when you put your attention there? Now move your attention down to your forehead, and how does it feel when you put your attention there? How did it change the way it felt when you put your attention there? Now put your attention on your eyes. Imagine they are like two little pools of water in the back of your head and you're just observing them. How do your eyes feel?

The Leader continues the focusing of attention on the rest of the face. Leader continues with mouth, lips, tongue, jaw, ears. "Now stop a minute and see how your face feels."

The Leader continues focusing the trainees on the body: the neck, shoulders, arms, outside elbow, wrists, feeling the pulse, the palms, the thumbs and fingers, feeling the pulse in the fingertips, moving back up the arm, the inside part of the elbow, the shoulder, chest— feeling the heartbeat—the solar plexus, hips, thighs, legs, ankles, feet, toes, soles of feet, back to heels, back of legs, thighs, hips, backbone—beginning with the tailbone—moving vertebrae by vertebrae up the spinal column, the neck, and to the crown of the head.

Leader: Go inside and find a word to describe your experience right now. Then say, "I am (your name), and I am" (whatever word you had). (Time allowed for this)

263

As you are ready, come back. Gently open your eyes and just let your eyes see whatever is there without analyzing it—for example, just noticing the shape of a nose. Just experience that without giving it any meaning. Now use your eyes to make contact and notice the difference.

Sharing

Cora: It's very strange to look without having eye contact. When I have eye contact, I feel I need to smile.

Clara: When I was just looking, I was noticing the outside of your ear. (To partner) It has such wonderful curves in it. (Others laugh) It was really neat to look at it. That was exciting to see that. Then making eye contact for me, first place—I said, "It's okay to be seen—to see me." Then, when it was okay to see me, I could make eye contact. I felt a softness in me. That was nice.

Gill: I found it really interesting to be given permission to look at somebody without having to put anything into it—to connect and then to shift—it was like a certain softness when making eye contact. It felt good.

Ned: I felt like I was staring at Clara.

Paul: Clara is so calm. How does she do it?

Clara: I thought we had known each other in another life.

Hello Circle Time Song

Leader: (To tune of *Frere Jacques*) Hello, Cora (all repeat). I see you sitting like this (all repeat). And over here is Ned (repeated). He is looking at Gill (repeated). And she nodded her head (repeated). And next to her is Paul, and he brought his hands today (repeated). He looked at his hands (repeated). Then he looked at me (repeated). And he smiled when he did that (repeated). Etc.

Saying Hello to Each Other

Leader: I'd like to say Hello to Ida. (Reaching over and touching her)

Trainees: (Respond to each other verbally or through touch)

Leader: (To Clara) Could you make a tune or a sound to go with what you are doing with your feet?

What we have been practicing this morning is creating structures within which children can relate to each other, just as you people first did.

Follow-the-Leader Circle Game

Leader: Do what I do. (Claps her hands, makes all kinds of sounds)
Trainees: (Imitate)
Leader: Now, you're the Leader (choosing a trainee), and game continues
until everyone has had a turn to be the Leader.

This game focused and energized the adults. They had a lot of fun doing it. The trainees had the experience of being in charge and creating something while at the same time being seen, heard, and touched. Just allowing their bodies to move or make sounds without thinking about it or making plans ahead of time gave the trainees a tremendous sense of freedom. They didn't really know what they were going to do until they had done it. It also binds the group together because it is a group process.

This particular group did what children do in this game. For example, they began imitating each other. When one person ended her turn by saying, "I'm done," the others started saying it, but saying it at a different pitch as if said by a small child. One trainee started by saying, in a very authoritative voice, "I'm in charge. Do what I do." When one person didn't follow, the one leading said, looking at her, "You didn't do it." It is a game that gives the trainees an opportunity to act out or express repressed wishes. They can be children again. Thus, this simple game is both an avenue for teaching adults how to play with children in a Developmental Play way and, at the same time, an avenue for providing adults with the experience needed to be able to do it.

When everyone had had a turn, the Leader took over the group by starting a sound—a soft, quiet hum—directing the group to find the right pitch for them to keep it going until they feel the sound going right out the window into the cosmos. This group sound was very beautiful and quiet. It brought the members back to their inner selves within the group setting. The trainees noted how the humming quieted them down after their loud noise-making. Some said they felt the vibrations in their whole body.

HOLDING HANDS EXERCISE

Leader: You need a partner for this exercise. (As before, partners are chosen, with one being the Giver and the other the Receiver.)

(Partners are sitting facing each other, and both have eyes closed during this exercise.)

Givers, what you are going to do in a minute is to reach out and take your partner's hands. First, however, get in touch with the quality of your partner's energy. Know that this person you are going to touch in a minute is a unique person; no one in the whole world just like him or her.

So when you are ready, move up so that you are touching and take your partner's hands and just hold them. You don't have to do anything else. Rest your arms on your knees so that you don't have to hold them up. Just feel the energy in your partner's hands in your hands, and feel your breathing. Notice if your hands get warmer, or colder, or sweaty. There are no rights or wrongs to this exercise. Feel the pulsing between your two hands? Just see what it's like to be with someone, to be present with someone, touching and not having to do anything at all. Just be aware of what your body is doing and feeling. (Time for quiet moments)

Givers, now, with your eyes still closed, get ready to say Goodbye just with your hands. Do something with your hands to indicate you're going to say Goodbye. After parting your hands, separate your bodies. Don't be touching now. Go inside and be where you are. What was it like to be the toucher, and what was it like to be the one touched?

Sharing

The Leader asked the Receivers to name one thing they liked best that the Giver did and one thing they would have liked the Giver to have done differently. The Leader then asked the Givers to share with their partners what it was like to be the Giver. (Time was allotted for this. Then they shared in the large group.)

Givers. (Gill) The most difficult part was not having to do anything, to not put any demands on me. (Cora) The most uncomfortable part for me was the letting go. It was hard saying Goodbye with my eyes closed. It's easier to say Goodbye with your eyes.

Leader: You got in touch with how hard it is to say Goodbye.
  Cora: Right.
  Clara: I had the same experience with Ned that I had with Gill—looking at her ears—experiencing his hands separate from him. It was really nice.
Leader: You liked his hands. Tell him.
  Clara: (To Ned) I liked feeling your hands, and I liked the feeling of your hands by themselves—neat.

Receivers. (Ida) I do real well when my eyes are closed. I really am shy. I'm just learning that because when I look in her eyes, I get threatened, or something. But when she held my hands and my eyes were closed, I was perfectly at peace. (Paul) Having Cora touch me—it was so soft and nurturing.

CRADLING

The Leader introduced the cradling by asking the trainees to keep the same partners and decide who would be willing to be the one cradled and who would be willing to be the cradler. (No one is forced to do this if it doesn't feel right for them. In this group, they all did it.) They are instructed to do it so that it is comfortable for both parties—the cradler with her back supported by the wall, and the one cradled to select her position without having to support herself.

The Leader sang Brahms Lullaby. (Time allotted for quiet time together)

GOODBYE CIRCLE TIME

The Leader invited them back to the circle. Snacks were passed around (with much laughter). They were asked for a one-liner:

Cora: It's easier cradling a child. I can put her in my lap.
Paul: I was surprised. I've done the cradling exercise before at other workshops, and I was not very good at being cradled. This is the closest I've come to letting myself be cradled. I was comfortable with it. It was more than I've done before. Before, I just leaned against the wall.
Clara: I'm a little scared about seeing the kids next week.
Leader: Next week, we will all be playing with the children. We'll play Pass-the-Child. In this game, you get to play with each child five minutes and then you pass her on to the next adult.

The Goodbye Song

To the tune of Goodnight Ladies, the Leader sings to each one, and the group repeats what she sings: Goodbye Ida (others repeat), Goodbye Clara (others repeat), Goodbye Ned (others repeat), and Goodbye Paul (others repeat), Goodbye Gill (others repeat), Goodbye Cora (others repeat), and Goodbye Vi (others repeat). We'll see you again next week (repeated).

COMMENTS

The second preprogram training accomplished the following:

1. The trainees got in touch with their own inner selves. Through the hand-holding and cradling, they became more aware of their own boundaries and who they are (Paul allowing himself to be cradled, and Ida aware that she was shy and could be at peace when touched with her eyes closed).

2. The trainees learned contactful ways to relate to children. The same exercises—the touching and the cradling—which enabled the trainees to know themselves and to create a sense of community could also be used with children. The trainees learned Circle Time activities to do with children. They learned, through doing a Circle Time, its form: the beginning (the Hello part), the middle (the playing part), and the ending (the Goodbye part).

3. Through the sharing and interactions with each other, the trainees created a sense of community that enabled them to become more aware of the richness of their inner life and the effect of this new awareness on their relationship with themselves and with others. This sense of community will provide a container for their work with the children and with each other.

SESSION 1: MEETING THE CHILDREN

PRESESSION TRAINING

The Leader begins the session by inviting the trainees to go inside to see where they are right now, to say a word that describes where they are at this moment, and then to make eye contact with someone. The Leader invites the sharing of any experiences that happened during the week.

The Leader guides the trainees through a centering or meditation that is focused on body awareness. They are asked to say out loud a word that describes their inner experience. This is followed by inviting them to say their name and "I am" (whatever word described their experience in the meditation). For example, "I am Sharon, and I am calm."

The Seeing Exercise

The Leader asks the trainees to get a partner, sit facing each other, and decide who will be the Giver and who will be the Receiver. (The roles will be reversed in a second play.) The Giver is to look at her partner and say three things she can see with her two eyes without using qualifiers. The Receiver is simply to listen and focus on what she experiences. Then the two share their experiences— what it was like to be the Giver, and what it was like to be the Receiver.

The Leader chose this exercise at this time for a specific purpose: to give the trainees practice in doing what they will be doing with the children in a few moments, and to relieve their anxiety by having them focus their attention on something concrete and specific.

Defining Goals

The Leader asks the trainees to close their eyes and get a picture of the kind of child with whom they would like to work and then to come back and write their answers to the following questions:

1. What kind of a child would you like to work with?
2. Why do you want this particular child?
3. What do you have to give to this child?
4. What do you expect to learn from this child?

THE CHILDREN'S HOUR

The very first meeting with the children included the following:

The Hello Circle Time Song. The children are seated on the floor, a child between two adults. The Leader sings this song to each child and each adult (repeated each time by the group). Children and adults have been greeted and know each other's names.

Follow the Leader. This game helps to put the children at ease by giving them something playful to do with adults. In it, they each have the opportunity to initiate and to follow.

Pass the Child. In this game, each adult picks up the child next to her, puts the child on her lap, and plays with that child until the Leader calls time (which is five minutes) and says, "It's time to get ready to say goodbye to your child." Then the child is passed on to the next adult, and that adult gets a new child. This is continued until every adult, including the Leader, has played with each child.

Snacks. During snack time, the Leader tells the children that they will come here every Monday (whatever the day) and play with us. One of these big people will be their play partner.

POSTSESSION TRAINING

Reactions to the Children. Following the departure of the children, the trainees returned for their session exhibiting a lot of nervous laughter. They said they found it very hard to be with these children even for five minutes. They wondered if they could last the thirteen weeks' play with them. They quickly found out that playing these games with real children is quite different from playing them with each other, beneficial as that was.

269

Choosing Your Child

The adults, or trainees, have the task of choosing the child they want. In this program, the child does not do the choosing. The Leader asks the trainees to write down, in order of preference, the names of the children they would like to have as a play partner. The Leader asks them to hold up their list. In some groups there are no conflicts. That is, each child is chosen by one adult only. In this group, two different children were chosen by two trainees. The Leader invites each of the two pairs to talk about their conflict. The Leader does not make the decision as to who takes which child.

Sharing Experiences of Being With Each Child

Paul: What bothered me most about Tom—he isn't clean. He's so needy.

Ida: I had James for a whole hour. (Group laughs)

Cora: Hardest was Tom. He wanted to go someplace else. Hard to keep him there with me. I wanted to say, "Okay, you can go."

Ida: James wanted to do physical exercises—jumping up and down.

Clara: The hardest part was when Celia ran away from me. When I started to cradle her, she looked like she was going to cry. When I just let her sit here, she took off. I didn't know whether to bring her back.

Gill: I was struck by how little ability they had to be in touch with themselves; for example, when I noticed their hands, it was like it was the first time they paid attention to their fingers, like it was a revelation to them— just the way they would look at the fingers and their hands.

Leader: To have the undivided attention of an adult is so new to them, it could be scary at first. How was Tom for you?

Gill: I felt his resistance—nothing personal. I felt he was out of control. I wasn't aware of what other people were doing in the room. I felt maybe I was the only one who couldn't keep him on the mat.

Others: (Laugh) You weren't the only one.

Clara: Tom—he would twist away from me. When I focused on his knee, it seemed okay for a moment, and then he would take the focus off his knee.

Leader: Like it's too much attention.

Paul: A lot of our kids are very different. At a very early age, these kids are very independent. They can't be dependent and feel their emotional needs. They just don't get their needs met. I'm worried about opening them up.

Ned (the teacher): The kids go home and say this is what happened.

270

COMMENTS

The first meeting with the children gives us a baseline from which to assess later developments. We have a beginning with which to compare the end—for the trainees, the children, and the three staff members who became anxious about the effect this program might have on the parents and children.

The trainees found these children very difficult because the children did not respond according to their expectations. These children were active, either moving away or playing a game of their own. The trainees didn't know what to do. They needed to become a part of their games before the children could relate to them. In addition, this Developmental Play way of interacting was new for both the children and the adults.

The Leader's experience with each child was one of playing with very young two-year-olds. The children responded well to being seen and touched when it was done in a way that was in tune with the child's own energies. Playing with them was like playing with babies.

SESSION 1 WITH CHILDREN

Today is the first time each trainee will be responsible for her child the whole session. Following the usual presession meeting, each trainee will meet her child at the door, take the child by the hand and go over to their designated place in the room, sit down on the floor face-to-face, and play. The Leader observes each child-adult pair and makes herself available to coach any trainee needing help. Below are examples of this coaching.

COACHING DURING THE CHILDREN'S HOUR

Paul With His Child, Tom

Paul was having a hard time with Tom because Tom was wanting to do one thing, and Paul was wanting him to do something else.

Tom: I want to lie down.
Paul: I want you to sit up here with me.
Leader: (To Paul) How about you letting him lie down and then just look at him and say what you see.
Paul: (To Tom) I see your face.
Tom: (Covers his face with a large piece of cardboard he found in the room)
Paul: (Tries to pull it off)
Tom: (Holds on to it)

271

Leader: (To Paul) Leave it there and say, "Oh, you went away."
  Paul: Where did you go?
   Tom: (Covers more of his body)
Leader: (To Paul) Put your hands on his stomach, feel his breathing and say,
        "Look how this boy can breathe!" Ask Tom if he can feel his stomach
        go up and down.
   Tom: (Little by little uncovers his body and face)
  Paul: (Looking at Tom) There you are!

Later on during the session, Tom was wanting to play with the water in the
sink behind where they sat. Paul did not want him to do that.

Leader: How about you letting him play in the water and then you take the
        towel, wet it, and wash his face and hands gently.
   Tom: (Allowed Paul to wash his face. He liked it.)

In doing that, Paul started a dialogue of touch with Tom.

Cora With Her Child, Celia

Cora had a similar problem with her child. Celia would cover her head with
her jacket, and Cora was trying to get her to remove it. The Leader suggested to
Cora that she simply reflect what she sees Celia doing such as, "Oh, you've gone
away." When Cora did that, Celia began to respond. Later, in Circle Time, Celia
volunteered a song that said, "I like Cora."

These are examples of on-the-job coaching: helping the trainee to begin by
simply observing the child and saying what she sees the child doing. This coaching
also gives the trainee permission to initiate contact, *not by telling the child what to
do, but by gently touching her to enable the child to experience her own body*—in
other words, to initiate the dialogue of touch.

THE FIRST CIRCLE TIME

As the Leader of the Circle Time, I, too, had to learn to make contact with
this group of children by paying attention to what they were doing at that moment. For example, one child got up and stood in the middle of the circle without
any apparent reason. I gave her act a purpose by asking her to pick another child
to stand up with her and to give her a hug. It was difficult for these children to follow instructions, so I followed them until they were able to respond to me.

Yet, as the Leader of the circle, I also provided these children with activities I initiated. However, I initiated them by doing them and not by talking about them. For example, we played "train" by holding the children with their backs to our fronts in a tight circle as we made train sounds going up hills, around curves, and down hills. By putting the children in the act of doing the game, they learned it. The children could allow themselves to be held close because it was fun, and their attention was on the game.

The way the children play these games can be used as a diagnostic tool. For example, while pretending we were on the train, I asked the children what they saw when they looked out the window. They said things like "a chair, a mat." When I said that I saw a cow, one boy then said, "I see a bunny rabbit." These responses show that these children are operating at a very concrete level; they also show the potential of being able to fantasize when the stimulus is provided.

For the cradling—another activity chosen by the Leader—I sang Rock-A-Bye Baby, and the adults sang it with me. The children loved this song. This song fitted these children. It was simple and concrete. (I always add to the ending, "And I will catch you.")

While snacks were being served, I asked each child what they liked best today. They all looked at Ned and said, "Ned," and Sam went over and hugged him. At that point, I said, "Maybe we could make up a song about that" and asked them to help me. The song was, "I like Ned. I like Ned. I like Ned." Celia then sang, "I like Cora," and Sue said, "I like Gill." They smiled and giggled as they said it.

The question, "What did you like best today?" is abstract. To answer it, the child has to search through her memories for some experience that stands out. To answer it, the child must have had a pleasurable experience of which she is aware. These children became aware that they liked their teacher, Ned. That is a concrete answer to an abstract question. When the Leader invited the children to make up a song expressing these feelings, they discovered a new awareness; namely, that they also liked their new adult partner. That response is still concrete, but it is a step in the right direction.

The children's ability to make this shift (from liking Ned to include liking their own partners) shows the potential for growth in these children when someone invites them to express where they are.

At the end of Circle Time, the children were relating to each other and to the adults. At the end of the cradling, when we sang Rock-A-Bye Baby, they were very quiet. The feeling of enjoyment was palpable.

The Children. The behavior of these children, shown by the type of games and activity they initiate (Peek-A-Boo, cradling) and the concreteness of their behavior, shows that we are dealing with developmentally delayed children. They are like babies. They never got their needs fulfilled as infants. These are the children with whom the trainees are learning to do Developmental Play therapy.

THE POSTSESSION

The four trainees whose children were present reported their experience from the first session. Gill said she was pleased with the work she did with her child, Sue (the one who was a cocaine baby). Sue just allowed Gill to do whatever she did—primarily, cradling. Clara said she was happy with her work because her child, Sam, seemed content to be with her after some "testing out" (her interpretation).

Cora: I could learn to set limits without being so authoritative.

Paul: I didn't like the feeling once when I pulled Tom up too hard. It wasn't right. I feel like I'm in a power struggle with Tom, and I don't like that feeling. I feel like I'm trapped. I shouldn't have to be in that position. I'm getting in touch with my own sexual abuse as a child. This program is much harder than I expected. I'm beginning to see that I need to give Tom more space, more choices to see what he needs or wants to do.

Ned: (His child, Aretha, was absent) I didn't know what to do in Circle Time when the kids came over and hugged me. Did I mess things up by hugging Sam? I didn't know what I was supposed to do. I felt better when he went back to Clara.

Clara: It's fine with me that you love him, too.

Ned: I want to share something. I love these kids. I feel like a father to them. I'm not just a teacher. I'm their friend. When Sam looks at me, I feel his love.

Leader: Would you just take time to feel that right now?

Ned: (Is quiet)

Cora: (To Ned) I'm moved by what you said.

Paul: I feel that way about him (Ned). I feel like a father to him, and I love him. I am proud of him.

COMMENTS

This first meeting with the children sets the stage for the quality of the work to be done with these children in this thirteen-week program.

1. The feeling of community created by the adults through their ability to take risks to share intimate personal feelings provides a safe place for them to know themselves and an avenue within which to do it.

2. This sense of community between the adults provides the children with the conditions needed for them to feel safe where they are.

3. The atmosphere of community provides the space needed for the adults to become aware of how their play with the child opens them to hidden feelings and to their own childhood experiences. For example, Paul and Cora got in touch with their anger and their need to control others. Ned got in touch with the love inside him.

4. The community sharing in the pre- and postsessions made the trainees realize that once they become aware of their own needs, they can give them up and look at the children's needs. They can then start taking charge by noticing the child, by helping the child experience her own body and her own existence through the dialogue of touch.

SESSION 2: PRESESSION TRAINING

Leader: After your first session with your child last week, what are your expectations this week?

Clara: I did all I knew last week, and I don't know what to do this week.

Gill and Cora: (Said the same) (Paul and Ida were absent)

Ned: I'm getting a lot of positive feedback from the parents. Sue's grandmother was very pleased with Sue (Gill's child, the cocaine baby). The grandmother said she talks more and said, "Thank you" when given something. I was surprised, however, at the negative behavior here last week from Celia. She doesn't act that way in my room (at school).

COMMENTS

The unsolicited report of the parents who noticed positive changes in the children after the introductory meeting is in marked contrast to the first reports by the trainees. The trainees found the children difficult, and they were also concerned about "opening up" these children—the effect it would have on them and their families.

The trainees' concepts of therapy is also revealing. They view therapy in terms of tasks or activities to be done. ("I did all I knew last week, and I don't know what to do this week.") They do not experience therapy as an ongoing interactional organic relationship process between two people—an "I" and a "Thou."

The presession and postsession trainings are designed to create the sense of community needed for the trainees to experience within themselves what it feels like to be in an "I-Thou" relationship with another adult or child.

The trainees' reaction to their first session with the children showed that they need help to be present, to see and to say what they see. To provide that help, the Leader asked for two volunteers to role-play—one being the adult and the other being the child. Gill volunteered to be the adult and Ned, the child.

A COACHING DEMONSTRATION

Setting: Gill and Ned are sitting facing each other. The Leader sits near Gill to coach her.

Gill: (To Ned) Good morning. You're smiling. (Takes his hand, rubs it)

Ned: (Looks at her face, smiles)

Gill: (Looks down at his hand; doesn't see his smile)

Leader: (Coaching her) What does his face say to you?

Gill: (Looks at his face) He's interested.

Leader: (Coaching) I see you looking at his face.

Gill: (Laughing) I want to make this complicated.

Leader: (Looking at Ned) He nodded again.

Gill: Mhm mhm. (Yes)

Leader: When he smiles, what do you see?

Gill: (Looking at Ned) When you smile, your whole face smiles. Your eyes are smiling.

Leader: (To Ned) And when you smile, I see your dimples and the lines around your mouth.

Ned: (Smiles more) Keep going.

Leader: (To Gill) Respond to him.

Gill: So you want me to keep going. You'd like me to notice you. You like being touched.

Ned: (Moves his other hand toward her)

Gill: (Takes that hand and looks at it) You're looking at me and smiling.

Leader: Now get ready to part. After you part, close your eyes and see what you feel.

Ned: It felt like a mother taking care of a sick child. It felt real caring, real gentle.

Leader: Look at her, and tell her you liked it.

Ned: (To Gill) I liked it.

Leader: (To Gill) What cues did his body give you?

Gill: His eyes are soft. He leaned forward. He smiled, and I felt him being really present. He was really with me.

Leader: You do know what to do next. You simply say what you are seeing and follow the child.

Gill: I think *I'm beginning to let myself see what I'm seeing.* I just recognized the things that get in the way of that—that I still want to put more value judgment on what I'm seeing than just reaching for what's there.

Leader: And what was there, in three words?

Gill: It was total acceptance.

Leader: He liked it.

Group: (Laughs)

Gill: It's so simple. Why is it so hard to do?

Leader: (To other trainees) What was the effect on you, watching this?

Claire: I learned that I could touch their hands and look at their face at the same time.

Cora: Last week when I said to Celia, "You brought your hands," she said, "I don't have any hands." She hid them in her coat. She wouldn't bring out her hands.

Leader: (Demonstrates with Cora) Your hands went away. They were here a minute ago.

Cora: I don't have any hands. (Keeping her hands behind her)

Leader: You don't have any hands? (Looking at her legs) You have some knees. (Touching them)

Cora: I don't have any hands.

Leader: (Looking for her hidden hands) Are your hands behind you?

Cora: (Starts moving her hands further away, giggles)

Leader: (Stops the demonstration) What's the effect on you?

Cora: What I was trying to do with Celia. I said, "You have arms." I wanted her to bring her arms out. If she did that, she would have to bring her hands out.

Leader: (To Cora) Did you notice in the role-play the effect on you when I changed my focus and started paying attention to where your hands might be?

Cora: I felt relieved. I felt connected to you—that you heard me.

Leader: *The idea in Developmental Play is not to make the child do something you want her to do. The idea is to enable the child to feel her bodily presence through touch, through feeling your body and your presence.*

As you talked about your interaction with Celia, it felt more and more like a power struggle. I felt that also in role-playing with you. When I changed to *your* focus (I don't have any hands) and started looking for your hands, I felt your energy change—and you were more with me, and I was more with you. In other words, the child is giving me cues as to what to do and where to go. *I don't have to figure out what to do be-cause the child is telling me, one way or the other.*

Comment. Celia played this Hide-and-Seek game differently from most chil-dren. For example, usually when I say, "You don't have any hands? Well, I see you have some knees here" (touching them), children will hide their knees by covering them with their hands. When I move to their eyes, they will cover their eyes with their hands, and we end up playing a Peek-a-Boo game. With Celia, you have to play a Hide-and-Seek game with her hands from the beginning. Celia needs to have her focus recognized. She needs to feel seen. She has a need to feel that she is in control of the interaction.

It's time to be with the children now (Children's Hour).

POSTSESSION TRAINING

Leader: Go inside and see what you are experiencing now after being with the children. How do you feel about your work, and how do you feel about your child? Then come back and share.

Clara: What's been coming up for me—I'm aware I'm wiped out. Am I doing something that's causing Sam's behavior to escalate? Am I doing some-thing that's going on there?

Leader: What's your answer?

Clara: Yes and No. The Yes is that I'm not doing enough to keep him focused, and the No part is he's tempting me. If I did more to pull him back in and keeping him focused, physically pulling him, then he wouldn't do that. He's tempting me.

Leader: So you're blaming yourself for his behavior. If you did something differ-ently, he'd behave differently.

Clara: Right.

Leader: Did any of the rest of you have that feeling?

Group: (All laugh)

Cora: I had an *extremely* difficult time keeping Celia on the mat. Everybody's telling me not to ask questions—just very difficult to keep her on the mat. She doesn't want to stay. I said that this is our special place. She wants to run back and forth, you know. Maybe I'm just not setting enough limits. Even when I did set limits, she wants to get up. My back hurts from trying to hold her down. Am I doing something to encourage this behavior to escalate?

Leader: In answer to your question, yes, you are doing something that stimulates this behavior, and what you are doing is something she needs. What you are doing is requiring her to relate to you and to be with you, and she is not used to that. She has periods of being uncomfortable. I don't think that she is testing you. You're making demands on her to relate. That's new. You are creating an environment that's new for her. You have to see that. There's a process that both you and your child go through. I saw some places where you and Celia came together. Sometimes you're so tired chasing after the child that you don't see when the child is letting you in.

Cora: I felt more of a struggle this week than last. We really struggled!

Clara: I was going to say the same thing.

Leader: Do you know why? The increase in the resistance is a sign that they are beginning to like it. The fighting it is evidence for that. They are sensing something new and something they want. We don't know the previous experiences of these children. You have to be patient. There's also another quality I think you are missing. Their resistance takes the form of playful Peek-a-Boo, Hide-and-Seek games, especially with Celia. Basically, these children are experiencing two feelings: one part of them wants the touching and closeness, and the other part tells me that it's a no-no. It may be a last stand before they surrender and let themselves have it. You have to understand that this is new for them.

Celia has a wonderful voice. When she said to me in Circle Time, "I don't like you. I don't care," I heard it. She can express herself, and that's what we want. She has an aliveness to her. In Circle Time when she said, "I didn't get nothin' out of this," I could feel her energy. What would happen to her if she said this in the outside world?

Cora: You don't talk back, little girl. Don't talk to me like that.

Leader: (To Cora) You need to initiate and give her something to respond to. For example, when I picked her up and held her a moment, I could tell she liked it. I didn't ask her if I could do it. I did it, and when she became uncomfortable, I kissed her on the cheek and put her down. This showed her that I listen to her and yet I do what *I* think she needs. After I have kissed her on the cheek, she can't undo it. It's already done. You have to learn to sneak it in—in small doses.

Demonstrating with Cora

Leader: (Reaches over and hugs Cora and gives her a quick kiss on the cheek)

Cora: (Pulled back)

279

Leader: Were you aware that you pulled back when I did that to you?

Cora: Yes. I didn't want to mess up my make-up. (Group laughs) Celia gave me a hug. She wanted to go over and give you a hug, and I told her she could do that later. Then, after she gave me a hug, I gave her a hug, and she didn't pull back.

Leader: When you invited her to give you a hug, she came over and did it. You need to invite her more, to initiate more instead of telling her what not to do. I could hear the anger in your voice when you were doing that—trying to hold her down.

Cora: I don't like to be physical with anybody—to hold her on the mat. I was pulling her. My back hurts right now.

Leader: Well, you can call on me to help you. That's why I'm here. I saw her lying there quietly, and you were saying, "Here's your head, here's your shoulder."

Cora: That was all right then.

Leader: They will allow that for a short time and then they resist, but then they will stay there longer and longer, and even ask for it. You'll see.

Clara: As you were talking, even in the Circle Time, Sam would get all over the place and want to be in everybody's stuff, but then he would come back. He came back and would put my arms around him. So I was getting both—he's out there and at the same time, he'd come back and take my arms and put them around him or put them on his knees. Yet he was in control of that.

Cora: I'm trying to learn a different method in place of being strong and stern. It was hard today.

Leader: Look at me, and tell me it was hard today.

Cora: I want you to see how rough it was, and I want to say also, it's not dealing with Celia that is rough. It's just the physical. I really feel like I was pulling and tugging at her. I don't like that. I don't like the way I felt.

Leader: Is there a feeling of anger in that pulling?

Cora: No. No anger.

Leader: So what was it you didn't like?

Cora: The tugging, pulling. I don't like to do that with kids. It's like fighting. One of the things I really like—the way I've dealt with things in the past—if I didn't chase her or force her to come back, she would come back to me. Ignoring that she's going away over there, she'll come back.

Leader: Try it out. And while she's away, you can talk about her: "I wonder where that Celia is." Did you ever get the lotion out and do the Slippery Hand game?

Cora: She asked for it, but by then there wasn't time.

Leader: She even asked for it. That's a plus!

Cora: She said, "Did you bring the lotion today?"

Leader: So she does remember what you did from week to week.

Cora: The week before she said, "Play what you played before," and I didn't know what she meant.

Leader: I'd start right at the beginning of the session with the Slippery Hand game. And you can do it with her feet.

Cora: Well, she had taken off her shoes and was brushing off the sand.

Leader: How do you feel now? Do you feel understood?

Cora: I feel understood. Actually, I'm looking forward to next week and trying it again. It's going to be a learning experience for me. And I think, in the end, Celia will grow, too.

Leader: Say to someone, in your own way, "I want you to see how hard it was for me."

Cora: (To Clara) I want you to see how hard it was for me. I also think it was hard for you.

Clara: I wanted to cover Sam's face with kisses and love him. It was wonderful. He played with my hands.

Cora: I felt like trading her for a new kid. (Laughs)

Leader: (To Clara) Can you understand her?

Clara: Yeah, I can—when he was grabbing my glasses and throwing things.

Cora: And she bit me one time—she did! I ignored it. She did that when she didn't want to be held.

Leader: How about you, Ned?

Ned: I was pleased. Aretha came to me without help. (Aretha is a nonverbal, withdrawn child with autistic-like behavior and little eye contact. Ned especially wanted her as his child.) I put the lotion on her. She loved it. And then, all of a sudden, she stopped. She kept looking at Celia (they are cousins). I would hold my hand out, and she would come and grab my hand, and she came back to me. I sat her down and started rubbing her feet. Then she started to walk. I held my hand out and she would hold my hand and then I would pull her back. Then she started Peek-a-Boo, and that was great!

Leader: That *was* great! Her Peek-a-Boo with you in Circle Time was great, too. In Circle Time, I had her do it, and then I had all the kids do it. It's using what the kids are already doing. What you did, Ned, is an example of how you use what the kid does.

It's using what they are already doing and making something out of it. (In Circle Time, when one child covered her face, I asked another child to go over, knock on the door, and see if anyone is home.) Just as Ned did, you create your own touching games.

Ned: I laid down and held her up in the air as if she's flying. Then I bring her down, and our foreheads would touch. She rubbed my nose. Then she started putting her hands on my face, and I'd say, "That's my nose. That's my eyes." Then I'd lift her up, and we would touch foreheads.

Leader: That's great. You followed lifting her up by bringing her back to you to be touched by you—so she feels her own body when touched by you.

Ned: This is cool. She wanted to flip and go backwards, and so she hung way over and she'd see me again. When she saw you all swinging Celia, she wanted to do that. I started swinging her by the legs, and when the time came for Circle Time, she didn't want to quit.

Leader: (To Ned) You are doing two things these kids need. They need to move—move their bodies and make noise and be touched. You cradled her later. She looked like a different child in Circle Time today. Her face looked as if there was a person behind it.

Ned: She wanted me to hold her hand. She leaned back against my chest (in Circle Time).

Leader: How did that feel?

Ned: That felt great.

Leader: So do you have a word that expresses how you were today?

Ned: Refreshing.

Leader: I get a sense that you were pleased with yourself. Correct?

Ned: Right.

Leader: Want to tell someone that?

Ned: I'm pleased with myself. Can I say something?

Leader: Sure.

Ned: (To Clara) I know how you feel when you said you'd like to kiss Sam. I know how you feel. Even when he "shows off," he's still got that playful part with him—I can understand it. It kills you when he does that, you know. I understand how you feel toward him. (Ned is self-conscious as he talks about Sam.)

(To Cora) I have never seen Celia act the way she did today—running away. I've never seen her act that way before—never. I've seen her do that in other classes, but not that bad. When Celia and Aretha hugged in the middle of the circle, Aretha started to hit Celia. I've never seen her do that. Never! They are really close. They never push. Nothing comes between them. I was shocked.

282

Leader: What does it mean to you7

Ned: I don't know.

Cora: Aretha may have acted that way because she didn't like the way Celia acted.

Gill: I wonder if Aretha was beginning to have a sense of her own. Is Celia the dominant one of the two?

Ned: Yeah.

Leader: I think they do it because this is a safe place. I look at any negative behavior that is new as very positive. The children feel free enough to be whoever they are.

Cora: Could we have them take their shoes off before they come in here? It takes so much time, getting the sand off.

Leader: That's part of the process—taking shoes off, brushing the sand off—all of it involves touching and caring. You can smell feet, count toes in the Slippery Foot game, and have a wonderful time.

Ned: Celia's the oldest, and I think they do that at home. She's got a little brother at home. They hold hands in the hallway.

Leader: Celia is a care-taker for the younger children. In this program, she can be a receiver of that care—and that's new for her. She's used to being in charge of others. She's not used to allowing herself to be a receiver, be the one touched and the one sung to. She is uncomfortable, and she moves away from it. She has to have time to get used to it at her pace.

(To Cora) You found that out. When you didn't run after her or yell at her to come back, she came back on her own and even invited contact.

Clara: I get that feeling from Sam. He tries to take charge. He wants to put the lotion on himself.

Leader: You have to let them do some of that—that's where they are.

Ned: Aretha, she wants to do it to me.

Leader: You allow that in the beginning, but then you say, "I have to put some on you." (To Gill) How about you?

Gill: I have mixed feelings. I feel like Sue (her child) is responsive to me, and she did a little more active stuff today. She wanted to rock, and she pushed me over and said the "magic" word to get me up. (See Appendix for the Magic Button game.) In that regard, she was more active. When you came around and mentioned how quiet I was, I wasn't aware that I was that quiet with her. That made me aware of how much that child needed to come out. I had a feeling that maybe I was keeping her there—both staying in our quietness. I can really relate to that. That was difficult for me, and *I touched a part of myself when we started doing more active things.* It was really very difficult for me, too—to be right out there, to make noise, to have an effect on her. So that's something I really have to work on. She loved it (Gill's voice gets louder as she talks). She really responded to that—hearing her voice, saying it loud, and saying it louder. Her little face just started to light up. So in a way, I was a little disappointed that I wasn't again really challenging myself a lot. I was more doing what comes naturally to me. I wasn't going into any pockets of myself.

Leader: I'm wanting you to see me as a coach—to try things out rather than feeling criticized that you're not doing it right. Sue is a very different child from the others. She needs to expand. She needs to get out and move her body so that she feels her body and feels alive. I might take her and do some movements—to jump so that she can feel the life in her body. When you started that active moving, she responded. Whatever you initiated—like moving your tongue—she did that. She needs you as a model. When you talk so softly, she does too. In Circle Time, she started to say something and no sound came out. You need to help her get the sound out.

Celia has such a wonderful voice. When she came out with, "I didn't like nobody," loud and strong, she had energy which gave life to what she said. I like people around me that have some life to them (group laughs). And Celia's got it!

Gill: When you said to her, "Stand up and jump and walk around," it's like I had the sense that, "Oh, I can do that, too." I almost felt like I'm rooted to the mat (Laughs; her voice is a lot stronger), and I can't get off my butt. I have to stay here.

Leader: You don't have to.

Cora: Actually, I feel that way, too. I wouldn't mind getting up and running across the room with her. I just feel that was real confining.

Leader: You do have quite a big space there. You don't have to sit all the time. You can stand up and move. You can make noises. In the Circle Time, when we were making noises, everybody was doing it except Sue. Everybody was making noises, and everybody was having fun. They all got in on the act when Aretha hid her face and we said, "She's gone away, and now she's coming back." They followed me, as the Leader, and we made up a story about Aretha. When they don't do anything, you make up something to make them feel present.

(To Gill) The cradling that you are doing with Sue is fine. From the reports of her grandparents, something is having an effect. It's just that she needs to be supported to be more active, also. She needs somebody that is active to be a model for her. Balance the holding with making sounds and moving to help her develop her verbal language and help her feel the life inside her.

The Gingerbread Cookie Game. To help the trainees with touching activities and games, the Leader taught them the Gingerbread Cookie game by demonstrating it with Clara (see Appendix).

Leader: It's time to close. Any last-minute things you have to say?
  Clara: No. (Imitating Celia in Circle Time) Nothing! I have nothing to say!
  Group: (Laughs; joined Clara; had fun) No, nothing!
Leader: (Taking her cue from the group, had each one, in turn, make some sounds or noises as a way to close and to feel their energy. All did it but Ned. They liked it and said that it was centering and the way the sound went out of the room was interesting.)
      (To Cora) So you felt your own life when you did that.
  Cora: Yes.
  Clara: It was so centering. I loved making that noise. It was so centering.
Leader: The main thing is just to feel the vibration as it moves up and down your body.
  Cora: (To Ned) I felt that way once. I wanted you to know that, but once you do it, it's wonderful.
Leader: Let's stand and hold hands (sings the Goodbye song). They go away laughing and in a friendly mood.

SESSION 3

POSTSESSION TRAINING

Clara was upset with the Leader during the one-to-one part because she didn't come around and say something to her—help her.

  Clara: Sam ran into my arms and immediately wanted to be cradled. He wanted me to hold him—a shift for this kid who was all over the place. I was going where he is today. My objection was that you were so busy with the others and you don't have a chance to come and see what's going on with me. Why don't you come over and direct me? So I felt like I'm not doing it right. Oh, you're so busy that you can't come over here and see what's going on (angry tone) and give me some direction because surely I'm not doing it right. So that's part of what's going on with me.

Paul: (Who was observing all because his child was absent) My perception— you were going so smooth. You were so attached; the touching was so natural—a real nice, healthy attachment.

Clara: It was almost like he was a baby! For this kid, that was in control— he's a little baby. He shouldn't be this way, a baby; he's acting like he's two. He's not supposed to be acting like a baby. That's part of what's going on!

Leader: I'm really glad that you put this all out. *First* of all, I didn't come over because I was observing you, and you were doing just what Sam needed— to let himself be cradled—and you were doing it and doing it well. Second , Sam is acting like a baby right now because that is exactly what he needs to do, where he needs to be in order to mature.

COMMENTS

Two important things stand out in Session 3:

1. *Clara's reaction to the Leader*. It was good that Clara could say how she felt about the Leader. In this atmosphere of closeness, participants tend to relive their own family experience. Clara's reaction to the Leader may be an example of this: namely, that in her family, she felt like the low man on the totem pole. She also felt that not being seen, she must be doing things wrong. Furthermore, you're supposed to act your age, not be a two-year-old when you're four. That is the message she got as a child.

   The Leader does not do processing or therapy with the trainees. This is not a therapy group. She does, however, help the trainee become aware of her own experience in the here and now and to share that experience in the group. That approach is demonstrated in the DP training throughout this chapter.

2. *Sam's shift toward allowing himself to be cradled* . To provide conditions the child needs in order to allow herself to be touched, held, or cradled is the first and basic goal of Developmental Play. It is the behavior that makes possible the evolution of all other human behaviors. The DP therapist not only allows the cradling, but she provides it when the child is unable to ask for it herself.

SESSION 4

PRESESSION TRAINING

Centering

Leader: Go inside for a moment. What is the first thing you are aware of? Is it a thought, or is it a body feeling? Where in your body is this feeling? Now feel yourself in your chair and your feet on the floor; when ready, come back. Say a word that describes where you are now.

Gill: The word is apprehensive, but the longer I stayed inside, the more that went dissolving away.

Cora: I have a slight headache, and I didn't realize it until I actually went in and felt the body parts and the feelings, and I didn't know it, actually.

Ned: I don't know.

Leader: When you went inside your body, what part were you aware of?

Ned: My chest.

Clara: I felt calm—nice to give myself space to be here.

Ida: Happy.

Paul: I think I'm aware of my chest feelings—just being here and not out there (noisy outside). Also, Tom's not back, so I need a new child.

Leader: Anyone have anything they want to report?

Paul: I had an insight in my private practice that's related to our work here. This was a mother, her son, and me. The three of us were together, and I noticed I'm doing therapy differently. When a kid walked in, I'd say, "This is what we're going to do today." I'm a lot more open and a lot more letting the kids direct where they need to be.

My desk is off limits, and this kid went over to my desk three times. After the third time, I picked him up and I just held him. He called me names. One of the things I noticed is that all the time he's struggling, his head was cradled in my neck. He wasn't fighting back. It was very different from the experience I had the first time. When I was a kid, I was abused. One of the things that was real clear to me this time is that I didn't get the old feeling—that old trapped feeling. It was real good. I couldn't have done that before—what I just did.

Leader: What kind of a feeling did you get?

Paul: It was healthy and clean, and I really believed I did the right thing. I've restrained kids for years and it never bothered me. But here I was, aware of the cradling as well.

Leader: So now you didn't feel abusing when you held him.

Paul: I never felt abusing. I felt trapped.

Leader: You said you felt trapped when with Tom, your child.

Paul: Yes.

Hello Circle Time

Leader: Hello, Gill. I see your long eye lashes. (Etc.) Would you sing to Ned?

Gill: Hello, Ned. You got your Sox hat on today.

Leader: Ned, would you sing to Paul?

Ned: Do I have to?

Leader: Yes. (Group laughs)

Ned: I don't feel up to singing.

Leader: You can say it then, or chant it.

Ned: (To Paul) I don't feel up to singing.

Leader: (To Ned) What did you see?

Ned: Him. (Laughing, pointing to Paul)

Leader: And how do you feel now?

Ned: All right.

Leader: (To group) What was it like to pick out something to see on the other person?

Cora: I felt on the spot. I got to do it right. There are only certain things I can see. Like I saw a mole on you, Ida. I didn't know the word for it and I didn't want to hurt your feelings. Is that a mole or a beauty mark? So I picked your earrings. So I kind of had a no-see rule.

Leader: So that's where your head stuff came in and stopped you from seeing.

Cora: Right.

Ned: I felt uncomfortable doing it. I don't feel like it today.

Leader: How do you feel being here as you are?

Ned: I'm here.

Leader: Do you feel more here than you did in the beginning?

Ned: Yeah. Definitely.

Leader: And how did you bring yourself here?

Ned: You made me laugh.

Leader: You participated. Is something bothering you?

Ned: Yes, but I don't want to talk about it here.

Leader: You can put it aside for now.

Ned: The reality is it will come back.

Leader: You're looking at me. Are you sad?

Ned: I've been sad for four days (he had broken up with his girlfriend).

Paul: I found it easy to pick out something to see because I didn't have to interpret. And that is so different from what you're taught in other modalities—which is very nice.

Leader: (To Ned) If you want, I'll talk with you after we see the children.

Paul: I have another question. I don't know when to end (in singing the I See game).

Leader: You just stop when you feel like it.

Paul: Then how do you signal "I'm done?"

Leader: You do it with your voice. You stop looking at her. Or you can do it verbally, saying, "That's it" or "I'm done" or you can say, "Now it's your turn" to the next person.

Paul: Okay.

Leader: To help you learn to say what you see, let's have a practice demonstration. I need two volunteers—one the Giver and one the Receiver.

Clara: I'll be the Giver.

Gill: I'll be the Receiver.

Demonstration: Saying Hello

Leader: (To Clara) Say Hello to her. You pay attention to what you see happening to her.

Clara: Hi, Gill.

Gill: Hi.

Clara: I see you put your hand out, and now you're putting your other hand out. You're putting out both your hands. (Taking her hand) Oh, and you have fingers, and here's a hill and here's a valley. (Moving her fingers between each of Gill's fingers) And now I saw you look at me. And you held your thumb up so I could come all the way down to your wrist. You're smiling. You like that touch, don't you?

Gill: Mhm mhm. (Yes)

Clara: I can tell. Oh, you turned your hand over. You've got two sides to that hand. And those fingers are standing up there for me to say Hello to them. I can say Hello to all those fingers at once, and I can say Hello to them one-at-a-time, like that. Hello, finger.

Gill: (Moves her fingers)

Clara: Look at that! They are talking back at me. Isn't that wonderful!

Leader: (To Clara) Can you say Goodbye now?

Clara: It's time for us to say Goodbye. I'm going to say Goodbye to this hand (taking it in hers and kissing it) and I'm going to say Goodbye to this hand (kissing it). Goodbye.

Gill: Goodbye.

Leader: (To Gill) Want to say what it was like for you?

Gill: (To Clara) Yeah. I really felt seen. I loved the way you focused on the hand, the face, just really all inclusive. I was real drawn by what you were doing—a lot of feeling—a lot of warmth and it felt good, and I felt real responsive. I was touched.

Leader: (To Clara) What was it like for you?

Clara: Initially, I was apprehensive—it was really nice. (To Gill) Oh, but you were just responding to me, opening your fingers and going and wanting me to touch you here and touch you there. It was really nice—to see your face looking at me and looking at your hands. It was nice.

Leader: (To Clara) One thing I noticed that I liked was when you said Goodbye: after saying Goodbye to her hands, you went up to her face and said Goodbye to her face. The face is where it is. The eye contact between the two of you was lovely. That put an end to it. You made contact there.

(To others) Anyone want to say what it was like observing?

Paul: (To Clara) You've got a hell of a lot of courage. You volunteer for everything, and you're willing to try anything, and it comes out so natural—just natural and warm. I really respect that. I wish I was more like that. The other thing was that I was real clear that I felt the Goodbye part because you did it so well. I was real clear that I don't.

Leader: (To Clara) What was it like hearing that?

Clara: That felt real good to hear you say that. (Laughing)

Leader: I liked it, what you did. I have one suggestion. Want to hear it?

Clara: Yes.

Leader: Several times you said, "Oh, you must like it." You might vary that. Instead of speaking for her, you might say, "Does your hand like that?" If she says, "Yes," ask, "Would you have your hand tell me that?" In that way, you invite some verbal response back from her.

Clara: (Turns to Gill and practices this with her, and both liked it)

Leader: **Time to meet the children.** The children seem to like the blankets over them when we sing the lullaby. (Paul said he had plenty of blankets)

POSTSESSION TRAINING

Trainees Report on Their Experiences With the Children

Ned: Aretha did a lot more talking today. She said she wanted to do the Swing. We did that. Then she wanted me to hold her hand. After I let her down from swinging her, she said, "Lotion." So we did that. She

290

likes it, you know, when "you're slipping away." She put so much lotion on I was afraid she'd hurt her head (when she fell back). (See Slippery Hand game in Appendix.)

Leader: That's great that she's talking and asking for something. But you can control that by you putting on the lotion—what you want to do anyway—to get her to experience being given to. You say, "I have to put the lotion on." You need to be the one in charge, and she needs to experience that also. Another observation: the minute Aretha moved away, you grabbed her; but when you gave her a little space, she walked away but turned around and came back on her own. They need some space for them to decide what they want to do. In the beginning, they don't do anything. They don't know what to do, so you're always doing something to them by touching them or noticing them in some way to get them to experience your presence and their own presence. In the DP approach, it is the adult that has to create the conditions needed for growth—not the child.

Ida: How can I set limits better for James?

Leader: First, how did you feel about yourself with James?

Ida: I think I had a better grip on what he was doing this time than last time. I don't know if I was doing it great. I was doing the best I could. I wasn't worried about what other people would say when I had to chase him. I just did what I had to do. I thought I needed to be doing something that I'm not doing in order to keep him more confined.

Leader: Would you be willing to make a feeling statement like, "I felt good when . . ."

Ida: I felt good when he allowed me to put the cover over his head, and he looked up at me with his sparkling eyes and smiled. I felt very good. I felt connected to him.

Leader: How did it come about that he looked at you?

Ida: Because I was doing what he liked, something that we mutually could do together.

Leader: What did you do?

Ida: We made a fort or a house, and he wanted me to cover the top, and before I covered the top, I would say Goodbye.

Leader: The connection was made by something you did.

Ida: Yes.

Leader: You looked at him, and you didn't let him distance himself. He makes the fort. He makes it in a relationship with you. So did you like that part that you did?

Ida: Yes, I did.

Leader: So would you pick out someone and tell them, "I liked that part I did today."

Ida: I'll say it to this lady.

Leader: Does she have a name?

Ida: I forgot her name.

Leader: You could ask her.

Ida: What is your name? (To Cora) Cora, I really liked what I did today in terms of getting the direct eye contact of James. That felt fine.

Leader: What was that like, sharing with her?

Ida: Aside from being embarrassed not knowing her name, it was very nice.

Leader: How do you feel about yourself now?

Ida: I don't feel embarrassed.

Leader: You also shared something that you did with James. How do you feel about that?

Ida: (Laughs) Truthfully, nothing.

Leader: You did something very well.

Ida: I didn't need to get reassurance from her (Cora).

Leader: Well, maybe you don't need it, but what is it like to have it anyway?

Ida: It was nice. (Said quietly) It was nice to receive the acceptance from her.

Leader: The effect on you right this minute.

Ida: Right this minute it was very nice. I'm feeling defensive.

Leader: That's okay to feel that. What I'm doing is trying to understand what you are saying. When you talk in generalities, I don't understand what you are saying. What I saw you do—I thought was a fantastic job.

Ida: Thank you. (Said quietly)

Leader: What I am working on with you is to help you find a place where you felt you had some skills. You have a very difficult child, and I thought you did very well.

Ida: Thanks. I think I did well. But I feel, though, that I could do better.

Leader: That may be true. All of you are beginners in this group. You're not supposed to do everything "perfect" the first time around. You need to acknowledge in yourself the part that you do well. Have you got one moment in that session that you can describe where you felt good, something that you did that was hard to do and you did it? Something you created that you liked?

Ida: When he was in his little house and every time he covered himself, I would say Goodbye; and then, after a few times, I put my hand in and I shook hands Goodbye; and then, when we did it once more, I say Goodbye; and his little hand came out without me asking him for it, and he shook my hand and said Goodbye, and then I covered him up. I feel very connected to him right now though we were doing this nutsy stuff.

Leader: What does that feel like? That's marvelous what you're telling me.

Ida: Oh, I feel very connected to him now.

Leader: What's it feel like to feel that connection?

Ida: It feels good.

Leader: You made the touching contact with him, and then he invited you back when he put his hand up.

Ida: That was very, very nice.

Leader: So that's an example of being aware of what you did and owning it. You made that possible for him to do that. You gave him what he needed. Would you choose someone and tell him you're pleased with yourself?

Ida: (Laughs) I'm going to pick Cora again. I do feel pleased with myself, and (said softly) I would just like you to know that (she's moved). And I connect with her because she followed me.

Leader: How did Cora look to you? Did she look like she understood?

Ida: She looked warm. She has a hard child, too. She understood.

Leader: So you answered your own question, "How do you set limits?" You did it by seeing him and giving him something to respond to.

(To the others) What was today like for the rest of you?

Clara: I felt left out because my kid wasn't here today. But it was really beautiful standing up there and watching everybody in the session interact with their children. It was like seeing a piece of music. It was really beautiful. With Sue and Aretha, I saw their faces like I had never seen them before. It was really neat. Their faces looked completely different. (To Cora) I could see Celia really softened to you.

Cora: I felt that, too.

Clara: And I could see James inviting you to play his way, which was very neat. (To Paul with his new child, Norm) And Norm—you're playing with him—your Three-Hands game. I could see him moving forward a little bit towards you, coming closer to you. And I kept thinking, what a change from Tom.

Leader: The Circle Time was fantastic. It was different as night and day. The kids could take turns. They did something that you could build on, like when we started the clapping and Celia made the sounds, and it sounded really jazzy. I love it when the children do something that you can respond to and build on.

Gill: (Talks more assertively; her voice is louder when she talks. Before it was difficult to hear her because she talked so softly.) Sue was more creative, which was kind of neat. I could just kind of feel her have a sense of her self, which was wonderful. She seemed to get such joy out of making noises and making those movements and having me to respond to her. There was a real spark in her eyes today. She was really there.

Leader: It was wonderful. She was making loud noises. (Before, when she opened her mouth to say something, nothing came out—no sounds at all.) She looked like she was having fun.

Gill: Yes. The barrier's not down completely, but I could feel it coming down. There was almost that fear of, you know, fear of feeling herself—feeling herself in the beginning—a real hesitancy in her to allow herself to be heard.

Leader: So when she makes a sound, she hears it. Her body moves, and then there's a sound.

Gill: And the joy she had in hearing it was incredible. I felt wonderful.

Ida: (Referring to Sue in Circle Time) When James was doing something, your little girl, Sue, turned and looked with very much alertness at him and me and our two kids, and she was totally present and involved in that whole thing, which before I had never seen—her eyes just opened up wide, and she looked at everything that was going on, and I never saw her do that before—like she wasn't afraid to acknowledge or look beyond herself.

Cora: As a matter of fact, she was looking at me, and I looked over at her and smiled, and she gave me the biggest smile. I just never saw her be so there.

Ida: That's it.

Leader: When a child smiles or laughs and starts to enjoy herself, that's the beginning of healing. And I saw it in Aretha. I saw it in Sue, and I saw it in Celia even more. (To Ida) And there were periods with James in the cradling when you had the blanket over him that he was really quiet. I'm wanting you to honor those moments and enjoy it with him even though it's not there all the time. Feel yourself relax with him. You relax, too. (To Gill) What did you do today that made the difference with Sue?

Gill: I believe that we are really bonded.

Leader: What specific things did you do?

Gill: I just responded to everything that she did.

Leader: An example?

Gill: She was really there. I touched one hand and right away the other hand would come out. She was really asking for it. If she made a noise, I would make a noise, too. I would say, "Let's do it louder."

Leader: Did she initiate making a noise?

Gill: Oh, yeah.

Leader: Okay. It would help others understand if you could say what she did and what you did.

Gill: She made a little noise, and I said (excited voice) "Oh, that's wonderful! Can you say it again?" She did it a little louder. I said, "Let's do it louder." I said, "Is it like this?"

Leader: Did you hear the difference in your energy pattern when you were saying it?

Gill: Yes. (Said loudly) I can feel it louder . . . louder (laughs as she herself hears the energy increase in her own voice when she used to be so quiet herself.)

Leader: You feel that in your voice, that energy and vibration.

Gill: Yes.

Leader: That's what she is feeling, too. It's the feeling of the body. It's the feeling of the vibration. It doesn't need any interpretation. Louder—so nice. So go ahead.

Gill: And she went from that—we made a noise and then she changed the noise and the sounds she was making, and I reacted to that: "Oh, you changed it, let's do that now." We did our faces next to each other, hands next to each other's mouth, and then she would initiate a new movement with it and, you know. She would crawl around, and then she spun around and she'd make a noise when she spun.

Leader: Your putting your face next to hers and making sounds are all creative things that you did to give her a different experience. Doing that makes her feel your presence. These children don't change until you provide the conditions that make it possible for them to change. Each time, write down the things that you do that make a difference. Anything else?

Gill: No. I want to relish this feeling. It's a nice feeling. (Gill's voice is so different from what it was in the beginning. She has a beautiful voice with a lot of resonance in it.) *It was the joy in this little girl's face*—the sunshine in her smile is right there—that I just want to carry with me.

Leader: I saw something else: her beauty when she came alive.

Gill: (Said softly) Yes.

Leader: I remember what Paul said last week when he said that last week she came in with more of anticipation than fear on her face. She came in glowing today. She looked really beautiful.

Clara: (To Gill) I saw you seeing her, and I saw her looking back for that.

Leader: (Closing the session) Just feel your breathing, and just acknowledge your own warmth. (Quiet) Just notice how the energy changes in you and around you. (Sings the Goodbye song joined by all; laughter at the end because the bird in the room sang louder, too, when they sang.)

COMMENTS

The reports of the trainees in the Postsession Meeting show that the training is beginning to pay off. The results are seen in:

1. The skill and confidence exhibited by the trainees.
2. The remarkable change in these very deprived children after only four sessions (one month).
3. The sense of joy and excitement experienced by both the adults and the children.
4. The sense of community expressed by the trainees.

Once the adults got in touch with their own inner selves through touching themselves and seeing themselves, they could see and touch their children. Once the adults got over their fear of initiating contact and giving the children something to respond to, the children responded. Once the trainees got over their fear of touching and holding a child, the children allowed themselves to be touched and held, and even invited it.

In an approach that is based on touch, as is Developmental Play, it is very important that the trainees get in touch with their own bodies, that they feel their own bodies, that they feel the energy in their bodies and in the bodies of the children they hold or touch. It is this quality of presence that makes the child feel real.

Presession Training

The Leader prepared the trainees to be with the children through exercises in which they practiced being present through meditation, touching and seeing another trainee, and sharing how they experienced what they did. For example, Ned got help to put aside his own inner needs so that later he could be present with Aretha. That presence was reflected in the excellent work he did with Aretha, a very difficult child. Gill got what she needed through the demonstration she and

Clara did, and that is reflected in the exciting work she did with her child, Sue. Paul learned a new way to touch. From his experiences last week with his child, Tom, he got in touch with his own childhood experiences of being abused and his feeling trapped when he held a child who didn't want to be held. He said he learned that he could "cradle" a child as well as "restrain" him.

Postsession Training

Helping the trainees be present as they report what they did and how they experienced what they did is the goal of the Postsession Meeting. For example, what did you do with your child today? What did it feel like being with your child today? What was the effect on you? What was the effect on your child?

Ida, for example, began her report by judging herself ("I needed to be doing something that I'm not doing in order to keep him more confined") instead of saying what she did and how she felt about what she did. When the Leader kept redirecting her to do that—to say what she did—she learned that she really did some very neat and effective things with a child who was very hyperactive. She also got support from the group. She ended up being able to relive her interaction with her child and feeling a connection to him, and him to her. She could begin to own her skill.

Gill's report showed clearly how her behavior and being present was directly related to Sue's behavior. That is, when Gill spoke louder, was more present in her actions, Sue immediately picked it up and copied Gill's behavior.

When Cora became more comfortable just seeing her child and taking the risk to touch her, Celia began looking at her.

The Children. The change in the behavior of these very deprived children was remarkable. Aretha, who exhibited some autistic behavior, responded to Ned and initiated behavior in the Circle Time group. Sue (born a cocaine baby), who wanted to talk but made no sounds, became very active, saying things loudly. Celia began making eye contact with everyone and wanting to be with Cora instead of running away. These behaviors were expressed with great joy and a sense of aliveness. When these children got what they needed, the change was like a miracle.

The children's behavior shows that they are well into the attachment phase of relating to their adult partner (the trainee). According to the parents' reports, this attachment behavior is already being transferred to their parents. The first month of Developmental Play therapy has provided these children with what they needed to become attached—the basic requirement for growing up. They were seen, touched, and held to let them know that they exist and are alive. This is Stage One.

SESSION 7

This session followed a three-week break for the holidays. However, you would never know that from the children's behavior. They began where they left off as if there had been no break. They showed they were glad to be there. It was a different story for the adults. They were not present.

PRESESSION TRAINING

The Leader asked the trainees to close their eyes and visualize their child and what they might be doing with that child.

Then the Leader asked for volunteers to practice seeing and saying Hello, one being the Giver and the other the Receiver. The two experienced the awkwardness they felt in this process of reconnecting after a break. After a break, the trainees had the tendency to interpret rather than say what they see right now. In Cora's case, she demonstrated saying Hello to Ned by touching his hands, but she moved quite fast. When the Leader coached her to take time to feel his skin to see where he is—to connect with him just through the touch—they began to look at each other and see each other.

CIRCLE TIME GROUP

New Behavior. The children were able to follow me, as the Leader. I began by moving my hands to music asking the children to "do what I do." They all did it. Sue and Celia did it so gracefully. Their hand movements were so beautiful. One of the girls suggested that the boys do it alone. So I asked Norm and Sam to do it, and the girls watched. Then I asked Celia to stand in the center of the circle and show us her new hairdo. She let everyone touch it. Then she wanted to show us how she could do a flip. Then Sam wanted to do his "trick." His trick was closing his eyes, which are kissed by Clara to make them open. The group watched with rapt attention as they wondered, "Is he ever going to open his eyes?" At the end of five kisses on each eye, he opened both eyes to the relief of the audience. Here Sam experienced himself in charge of himself and the center of attention. When he opened his eyes, he looked at everyone with a big smile. He felt truly seen. He could take as much time as he needed.

When we got ready to say Goodbye, Celia spoke up and said, "I'm not coming next time." This statement is evidence that Celia also reacted to the break. She is going to say she is not coming before we could tell her that we won't have any more play time. This reaction shows that her relationship to Cora and to the group is important to her. Just before ending the Circle Time, we always cradle the children and sing them a lullaby—in this group, "Rock-A-Bye Baby." The children in this group wanted to be covered with a blanket as they were cradled and sung to. They loved that. Sometimes in the beginning, being cradled under a blanket was the only time some really relaxed. It was like being in the womb again.

Stage Two. The fact that the children are beginning to ask for what they need reflects their attachment to their partner. They can ask for something because someone is present to see, hear, touch, and listen to them. The attachment leads to experiencing their partner as separate from them. Experiencing the adult as separate leads to the ability to engage in a dialogue and to ask for what they need. The children show this ability to speak up for what they want in the next session.

SESSION 8

PRESESSION TRAINING

The Trainees Asked Questions About Last Week

Paul: When you told me last week to ask Norm if he brought any kisses when he came back after running away, I was conflicted. I didn't think the child was there to give to me.

Leader: What happened when you did do that?

Paul: Norm liked it, and he offered me several places, like his fingers, that he wanted kissed. He let me put lotion on him.

Leader: How was that for you, doing that?

Paul: I enjoyed it. I had a good time.

Leader: What is wrong with you creating something both you and your child enjoy?

Paul: I don't know. In real life I have a hard time letting myself enjoy something.

Leader: By enabling Norm to find a way to contact you, you found a way to contact him. Is it true by doing so you found a new place in you—a place of enjoyment in really connecting with a child?

Paul: Yes.

Leader: It's because you enjoyed what you and he did that he was able to enjoy it. With you, Norm is experiencing himself as a fun person to be with.

The intent of asking Norm if he brought any kisses is not to have him take care of you but rather to give him a way of contacting you—giving him something to respond to. Asking him for kisses brings him into a dialogue of touch through feeling his own body. Norm is an extremely quiet, depressed child. He doesn't seem to know what to do or have the energy to do it. He needs someone to touch him so that he feels his body, the life inside him, and feels himself touched by that person. By asking him for kisses, you give him something to respond to. He responded by inviting you to do more touching. Norm said nothing verbally, but he communicated through touch.

Clara Asked About Sam's Biting Behavior. Clara wanted to know what to do about Sam's biting her and his need to put everything in his mouth. I recommended two things: (1) that she stop him from biting her by holding his head away from her when he bites; and (2) that she help him do things with his mouth such as making sounds, blowing, making raspberries on her hand, on the cheek (she does it to him and then he does it back to her), moving the tongue in and out. She could also bring some crackers and have fun eating them in different ways.

Nearly all young children go through a biting stage. The child discovers the world first through his skin and through his mouth. Biting is quite a normal behavior at that early age—around two. At the same time, the child should not be allowed to bite another. The child is becoming aware of his mouth. You can help him with this awareness by doing other things with his mouth besides biting others. This biting behavior shows that Sam, although very bright, is functioning developmentally at about age two.

Ned Has Concerns About Aretha. Ned described Aretha's behavior when she gets off the bus for school in the morning. In the beginning, she never looked at him or smiled. After starting the DP program, she changed and would look at him and smile. Last week she didn't look at him, and he was afraid that she would be back into her old unrelating behavior today in the session. Because Aretha was that way in the classroom, he was anticipating that she would be that way in the DP group. He was preparing himself to be disappointed in her and in his work with her.

Cora Reports Her Concern About Celia. Cora brought up Celia's statement last week, "I'm not coming next week." The fact that Cora brought this up showed her concern for Celia and also her attachment to Celia. That is a new feeling for Cora because she did not really like Celia in the beginning.

POSTSESSION TRAINING

Trainees Report on Their Work With the Children

Paul: Norm was very different. He allowed me to set limits. I kept him with me and didn't let him run around. He was a lot more verbal.

Ida: I felt we were back to square one. (James was absent last week) Even though he was running all over the room, there was a lot of stuff he liked. He liked kisses.

Leader: (To Ida) How did you feel about yourself, the way you worked with him?

Ida: In the beginning, I thought I was bombing out; but once I got into it, I felt I was very present.

Leader: After a child misses a session, they nearly always go back to some old behavior at first. I saw you take charge. For example, when he was in his house (a cardboard box) all covered up, you kept contact by saying, "Knock, knock, are you in there? Could you stick your hand out so I can see?" I also saw him take a stick and hit you.

Ida: I told him not to, but I didn't physically stop him.

Leader: You need to stop him physically. Any physical violence, you stop instantly. He's probably been beaten himself, which is why he does it to you. Because he was absent last week, he didn't see you. His behavior shows that. He missed you. In Circle Time during the cradling, when we sang the Rock-A-Bye Baby song and you were holding him with the blanket over him, I saw him be relaxed for a few minutes for the first time. I don't think he experiences his body relaxed like that very often.

Ida: He said, "This is stupid" and he wanted it off. So I took it off, and then he looks around and sees everyone else is doing it so he wants it on. He said he wanted to do the Gingerbread like you all were doing, and then you did do it to him. When he was cookin', he said he wasn't done. (He heard Celia say that and copied her.) I liked what I did with him.

Leader: Will you pick out someone and tell them that?

Ida: (To Paul) I did like what I did with him today.

Leader: James is not only a very deprived child, but he is also very disturbed. (To Ida) I hand it to you for hanging in there with him.

Cora: I have to admit initially I was dreading this hour, the half hour. My energy felt like I was drained, and she started off with a bang.

Group: (Laughs)

Cora: Celia did a lot of running around and running away at first. I took her over to the sink and did the foot washing. Then she calmed down. She wanted to be cradled a lot today after we did the lotion and Slippery Hand game. She asked for that—the Slippery Hand game. Then she asked to be made into a Gingerbread Girl. Usually she wants me to hurry and bake her so I can eat her up, but today she just did not want to be done. "I'm not done yet, I'm not done yet." She lay there while I cradled her, and she was never done. (Little laugh) She told me I forgot to turn the oven on, and then she said, "I'm still not done." Then, when she heard it was Circle Time, she wanted to do the cradling first. First thing she said, "It's cradling time."

Leader: Today two children, Celia and Sam, asked for the cradling in Circle Time before I had hardly started the Hello part.

Paul: (To Leader) I saw Celia make a pouty look when you said Cradling Time, and then she relaxed.

Ned: Aretha was into it today. (Laughs) When you asked me what I liked best today, she answered.

Leader: I asked you first because I didn't think she would respond.

Ned: It shocked me, too. (Laughs) Yeah, I was very pleased today.

Leader: Were your earlier concerns unfounded?

Ned: I was surprised.

Leader: Then what she does in your classroom, where she has to share you with other children, does not always reflect what she does here when she has you all to herself.

Ned: She kissed me. She kissed me on the hand. I mean the real thing. I was happy. (Laughs)

Leader: She never kissed you before?

Ned: No. She just blew on me.

Leader: That's really neat. Kissing is a learned behavior from contact with others. She's learning to use her mouth and lips as organs of communication—dialogue through touch.

Ned: When she threw these paper towels at me, I would say, "Give me one." Then she'd give me more kisses. She washed my face, too. (Laughs) She was playing with the water. She started washing her face, and then I tried to go around and wash her face. She didn't want it, but she washed mine.

Leader: For her to do anything is great.

Ned: Yeah. I let her do it.

Leader: Do you want to tell someone how you feel about your work?

Ned: (With a big grin on his face) *It was awesome.* I'm completely satisfied. (To Paul) I'm completely satisfied. (Looks embarrassed) *I'm so happy, I can't talk.* She also started scratching me and slapping me.

Leader: I'd stop that by just taking her hand and have her hand touch you gently.

Ned: I did.

Clara: Sam was asking a lot more from me today. As soon as I put lotion on his toes, he said, "Go in between my toes." He asked me to touch his face and do the Gingerbread Cookie.

302

Leader: Did he say, "Touch my face"?

Clara: He'd put his face up so I could touch it. He would give me a raspberry, and I would rock back and give him a raspberry. Then I'd give him a kiss, and then he'd do it to me twice. He put a raspberry on my cheek. He initiated that. There were a lot more times when I was picking him up and holding him that he really let go. That was nice. For whatever reason, in Circle Time, he started scratching my face. I said, "You can touch my face, but you can't scratch it."

Leader: So you helped him distinguish the difference. Sometimes I don't think they know the difference. Also, when they hit or scratch, they feel the energy in their body and that feels good. Then again, this bit of aggression may represent some discomfort or that they don't know what to do.

Clara: Sam said, "I'm going to scratch you." He went like this (demonstrated), but he didn't scratch me. He said, "In Circle Time, I'm bad." He asked me to cradle him all the way to the cradling time in the circle, and then when we did it, he didn't want to. He asked me why I came. I said, "I like playing with you."

Leader: He asked you why you come?

Clara: Yes. He said, "Why do you come?" Sam said he didn't like it. He didn't like to play. He doesn't like to come. He wasn't going to come back. (Laughs)

Cora: One of the things Celia asked me was I coming back next week. I said, "I'll be here next week, will you?" She said, "No, you can have Sue." (Gill, Sue's partner, was absent and the Leader took Sue in Circle Time.)

Before Christmas, Celia asked me if I had any kids. I said I had a daughter. This week she wanted to know if I make her into a Gingerbread Girl. Do I do this with her? Do I do that with her? She wanted me to take her a cookie (from our snacks at the end of Circle Time). She asked about my Martin Luther pin. Does that man sleep with me? I said, "No." She said, "Well, does he sleep with another woman, then?"

Ned: I knew as soon as she walked in she was going to do things—the way she looked right at me even though she didn't respond with smiles or words. Aretha talked a lot today. All the time I was holding her, she was talking about her brother and sister who used to be in my class. All of a sudden, she said, "I'm going to tell my Daddy on you." I said, "What are you going to tell him?" She said, "He goes with Big Mary. I'm going to tell my other Daddy." I said, "Oh, so you got two Daddies?" She said, "Yup."

303

Cora: Celia couldn't understand why I had only one child. She said, "Do you have a little boy, too?" I said, "No, I only have one baby." She said, "Why?"

Ned: Very seldom are any of our children "only children." They average four or five with different fathers.

Gill: (Was absent today) Sue only came for Circle Time.

Leader: (Held Sue in her lap as she led the Circle) I think it's important to take time to own your own feelings and share how you felt about your work.

Clara: I was really touched; I felt good about it.

Paul: (To Clara) You work very naturally.

Leader: (To Paul) Did you tell someone about your work?

Paul: It was a struggle today.

Leader: Pick out someone, and tell them that it was a struggle.

Paul: (To Ida) You understood that it was a struggle. (Others laugh)

Cora: Even though I dreaded it in the beginning, it worked out well. I could see the caretaker in her.

Leader: That's why it's important that she experiences herself being taken care of by you.

Cora: She fights it but she knows she loves it.

Clara: Sometimes I'll be doing nothing, and Sam will say, "Ow, you bit me." If I say, "No, I didn't," he'll keep doing it. If I say, "Oh, I'm sorry," he'll say, "Okay" and stop.

Ned: *It was so wonderful, I can't talk about it.*

Ida: Sue is a whole different person. She couldn't say she was sad in Circle Time because Gill wasn't there.

Leader: Children first experience feelings with their bodies. Only later can they give them form through verbal language.

Ned, the Teacher, Talks About the Children (All Age Four)

Sue. Sue was premature and a cocaine baby. Since birth, she has lived with her grandparents, who are good to her. Grandfather speaks highly of her.

Celia. She lives with her mother in the "Projects." She has a younger brother age three. You can count on her in class. She talks. She's not wild. She's outgoing. She asks questions, and she looks after the other kids. Her mother and Aretha's mother are sisters.

Aretha. She is the youngest of several children, and her mother is pregnant. They also live in the Projects. She was very quiet, but she began to look at me when she got off the bus, and so I wanted to work with her. She was a challenge to me.

Sam. He has a lot of aunts. He lives with his mother, but his grandmother looks out for him. She doesn't approve of the mother's boyfriend. His grandmother cares about him. He's the smartest kid in class. I use him a lot to help the other kids. Once in a while he gets stubborn and won't do anything. He puts everything in his mouth—shoes, socks—while watching TV. He talks about his cousin.

Norm. He lives in a foster home. He has been in several foster homes. He has a little brother whom he looks after. He's real bossy. He likes to stand and walk around the toys and say, "I want that." He's open in class. He asks questions. The foster home wanted him in the DP group. Norm is very different in the DP group—silent and depressed. Not only does he not initiate anything, but he has a hard time accepting any attention. He's a totally different child in DP. Amazing!

James. He lives in the Projects and has a younger brother. There are no doors or windows on their building. The mother said, "How can I keep my kids off drugs in this place?" James is a caring kid. He's real open in the classroom. He shares with the others. When his mother visited school at Christmas, she never looked at him until time to go. Again, like Norm, James' behavior in the DP group is very different from his behavior in school. In DP he is very tense, hyper, and has to be moving his body constantly.

THE CHILDREN IN CIRCLE TIME

The children were very noisy and active. They all wanted to talk at the same time, and they all had something they wanted to do. As the Leader, I got them together by having them follow me doing the hand movements to music. They all did it, including Aretha, who usually doesn't. In the middle of doing this, Celia said, "It's cradle time." I said, "almost" and went on pointing to individual children, commenting on how well they were moving their hands.

Leader: Look at Aretha. She's doing it.
  Sam: I did it.
  Celia: Did I do it?
Leader: (Laughs) Yes, you did it.
  Ned: Aretha wants to still do it.
Leader: (To Aretha) Okay. You are the Leader.
Aretha: (Leads by putting her hands under Ned's hands and pushing them up. Other children follow her.)

Sam: Can we do the Rock-A-Bye Baby? (While Celia was in the middle of doing a flip)

Clara: (To Sam) Watch Celia.

Leader: (To Cora) Help her stand up and take a bow.

Sam: (To Clara) Make me a gingerbread cookie.

Chil-
dren: (All the other children had to be made into a gingerbread cookie, including James, Norm, and Aretha. The Leader did it to Sue because Gill was absent.)

Sam: (To Sue, after the Leader finished eating her up) Did you get all eaten up?

Sue: (Looks at Sam and laughs)

Leader: It's cradle time. Get your blankets. (The children loved being wrapped in a blanket as they were held while Rock-A-Bye Baby was sung—their ritual—and it had to be the same each time. When the Leader sang Brahms Lullaby, they wanted Rock-A-Bye Baby played from a recording.) Before we have snacks, tell me what you liked best today.

Ned: (Before Ned could respond, Aretha does. Aretha makes a raspberry on Ned's cheek.)

James: Nothing. (His answer)

Ida: I liked best what he did just now. He took my hands and looked at them. Then he showed me where he had a little sore, which I tried to kiss (kissing it)—I got it.

Sam: Making a gingerbread cookie.

Clara: I liked it best when I put a raspberry on Sam so we could rock back, and then I had to put a kiss on so we could rock back up.

Celia: She made me into a gingerbread girl, and then I was done.

Cora: I liked it best when she was in the oven, but she would never get done. I had to cook her for a long time.

Norm: (Whispers and points to Paul)

Leader: Turn around and tell him.

Norm: Nothing.

Leader: Was it when he washed your feet?

Norm: (Nods yes)

Leader: Turn around and tell him, "I liked it when you washed my feet."

Norm: (Says it, but it's barely audible)

Paul: I liked it when you showed me some kissable places.

Leader: (To Paul) Can you find one right now?

Paul: I think I see one right there. (Kisses him on the cheek)

Norm: (Turns his other cheek for it to be kissed)

Leader: Oh, there's another one. (Paul kisses it) (To Sue) You were only here
for Circle Time. What did you like best in Circle Time?
Sue: Ned.
Leader: Turn and tell him.
Sue: (Whispers) I like you.
Ned: I like you, too, Sue. (Said very warmly)

After the children and others left, Ned carried my tape recorder to the car
and spent a few moments with me. He said, "I felt real skilled today. I felt real
confident in myself today." I said that I could see that, and I was glad. I asked him
if he would like a hug. He said, "Yes," and I could tell that he liked it. He said to
me as I got in my car, "Drive carefully."

Ned's pleasure and excitement over discovering this new part of himself
touched me. He is a young teacher and not a therapist. It was moving for me to
experience this new place with him. It was an "I-Thou" experience for both of us.
I felt the energy connecting us, and neither of us had to do anything. Each of us
was simply present.

COMMENTS

Session 8 shows another shift in the children's behavior toward relating
more intimately with their adult partners and toward experiencing themselves as
more real. They have a sense of having an "I." Their behavior is directed from
the inside out rather than from the outside in. We will look at what the adults did
that made this difference in the children's behavior and what the Leader did with
the trainees that enabled them to provide the children with what they needed.

HOW THE LEADER WORKED WITH THE TRAINEES

The trainees began the Presession by asking questions about their children.
Paul began by questioning the Leader's suggestion that he ask Norm if he
brought him any kisses. He said, "I was conflicted about doing that because I
didn't think the child was there to give to me."

The Leader tries to answer a question by providing the trainee with the experience he needs to be able to answer it for himself. That means directing the
trainee to experience a relationship—to be in relation to himself and to his child.
As with the children, the Leader starts with where the trainee is.

To begin with, Paul had a difficult child. Norm, his second child, was very
quiet, depressed, and offered little to which Paul could respond. Tom, his first
child, had a mind of his own and wouldn't do what Paul wanted. Paul said he

307

liked Norm, but Norm did nothing—a very different behavior from his acting out in the classroom.

Paul himself tends to look at therapy in terms of tasks rather than as a relationship process. To do that, he has to get in touch with himself. He has a hard time giving himself credit for doing something well, doing something new, or enjoying himself. Therefore, the Leader dealt with Paul's question by having him relive the scene with Norm.

When the Leader answered Paul's question by asking him to describe what it was like for him to do it (ask Norm for kisses), Paul discovered that not only did Norm respond, but he, too, enjoyed this contact. Paul's enjoyment is experienced by the child and says to the child, "You are a fun person to be with." This interaction was healing for both adult and child.

The effect of the Leader's work with Paul is shown in Paul's approach to Norm during the Circle Time. The Leader uses the Circle Time to coach the trainee and to continue the process started with the adult in the Presession—for example, when Paul answered the question, "What did you like best today?" by saying to Norm, "I liked it when you showed me some kissable places." The Leader invited him to experience this act in the here and now—"Can you find one (a kissable place) right now?" Norm responded by turning his other cheek to be kissed after he allowed the first kiss.

In the Postsession training, Paul said, "It was a struggle today." Paul did two new things today. He set limits, and he provided contact for his child—both necessary for a child's growth. That is hard work. It is not easy to do. He was also experiencing himself in a new way: feeling pleasure and enjoyment in his contact with his child and feeling pleased with himself that he could set limits without feeling he's "restraining" a child. In other words, Paul is experiencing himself in a new way, and "It's a struggle." It is the quality of the energy experienced by the adult that makes the difference in the child. The Leader helped Paul get in touch with his own alive, inner self, and that quality was passed on to his child.

At the end, Paul could answer his own question, "Why do you ask a child if he has any kissable places?" The answer: that is one way to give the child something to respond to, and that is one way the adult can experience the child and help the child experience the presence of the adult. The child experiences himself doing something that results in contact and a touching relationship.

WHAT THE ADULTS DID WITH THE CHILDREN

The effect of the Leader's work with the trainees is reflected in the work they did with the children. All the trainees, in this session, did something to which their child could respond. In other words, from the moment the children entered the play space, the trainees made their presence felt by their child. The child could not get rid of her adult partner no matter what she did.

The trainees did this, not by making the child do or say anything specific or by telling her to do anything specific. Rather, they made their presence felt through seeing, noticing, touching, and inviting contact ("Did you bring any kissable places?").

Ida did not allow James to isolate himself by hiding in his "house." She was constantly present to him: "Are you in there? Stick your hand out so I can see you."

Cora responded at once to Celia's wild running around by taking her over to the sink and washing her feet. That contact resulted in an immediate change in Celia, who began to relate to Cora in ways she had never done before.

Ned said that when Aretha threw paper towels at him, he said, "Give me one" (a kiss). She gave him kisses—real kisses this time instead of just blowing on him. She, too, did things she had never done before.

Clara always did initiate contact with Sam. Now she is reaping the results as he is asking for touch in ways he never did before.

Gill was absent. Sue came only to the Circle Time.

THE EFFECT ON THE CHILDREN

All six children began showing behavior that normal children go through in the process of growth, albeit these children are doing it at a later age.

First, all the children showed this longing for, and enjoyment of, being held, cradled, and touched—the basic requirements for human development. Furthermore, these children communicated this need both nonverbally and verbally. For example, Celia asked for the touch in her request to be made into a "gingerbread girl." She also asked for a quiet cradling where she doesn't have to do anything—just to be held quietly in the arms of her partner. She kept saying, when in the oven, "I'm not done yet." To let herself be a receiver of nurturing care is a tremendous gain for a child like Celia, who feels she has to take care of others. To let someone else take charge so that she can be the receiver is very healing for her. It is also through the experience of being held in this quiet way that the child discovers her inner or core self because she is not distracted by outside events. Celia also asked, in Circle Time, to do the Cradle Time first.

Sam asked for more touch: "go between my toes, touch my face, do the gingerbread cookie." He also said in Circle Time, "It's cradling time." Aretha, who did almost nothing in the beginning, began initiating contact with Ned, giving him real kisses instead of just blowing on him. She would not let him wash her face, but she would wash his face. Norm, at Paul's invitation, also gave kisses and asked for them. For a few moments in Circle Time, James allowed himself to be relaxed during the cradling. All of the children asked to have the gingerbread cookie done to them in Circle Time. Sue loved having the Leader make her into a gingerbread cookie. The Gingerbread Cookie Game is a total body massage.

Second, like Mira (Chapter 5), these children had to be allowed to be wherever they are developmentally before they could move on. The first stage was allowing the cradling and the touching. The second stage was their use of the body for communication, as did Mira. Sam said to Clara, "Ow, you bit me." She did not bite him any more than I "hurt" Mira when she said I was "hurting" her. It's simply a form of body language. Like Mira, these children would hit or scratch the adult. In doing this, the child is not usually conveying anger but feeling something and not knowing what to do with it. Hitting does make them feel the energy in their body. They may be trying out what was done to them or what they were forbidden to do. I do not allow children to hit, slap, or scratch me. I stop this action physically with my hands, saying, "No hitting," etc. I do listen to what they have to say, but *usually* I do not interpret their body language because it's not meaningful to them at this stage.

Third, as with Mira, these children added verbal language to body language. For a child who didn't talk at all or make contact, Aretha's change was dramatic. She talked about her siblings and said to Ned, "I'm going to tell my Daddy on you." She answered his questions and gave a picture of the many people who live in her home. She had total trust in him to come out with all this family information.

Sam and Celia used verbal language to get information about the world from their adult partners. They asked "Why" questions: "Why do you come" (here to play with us)? Celia also asked Cora why she has only one kid and does she do the things with her kid that she does with Celia. She asked about the men in her household and who sleeps with whom. Sam was the most advanced, both intellectually and developmentally. He used verbal language to assess his own behavior ("I'm bad in Circle Time"). Very unusual.

Celia and Sam were also advanced in their awareness of and alertness to the world about them. Although they did not verbalize it, the break over the holidays made them aware that this program may not go on forever. (The children were told in the beginning that it would go so many sessions.) In Session 7, the one following the break, Celia said in Circle Time, "I'm not coming next time." In Session 8, Gill's absence aroused more awareness, reflected in Celia's remarks, "Are *you* coming back next week?" Cora said, "Yes. Will you?" Celia said, "No. You can have Sue." When Clara told Sam she came because she liked to play with him, he said, "I don't like to play. I don't like to come. I'm not coming."

Last is the growth in these children's ability to relate to each other and to enjoy each other, as demonstrated in their behavior in Circle Time. They pay attention to each other and copy each other. In the hand movements to music, they had the experience of being both a leader and a follower. When Aretha wanted to be a leader again, they all cooperated and let her do it. They responded more to the Leader and wanted her to see them perform. Celia asked the Leader, "Did I do it?" Sam stated, "I did it."

The children influence each other. For example, when Sam wanted to be made into a gingerbread cookie, all the others had to have it done to them, too. During the cradling, James said he didn't want the blanket on him; but when he looked around and saw all the others with blankets over them, he wanted it then, too. James had a hard time letting himself be nurtured.

One of the most charming moments was the interaction between Sam and Sue following the Leader having made Sue into a gingerbread girl. The Leader ended this play with "eating her all up," which she enjoyed. Sam was watching. He looked at her and said very warmly, "Did you get *all* eaten up?" Sue looked at him and just laughed.

THE EFFECT ON THE TRAINEES

When the children respond to their partners as they did in Session 8, the adults feel seen, too. There's a connection between child and adult—a flow of quiet energy between them. The child lets the adult in. The adults sometimes experience this as the child lets them love them.

Clara and Ned experienced this contact. They felt really touched by their respective child. Ned used the word "awesome" and said he had no words for this feeling: "I am so happy, I can't talk."

What is going on here is that this connection with the child stimulates the adult to experience her own inner self. She experiences this quality of love as inside her as it was when she was a child. Her inside voice says, "You are lovable."

One psychiatrist said that when the therapist feels that she likes a child, then the child is ready for termination. As the Leader of this group, I felt this affection for Celia. She was so alive and so present. She stated clearly where she was. She had a beautiful voice and was very creative. She had the quality of wholeness. She was present with you. I had this feeling of love toward her. I enjoyed her, and I'm sure I showed it in the way I looked at her and in the tone of my voice. I let her see my enjoyment of her. It is the experiencing of this quality of presence and connection from some adult that heals the child.

SESSIONS 10 THROUGH 13

Up to now, the trainees have been learning how to provide the children with what they need to become attached, that is, to relate to their partners as healthy children do with their parents. The children, in turn, responded by allowing themselves to be touched, seen, and held. In addition, the children created activities and games to get touched and seen. They asked for the touch. They have become goal-directed, organized children. That is Stage One.

The children's growth toward being organized and speaking up for what they need calls for a different approach from the trainees: namely, to back off from being so active (as they needed to be in the beginning) and just observe. They need to respond more to the children's behaviors and do less initiating. The children are able to do the initiating. Now they need someone on whom they can practice being on their own. This is the task for the trainees in Stage Two.

SESSION 10

Presession. To help the adults who had difficult children and who had a hard time staying present, the Leader had them focus their attention on feeling their hands when they touch. The Leader had them practice this in pairs, one being the toucher and the other being the one touched. They were instructed to feel their hands touching and to say to the other what they feel. This helped them be more present regardless of what the child was doing.

Paul was eager to share his weekend experience with his grandchildren.

Paul: I recognized that I dealt with them very differently than I used to. I mean, noticing them came out automatically. I was real pleased about that. That's my whole big thing. (Laughs)

Leader: Would you pick out someone and ask them to see how pleased you are with yourself?

Paul: (To Gill) Do you see how pleased I am with myself?

Gill: You look glowing.

Leader: You were surprised how automatically it came.

Paul: I was surprised how quickly I recognized it.

Leader: What was it like sharing that with us?

Paul: I couldn't think what category to put it under. I was happy about it. I knew last night I wanted to. It just felt good. It was good.

Leader: What did it do to the experience to share it?

Paul: It underscored it.

Leader: You are experiencing yourself in a new way—like having fun.

Paul: Yes.

SESSION 11: THE BEGINNING OF THE TERMINATION

The trainees were informed that today we would have a brief circle first to tell the children that, "We play today and two more times, and then we have to say Goodbye." The Goodbye part is as important as the Hello part. It is the Goodbye part that makes everyone appreciate their relationships. These children rarely, if ever, have the opportunity to prepare for an event because no one tells them or even seems to know ahead of time themselves. In Developmental Play, the children will have three sessions in which they can express their feelings and come to terms with the parting.

Presession Training

Ned: (Interrupts talking of group) I have something to say. Last week when you asked us how Developmental Play influenced our lives and all, and I didn't say anything, remember? Now I do want to say something. Working with kids, I'm always picking them up and touching them. When we first started, you know, I realized how much touch meant. But I see it more as an adult kind of subject in the way I treat my cousins and my girlfriend.

Leader: So how do you see yourself differently?

Ned: More sensitive, more caring. I express myself a hell of a lot more than I used to.

Leader: How is that for you?

Ned: (Loudly) Oh, it's good!

Leader: How was that to share it?

Ned: It felt good—a relief, I guess. What I was thinking but I didn't want to say it last week because I didn't want to be taken wrong, you know. (Laughs self-consciously)

Leader: Why afraid you'd be taken wrong?

Ned: I was thinking of touch. (Laughs) How I touch my girlfriend, you know, face and hands.

Leader: So sometimes it arouses sexual feelings in you.

Ned: Yeah (laughs), but to me it's more like caring. I can feel it more. I don't know. I'm a touchy, feeling kind. Yeah, before it was (?) and now I see it as much more caring and being sensitive. I wasn't thinking of it as sexual . . . I can just look at a kid's face, and I've always done it, but I see more. I see it differently now, and more caring and more sensitive. It makes me feel good. Like I'll walk around the staff here and put my arm around them and say, "How you doin'?" You know. It makes me feel good.

Leader: So you feel more open with others.

Cora: I was thinking how did Developmental Play help me with my daughter, and I thought how does it when you asked me. *When I touch her, I see more of her.* I am more aware of her. *I feel myself touching her.*

Ned: I respect Aretha more and others—their feelings—than I did. Before, I didn't give a shit.

Leader: I sense your excitement about the changes in yourself. It's wonderful for me to be a witness to that in you.

Ned: Thank you. I feel so much deeper, so much stronger inside me. I've always been big on loving and caring and all that stuff, but (loudly) now, Jesus—my God—like a whole different universe!

Leader: You're a different person.

Ned: Yeah, exactly! (Said loudly) I don't know. It excites me. It's like—I don't know. I have so much more respect and care for others.

Leader: Would you pick out someone here and say to them to see your new self in whatever way you want to say it?

Ned: (To Clara) See me.

Clara: I see you. It's like an awakening.

Leader: We have to get ready to see the children. How about you all closing your eyes and just say Hello to your self—maybe a new self. Just be with your body self, and you don't have to do anything.

Postsession Training

Leader: (To trainees) Take a moment now to see how you feel right now. How did you feel that you did with your child? How did you feel your child did?

Cora: I felt good with the interaction with Celia today. She let me cradle her a lot today. You know, I just held on to her. She wanted to be covered and for me to hold her while she let me cradle her. She was a little active during Circle Time. Something else I noticed. When you came over, she didn't want you to be with us, and that felt good. (Laughs)

Leader: This relationship is just private.

Cora: Just us.

Leader: I sensed that. Girl children at about this age develop this very private, intimate relationship with their mothers. It's as if they are the only ones in the world, and no one can intrude.

Cora: She called me Mommy a couple of times today.

Leader: Her getting burnt in baking her—whose idea was that?

Cora: I think it was hers. She said it's not done and it's cold and she wants to stay in the oven. One day she said she was burnt and I had to make her all over again.

Leader: What is she communicating to you with this body language?

Cora: She still wants that contact—"Do it again."

Leader: Did she say anything about her house again?

Cora: Yes, she did. "I'm not going home. I want to go home and go upstairs and play with my toys." I don't get any meaning out of her saying, "I'm not going home."

Leader: Today in Circle Time she said, "I want to go home." I think it has to do with telling them we stop after two more sessions. So they say it before the last session to prepare themselves.

Clara: Sam asked me if I was scared when I took him to wash his feet. We had this communication:

> Sam: Are you scared of me?
> Clara: No.
> Sam: Why aren't you coming back?
> Clara: Because we're going to be done . . .
> Sam: Ow! You hurt me. (Clara washing his feet)

Leader: That's another step in the child's growth. They express feelings and reactions with body language ("You hurt me.") They don't say what older and more mature children would say ("I'm mad" or "I'm sad.") It's best to let them say it in their language.

Clara: I was struggling today.

Leader: The whole group heard Sam say to Clara in Circle Time, *"I want you to come back."*

Gill: First thing Sue said when we went back to our corner, "Why are you not going to come back after two times?" I said, "Because the play time is over." Then she went back in her corner, and in the play she was more independent. When I tried to help her, she said, "I can do it myself." In Circle Time, when a couple of kids said, "I'm not coming back," she turned and said, "I'm coming back next time."

Paul: Norm said he was coming back.

Clara: When we sang the Goodbye song in the Circle Time and ended it with "See you next week," Sam added, "And one more time."

Leader: These comments show how well these children are organized and how important this program is to them. In this program, the children have the opportunity and the time to figure out what they are going to do

315

about the parting. In this program, they also have the opportunity and time to experience the loss and to deal with that loss. This is probably a new experience for them because I doubt if they have ever been told about an event ahead of time.

Clara: When you spoke to me in Circle Time, I felt so hurt. I thought I had been so bad and I realized that, "Oh, I'm not bad. She just told me what to do." I realize that's what I'm doing when I set limits—maybe that's what the kids feel. It was like this weight on my chest. If I feel that way, I think the kid's going to feel that way. That's why I'm having a hard time setting limits.

Leader: How are you feeling now?

Clara: I'm thinking I shouldn't feel that way.

Leader. But you are. Why don't you tell me?

Clara: (Long pause) I want to say I wasn't bad.

Leader: Want to hear my side?

Clara: (Long pause) Yes.

Leader: I wasn't saying you were bad. I was saying you don't have to be responsible for Circle Time.

Clara: I know, but you set limits for me.

Leader: How do you feel about me now?

Clara: Better.

Paul: I'm glad it's over today.

Cora: (To Paul) Norm was stubborn today. He didn't want to do anything. He pulled away.

Leader: I saw Norm as being more present today because he is actively resisting. He is *choosing* to resist, and that's very different from being passive and not doing anything, not caring, as he did before. He is watching what is going on.

Paul: Yes.

Leader: Norm is present. He's looking at everyone. When he does come out with something, it's because it comes from him and *he* wants to do it. He is not doing it because someone told him to do it. For example, in Circle Time when I asked him to do something, he said, "No." However, he spoke up on his own and said, *"I want my turn."*

Paul: I think he got upset when Aretha pulled everybody into the circle except him. She looked at him and then didn't invite him. His face changed. She looked at him, and he shook his head.

Leader: What is new here in Norm is an awareness of an inner self—a part of him that feels and sees and wants to be seen.

Cora: Celia will let me hold her in the cradling position in the one-to-one, but in Circle Time she faces the group so she can see everyone.

Leader: I would try to turn her around and say we cradle this way. With her eyes open looking at everyone and sometimes talking, she doesn't get the benefit of the cradling. She needs to learn to trust the group—that she will be okay with her eyes closed, just being with you. I invite you to try that.

Paul: I'm tired.

Leader: This is hard work, especially the Goodbye part, both for you as well as for your child. And you have to help your child say Goodbye. That's because this is a relationship process, and you are part of the relationship. *You have to say Goodbye, too.*

COMMENTS

Two events stand out in this session. First, witnessing Ned give birth to his new self was a very moving experience. In the actual sharing of his inner experiences, Ned became aware that he had a nurturing self. At that moment, it was as if the sky opened and he saw himself in an entirely new way—almost like a religious figure. It is very unusual for a young man in his early twenties to get in touch with this loving inner self. It is this quality of presence that is conveyed to the child, and it is this quality of presence that the child needs to experience her own inner self. It is this loving presence that he is in when he works with his child, Aretha, that accounts for her dramatic change.

Second, the announcement of the impending termination set into motion feelings and reactions that the children used to organize themselves in a very goal-directed way. The children responded in two ways: they increased the desire for touch, and they shifted into relating through language as well as through touch. In their verbal language, these children acted like normal children: asking why the adults are leaving; is it because the adults are afraid of them; suggesting that the children think that they have done something to make the adults leave. Sam said he wanted Clara "to come back." Sam reverted to body language when Clara told him about the termination ("Ow! You hurt me"). Some children said they are not coming back next time. Sue and Norm said they were coming back next week. Although it was hard for Paul to see, Norm was definitely coming out of his shell. In terms of new behavior, Norm and Aretha were the stars in this Circle Time.

These outbursts of talking show that these children have a backlog of experiences that they can utilize to organize themselves provided they are given the time to do it and provided they have a relationship with someone who listens and relates to them.

The announcement of the impending termination also had an impact on the trainees, felt in the amount of energy they had. They said they were "tired," it was "a struggle today," and they were glad when the "hour was over." The children's responses, which were all attachment responses to them, are forcing the trainees to deal with the Goodbye also.

SESSION 12

Presession Training

Paul: I was surprised at how much the children reacted last week (session 11).

Leader: Last week you saw how the announcement of the impending termination mobilized these children to make use of their new sense of independence and their ability to empower themselves as resources for dealing with the upcoming Goodbye. They all demonstrated that they have an inner self, a core self that organizes and guides them. They can, and want to, do things for themselves. (To Gill) When you played in the water with Sue, she said loudly, "This is my water" (said by a child who couldn't get any words out in the beginning). (To Paul) Norm, who never says anything, spoke up twice saying, "I want my turn" and "I'm coming back." (To Cora) Celia is creating her own form of the Gingerbread Cookie to get her needs met. (To Clara) Sam said to you, "I want you to come back." In other words, the children are creating their own worlds—new ones for them.

Cora: What do we do when the child doesn't want our play time to end?

Leader: You could suggest in the one-to-one that they might play these games with their parents.

Paul: These parents are so little available. I don't know if these parents have it to give to them.

Leader: In the interviews that you're going to do with these parents at the end of the program, I think you'll find new things are happening already.

Cora: I wouldn't be surprised at all if the parents said they hadn't noticed any difference.

Paul: Again, there is so much deprivation in the environment, in their houses. They're not going to be emotionally attached because that hurts too much. Norm has been in several foster homes.

Leader: These children are already attached to you trainees. How much of this ability to become emotionally attached is transferred to their parents we will have to wait and see from the parents' responses in the interviews to be done next week.

The Leader moves the trainees out of their heads into experiencing themselves. She demonstrates with Cora to illustrate again that you begin with a child by noticing and touching her.

Leader: (To Cora) Hello, Cora. I see you brought your hands today and you smiled, and when you smiled I saw your teeth. You must have brushed your teeth because they look so white. (Holding her hand) Your hand is so warm.

Cora: Your hand is cold.

Leader: You're good at saying how my hand is. You felt it. And you got all your fingers (touching each one), and now you're here looking at me—so, Hello. What was that like?

Cora: It felt good. I didn't have to do anything. I knew you were seeing me, and it felt comfortable.

Leader: (To group) Your reaction to this interaction?

Paul: You were right there.

Leader: Doing this with Cora helped me to focus also. I had no idea what I was going to do. I used my eyes first and said the first thing that I saw. (To Cora) I took your hand and said how it felt. Then you, Cora, said something and I responded to your cue. Doing this with you, Cora, made me feel focused and centered. Now I'd like each of you to find a partner and practice this Hello.

Following this exercise, the Leader initiated the Hello Circle Time, each taking turns singing to the person next to them.

Leader: How are you now?

Group: Present. We feel more together.

Cora: I want to say something about getting into my quiet place. Doing that means not listening to my critic that's telling me how I should respond and what I should be doing. So that's what it means to me.

Postsession Training

The Postsession of session 12 was devoted to viewing the previous session—session 11—which was videotaped. This was the session in which the children and the adults were told that the program would end after two more sessions. The Leader had each trainee look at her part of the tape and say how she thought she did and how she thought her child did. What did the trainee learn about herself? The Leader first asked the group what changes they noticed in the children.

Cora: The touch and the cradling.

Leader: Yes, and something was added.

Paul: The attachment and the cooperation between the children.

Leader: Yes, there was a dialogue.

Cora: Celia is asking for the touching. She's not fighting it anymore.

Leader: There's one other—the enjoyment and the pleasure these children experience. That experience of pleasure comes from feeling their bodies being touched and from the way you touch and the pleasure you get in doing the touching and seeing. In other words, it's okay to allow yourself to experience the beauty of working with these children.

Cora: (After viewing her part of the videotape) Celia invited touch many times. She asked me to make a gingerbread girl. She asked me to cook her slow. Then she asked me to cry. When we first started doing this, she'd never be done, and I'd say, "Oh, I'm so hungry and I want you to be done," and so now she's saying, "Cry." Then she said, "I'm cold," and then she's ready for me to eat her. "Eat me. Do it again."

Leader: Look at all the times she invites you in. It's important that you see this, feel this.

Cora: I see the love that's there, too.

Leader: Would you choose someone and tell them how you feel about your work?

Cora: I feel good about Celia. I see a lot of growth in her and in myself.

Clara: I was smiling watching that. (Cora's tape)

Cora: She wasn't fighting me. She was accepting me. I actually see her smile. She looks like she's enjoying it.

Leader: Her laughter is quite loud. For a child to hear her own laughter is quite tremendous. In doing that, Celia feels her aliveness. She has a voice in the world. (To Cora) You did another thing. You said, "Come on. You can do it louder." Then you put your cheek against hers, and you sat there a few minutes really being quiet so she had time to feel your contact. After that, she reached up and touched your face. So there was a quiet touch, and she gave it back. Your work had rhythm. You did it loudly, and you did it softly.

Ned: (After viewing his part of the tape) I'm pleased. It was successful.

Leader: What did you do to make it that way?

Ned: I don't know. (Laughs) I don't know.

Leader: You impinged yourself on her all the time so that she felt your presence. Whatever she did, you made her experience it with you. You were part of her experience. You kept guiding her. Her laughter was fabulous.

320

Ned: I intruded more in the hand washing when I was taking the soap off. She (Aretha) gets real funny about that. She won't let me go in there and wash her face, but if I say, "Let me get the soap off," she will. That was kind of a first. She didn't fight me after that.

Gill: (After watching her tape. Gill and Sue were playing with water in the sink. Gill had her hands in the water, also. Suddenly Sue looks up and says, in a loud voice, "Hey, that's my water.")

I didn't even remember her saying that, so I'm glad I've got this on film. (Gill's voice here was also strong and clear; in the beginning, you could barely hear her.)

Leader: Did you hear your own voice just now, how strong it is?

Gill: Not until you mentioned it.

Leader: What is the significance of what Sue did?

Gill: She's showing independence—separating from me—showing she can do it herself.

Leader: Also notice the strength of her voice when she said it.

Cora: And her facial expression there.

Leader: (Replays that scene)

Gill: I feel I'm hovering (laughs) over her. It was wonderful to see her take charge and speak up for herself. I loved hearing it.

Leader: Well, you were in there with her, so she had something to resist. If you hadn't been active, she wouldn't have had anything to resist.

Gill: The confidence in that voice when she said it. Great!

Leader: For a child who didn't have any voice in the beginning—for her to come out and say loudly, "This is mine"—that's quite remarkable.

Paul: (After watching his tape. Norm is looking at the microphone: "What's this?" Paul: You going to talk? What are you going to say in the microphone? Taking his hand, "Pull hard, that's it. Now come back. How hard can you pull? Wow, that's strong! Can you pull back now?" Every time Norm came close in this game, Paul hugged him.) I was ready to have him go and play in traffic by then. (Little laugh)

Clara: Sam and I were like that once. (Being supportive of Paul)

Gill: Norm's smile was so real. He was enjoying it, whatever it was you were feeling. He was enjoying it.

Leader: (To others) What did you notice Paul doing? What did you notice Norm doing?

Cora: I noticed Paul turned it into a game where he pulled Norm into him.

Leader: How would you have felt if you had been Paul?

Gill: Tired. Exhausted.

Cora: Frustrated.

Leader: (To Paul) You were very skilled in what you did, and it was hard work. There wasn't one minute that you had to yourself because he was doing something you had to attend to. There wasn't time for you to be in your head. You said, "Pull, and now can you pull yourself?" What you constantly did was to give Norm something to respond to. You gave him a direction. ("Pull. Now come back.") There was a rhythm to it and moments in which he enjoyed it.

Paul: Yes. There were moments that he enjoyed.

Leader: Where were they?

Paul: Mostly when I was bringing him back, when I caught him and rolled him up in my arms and hugged him.

Leader: You cradled him in your arms and your face was close to his, and these were the moments where he smiled and his body relaxed.

Paul: Yes.

Leader: You had a nice flow. You didn't hold him in a vise. You hugged him and then let him go. You had a rhythm. You tried to make it comfortable for him. He wanted to pull, so you let him pull. Then you pulled him up close, and then you let him go. Then you turned him around. There was a constant moving, and you were in charge the whole time. You were paying attention to him. Your reaction to what I just said?

Paul: I feel impressed that I did it.

Leader: And you weren't abusing him.

Clara: Did you know you were so skilled as Vi just said?

Paul: No.

Clara: (After looking at her tape. Sam was telling her what he wanted and where he was, both with words and with his body. He wanted his feet washed, to which Clara did not respond. He put his thumb in his mouth—Clara pulled it out. He said, "I want to lie on the mat," pushing her away. Clara pulled him up, held him, and kissed him all over.)

Leader: (Called her attention to what she was doing and shared with her how that would feel if that were done to her.)

Clara: I did what you told me to do, and now you're telling me that's wrong. (Very angry; crying)

Leader: I was trying to help you see that Sam is in a different place. My intent was not to make you feel wrong.

Clara: (Very angry) That is easy for you to say. (Calming herself) What I needed to do was use my own intuition. Instead of grabbing him and bringing him to me, I should have let him do what he was doing.

Leader: So what would you do now?

Clara: I would let him be before I brought him back to me.

Leader: Where are you now?

Clara: I was in a lot of pain. I feel proud that I could do this.

Leader: I feel proud of you, too.

COMMENTS

The training sessions in session 12 were devoted to looking at and reviewing what happened in session 11, at which time the children were told the number of times left to play in this group. The children's behavior in session 11 has to be seen, in part at least, as a reflection of their ability to handle the stress of having to part and separate themselves from an intimate relationship—a relationship in which they got some of the things they needed in order to mature, maybe for the first time. The video recording of the previous week's session also showed the reaction of the trainees to having to say Goodbye. The Postsession was used to have the trainees look at their work on the tape and to respond to what they saw.

The children's reaction to the impending termination was reported and assessed in session 11. All the children showed new skills and new behavior in dealing with the upcoming ending. They did extremely well considering where they came from in the beginning.

Here we will focus on the trainees' reaction to the ending as it was demonstrated in the way they worked with their child as seen in the videotaped session 11.

Just as the children have to deal with their attachment to the trainee, the trainee has to deal with and own her attachment to her child. Otherwise, there is nothing for the trainee to say Goodbye to.

Through the termination process and the responses of closeness from their child, the trainees become aware of the quality of their relationship with their child. Through their Goodbye approach to their child, the trainees often relive their own childhood experiences relating to parting and thereby become aware of a new part of themselves.

We will begin with Paul. After looking at his work on the tape, Paul laughingly summed up his experience with, "I was ready to have him go and play in traffic by then." Paul's statement shows that he dealt with the Goodbye issue by distancing himself from feeling connected to his child and distancing himself from acknowledging his own skill in dealing with a difficult child. Even looking at himself on the tape, he could not see his skill until it was pointed out by the Leader and others in the group. All he genuinely felt was "a struggle."

Anyone looking at the tape could see that it was hard work—hard, physical energy as well as emotional energy. However, it was just the intensity of Paul's energy that this child, Norm, felt and that changed Norm's behavior. Norm felt really cared for. He could not deny Paul's presence even though Paul, himself, was out of touch with the value of what he did and his accomplishment.

In looking at her work on the tape, Cora, who didn't want Celia for her child in the beginning, showed in her work that she felt connected to Celia and that she enjoyed her. This was expressed in her statement, "I see love there. I see a lot of growth in her and in myself."

Cora's work on the tape showed her growth in her ability to move away from her demanding behavior that Celia do this or that and to see the playfulness in this child. It was through playful touching games that Celia communicated her needs and through them, she would let Cora give to her. In these games, Cora became a participant instead of an authority figure. For example, in the "Gingerbread Girl" game, Cora added her own spontaneous responses ("Oh, I'm so hungry, and I want you to be done.") Celia, in turn, accepts and uses this fantasy of Cora's when she said to her, "Cry. I want you to cry." And Cora would pretend to cry.

This little excerpt of the interaction between Cora and Celia is an excellent example of how the concrete touching dialogue provides the conditions needed for the emergence of abstract symbolic thinking. That, in turn, leads to relating through language and fantasy.

In looking at his tape, Ned became even more aware of his love for his child, Aretha. He said he was "pleased" with his work. He saw how well he was in tune with the rhythm and energy of this child. He helped her feel seen and touched in a way that was acceptable to her. If one thing didn't work, he would try another, always being guided by the child. For example, when she initiated washing her face, she didn't want Ned to do it; but when he said, "Let me get the soap off," she allowed him to touch her. He saw how her face and her laughter (which was very new) expressed the pleasure she felt being with him. There is definitely a relationship between this child and her therapist (trainee). When she is with Ned, she feels "being-withed." When Ned is with her, he feels the love inside him.

The videotape shows that the children of Paul, Ned, and Cora are working at the Attachment Stage. For the children to master this stage and move on, the adults working with them must also experience their emotional connection with them.

The children of Gill and Clara are working at Stage Two—the Separation Stage—in which the child empowers herself to do things on her own. At this stage, the child does not need the adult to provide all the structure. The child can and wants to create her own agenda for the day. This striving for autonomy was demonstrated on the tape by both Sue and Sam. At this stage, the child needs support to do things on her own.

Gill said that she learned a lot from watching herself with Sue on the tape. First, she said she didn't remember Sue saying, "Get your hands out of here. This is my water" (when they were playing in the sink). Second, she thought it was wonderful that Sue said it, especially the firmness and the loudness with which she said it. Everyone in the room heard her. Gill said she was pleased.

Where was Gill during the session that she didn't remember this remarkable shift in Sue's behavior? Gill said, "I was in my head trying to figure it out. I wasn't present. I was trying to do it right. I was afraid if I just let it flow, it would be more her stuff. I was aware of her voice being strong—very strong. If I had one word to describe her, it would be confident. It left me a little confused and not sure-footed. I didn't have fun last week. I felt like I was in my head trying to do it right. By my not having fun and my not being able to let go and be present, I'm also more aware of just being—what it means to be. I had to experience not being present to learn how to be present."

Gill used the word "hovering" to describe her behavior seen on the videotape. Gill was working with Sue as if she were in Stage One. Gill said she didn't think Sue should be doing her own "stuff," and Sue was doing her "stuff" when she was studying her hands as if seeing them for the first time. She had such joy on her face. Gill saw how she distracted Sue from this experience by calling her attention to her feet. Like Paul, Gill dealt with the Goodbye process by not being present and not feeling connected to her child. From that place, Gill could not recognize Sue's autonomous behavior—her "stuff." Gill, however, assessed her new awareness as a learning experience.

The videotape is a very valuable tool for helping the adults get a new experience of themselves in their work with a child. It is a different experience from being in the interaction itself. Gill said she was glad she saw the film because it gave her a new experience of her child. However, if the trainee is not able to experience her own presence, she is not apt to experience herself being present from viewing the tape. This was true of Paul. It was also true of Clara.

Clara's work with Sam, as shown on her tape, demonstrated the same issue: namely, that Clara was working with Sam as if he were still in Stage One when he had clearly communicated that he had moved to Stage Two. For example, Sam, in pushing Clara away, said he wanted to lie down and he put his thumb in his mouth. Clara did not allow him to do this. She took his thumb out of his mouth, picked him up, and kissed him all over.

In the beginning, Sam needed to be noticed and picked up and held. As shown in the reports, Sam learned to love this contact and often asked for the cradling. Clara was very skilled in providing the cradling. At this point, however, at the Goodbye time, Sam simply wanted some space by himself to get in touch with himself separate from Clara and at the same time be in her presence. He needed his therapist simply to be a witness rather than a participant.

Like Gill, Clara was not aware of her clingingness to her child even when she looked at the tape. Clara's energy was focused on pleasing the Leader and doing it "right." From that place, it would have been impossible for her to be present. Only after expressing her anger and sharing her pain could she allow herself to see what she was doing on the tape. Only then did she feel that she could allow her own intuition to guide her, that she could do what felt right to her. Like some others, Clara dealt with the first phase of the separation by staying in the Attachment Stage (where her child was not) and by not being present.

In summary, you have seen and perhaps experienced what it's like to be a Leader of a group of trainees who are beginning the process of saying Goodbye for their child and for themselves. You have seen and perhaps experienced what it would be like to be a trainee helping a child say Goodbye. You have seen and perhaps experienced what it would be like to be a child having to say Goodbye to an intimate relationship with one person.

As you can see, the Developmental Play training program has two parts: (1) Helping the adults develop ways of being with a child through noticing, seeing, touching, and responding to the child's cues to enable the child to grow by becoming attached and then by becoming separate; and (2) Helping adults really be present as they contact the child, and helping adults understand their reactions to what they do with a child without having to do a piece of work on their childhood experiences and memories. The Leader focuses them on their here-and-now experiencing which they are asked to share with another.

The part that is omitted in most training approaches to play therapy is the second part—the work with the adults. As said before, it is the quality of the energy and the presence of the adult that is healing, not the technique.

SESSION 13: THE LAST SESSION

Presession Training

The group began this session by defining Developmental Play after having experienced it for fifteen weeks.

Cora: It's learning to get in touch with kids while playing with them— learning where they are—actually seeing them and not just playing with them.
Leader: Being conscious of what you are doing.

Cora: Right.

Leader: Being conscious when you are connected with them and when you're not connected with them.

Cora: Being with them. When I say that, I don't just mean physically being.

Leader: So there's a dialogue between the two of you—so you get back from them as well as you give them something, and being aware of it. The biggest part is being aware of touching a child. You feel if the child is pushing away. You're aware of it. You don't ignore it. If the child is coming toward you, you can feel it. When you get stuck, you can feel that also.

Cora: That's where a couple of weeks ago you asked me if I noticed any change in myself with my daughter (two years old). Now I thought about it. While I'm with her, I feel I am more present with her than I was in the past.

Leader: You feel more alive (demonstrating). I never noticed you (to Cora) wearing those shoes before, and that's true (said as she realized it and group laughs). I feel myself when I focus on you. I make contact with you and I get a response back from you. That gets me out of my head as well as gives you (Cora) something to respond to.

Working with a child makes you aware of your own issues. As we go through this Goodbye process, I'd like all of you to think about what you became aware of in yourself as you worked with your child.

With one more day to play, where do you think your child is in this Goodbye process? How is your child dealing with the Goodbye?

Cora: Sue's more attached. She wants to be hugged, kissed, and cradled. She's more calm. I don't know if that's a step in the program or a part of separation.

Leader: What's that about?

Cora: Part of Goodbye.

Leader: What part is it?

Cora: Letting me know she's going to miss me. I don't know.

Leader: Do you have a memory of saying Goodbye to someone close, someone that you're not going to see for a long time?

Cora: (Laughs) Yes.

Leader: What did you do?

Cora: Spent more time then with them.

Leader: What's underneath that?

Cora: Holding on to them and not wanting them to go—making a memory.

Leader: Right. That's one thing children do—build memories. Their behavior in this group shifted the day I said we have two more times to play. They moved into a new stage, different from the way they were in the beginning where you had to do all the initiating. Now they ask for what they want (for example, "Give me more kisses"). This builds up memories. Another step that's new that you saw last week, and we talked about it—the move toward independence.

Cora: I don't see that in Celia at all.

Leader: Last week she came over and asked me to swing her.

Cora: Okay.

Leader: What you might look for is behavior that says, "I don't need you. I can do it myself." Another behavior that appears during the separation phase is wanting to be by themselves while you just observe—just be there. You don't have to do anything. That was where Sam was last week. He said very clearly that he wanted to lie down. He wasn't rejecting Clara. He wanted her to be present, but he wanted some time just to himself to capture his sense of self in this place. Another example of that from Sam was during Circle Time last week. He simply laid down in the center of the circle and was quiet. Then James spoke and said, "He's dead." Remember that?

Clara: Yes. He said, "I'm sick."

Leader: He just wanted a quiet moment by himself and yet be the center of attention, and he was. Interestingly, all the other children were quiet, too, as they observed him. For these children, being sick may be the only time they get some attention. Whenever a disturbed child (and James was) uses the word "dead," he feels alive. That is, once the child experiences herself alive, she knows what dead means. Sam's behavior definitely shows the presence of a core or inner self that guides him and makes him capable of feeling.

Then there's that wonderful scene where Sue is playing in the sink with the water. She holds her hands up and looks at them, studies them as if seeing them for the first time, the way infants do. There was such joy on her face. She was playing without needing anyone to say anything. The tendency is to want to make comments, or call the child's attention to what she is doing, or to call her attention to something she is not doing. All that distracts the child from experiencing her own body and her own boundaries. No words are necessary. Just be present, observe quietly, and enjoy what you are seeing.

Paul: That's not where Norm is.

Leader: Right. And he started in the program late—four sessions late.

Paul: Norm and I are still working on boundaries.

Leader: Right. He's still working on Stage One, the Attachment part.

Paul: I think it's most interesting that the most difficult part I have in therapy is the termination process.

Leader: So you, too, have to say Goodbye. What memories do you have saying Goodbye to someone close?

Ned: Yes. I want to say something. In school last week, Aretha was lying on her mat. I was at my desk, and she looked at me and said, "Ned, I got to use the bathroom." I realized that is the first time she has ever called me by my name. Usually she says, "I got to pee." This time she said loudly, "Ned, I got to pee." (Laughs) She was so confident. It just came out. She never used my name before.

Leader: What was that like for you?

Ned: Hell, it was good. (Laughs) It's the truth. (Said softly)

Leader: What else?

Ned: I felt she made a big step—more open.

Leader: When she looked up at you and made eye contact and said, "Ned?"

Ned: I don't know.

Leader: Did you feel recognized, accepted?

Ned: Yeah.

Leader: Like she knows who you are.

Ned: Yeah!

Leader: You can feel that energy between you and her when she looks at you. She's present, and you're present. You feel connected. She gave something back to you—a wonderful feeling for you. I'm glad you spoke up and shared this. It's too bad Aretha was absent from the DP program last week, especially when we're working on saying Goodbye.

Cora: I've noticed a big change in Aretha. In the beginning she just sat there, not participating—not being there. Now she wants to take control of the Circle Time. She stands up and gives that quiet half-smile.

Paul: I see the biggest difference in the kids in their day-to-day activities. In the beginning, Sue was invisible to me. She's not anymore. She makes herself visible. She sets it up that way. She'll come in and smile and say, "Hi."

Leader: Now when you look at her face, there is somebody behind those eyes.

Paul: She doesn't look as scared or lost.

Leader: There's this joy on her face as she focuses her attention on someone.

Centering. We have to get present now to meet the children for their last session and your last session with them.

So close your eyes and focus on your breathing. Feel yourself breathing, in and out. Feel the rhythm of your own breathing which is not exactly like anyone else's. See what part of your body starts to let go first. Is it your head, your eyes, your face, your shoulders, your hands, your solar plexus? Feel this flow of energy down your body out to your legs and feet. Where do you feel energy spots in your body? Is the energy going in or coming out? Be there now without doing anything. (Pause) Put a word out that says where you are right now.

Group: Slowing . . . calm . . . relaxed.

Leader: What would it be like today to be with your child from this quiet place? Where you feel you don't have to work so hard? You can just really let yourself see your child whether she's smiling, crying, enjoying herself, or showing you she can do something you can't do. How do you let yourself know and show you love your child?

When you get ready, open your eyes, come back, and make eye contact with someone. Say Hello with your eyes. You don't have to do anything to say Hello but feel the quality of the energy between you and the other one. (Pause) Anyone wanting to say anything at this point?

Paul: I didn't feel real good when I realized I couldn't feel very connected to Norm. When you said what would it be like to say Goodbye to your child—when I thought of Norm, I felt relieved.

Leader: What's that like, to speak the truth?

Paul: Kind of sad, I think. (Long pause)

Leader: Just feel your sadness . . . You, like him, got cheated out of having the same amount of time as the others because of Tom leaving and Norm starting four weeks late. I feel sad, too, because I see Norm wanting this relationship with you. He said, "I'm coming" (next time).

Clara: For me coming from my quiet place, it felt good and very sad. (She sounded and looked sad)

Leader: Just allow the sadness.

Cora: When you said they are getting more independent, I wondered how Sue is going to react, whether she's going to be rebellious or that part where she says she can do it herself—I don't need you anymore. How is she going to react? I'm curious—anxious, actually.

Leader: What is your anxiety about?

Cora: I don't know.

Leader: I think it's good that you are acknowledging your anxiety. What do you need?

Cora: Just do it.

Ned: What happens if I cradle Aretha and she doesn't want it? When I try to do it every week, she starts whining.

Leader: You can try doing it as much as you feel comfortable. If it doesn't feel right to you, don't do it. I put it out to the child, saying that this is our time to be together; and as I say it, I am moving her into it. I focus her on her body.

Ned: In the room, I can do that.

Leader: In Circle Time and also in the one-to-one, I would try to turn her around so that she is not facing toward Celia (her cousin). Aretha may have some catching up to do because she wasn't here last week. It may be harder for her today.

Postsession Training

Paul started this session, following the meeting with the children, by expressing his anger at several people, including the Leader, as well as his own staff who took over the care of these children following the DP program. Aretha had a heavy crying spell right at the end of the Circle Time, and she continued to cry afterwards when the children had to go to lunch. He did not feel people handled Aretha adequately. He then took Aretha into another room, and she quieted down. This, in turn, set up feelings in Ned because he felt Aretha was his child and he could have done that if he had been instructed to do so.

Clara: I don't know why she was crying, but her crying felt very painful to me. I just stayed with Sam.

Cora: Just observing her—Ned said she was crying because he was cradling her, but he tried to sit her up and she flayed back. I wouldn't have known what to do.

Ned: When she started crying, she wasn't fighting me anymore.

Leader: What was that like for you?

Ned: I felt like I hurt her, but I didn't. I know I didn't physically. Maybe I did emotionally. I'm wondering if it's me or it's . . . I don't know.

Leader: What was it like for you, going through this?

Ned: I hated it. I felt like I was the cause. I'm supposed to be the person to hold them when they're upset. I shouldn't be the one who causes the upset. Whatever I did, it didn't do any good.

Leader: Are you angry with me?

Ned: No, but I thought there was more to do than to take her to the cafeteria (which followed the program).

331

Leader: I told you to do it because we had to leave, and I thought maybe she would calm down on the way to lunch, but that didn't work for me, either.

Ned: I was confused trying to figure out what was going on. She started fighting me holding her, but once she started crying, she stopped fighting.

Leader: If this is the first time you've ever done this with a kid, it's very hard because you don't know if you're doing it right or not.

Paul: Are you mad at me?

Ned: I'm not mad at you at all, but I wanted to do what you did (carry Aretha to a private room and hold her), but I didn't know if I was helping or hurting.

Gill: If this is the first time she's allowed the cradling, her crying may be a feeling of helplessness because you said she was relaxed. The next time maybe she will be able to trust.

Ned: Kind of what I felt and it kept going.

Paul: But you don't have any control over her. Had you not been able to reach her, she would not have had this response. So it was because you did things right that she brought this about.

Ned: When she was on the floor, I pulled her back.

Cora: Then she laid in your arms.

Leader: (To Ned) I had a sense that something in you changed and that you felt it was all right for you to cradle her. You said, "I'm getting braver." When I smiled at you and nodded to you to go ahead—do what you are doing—something in you said, "It's Okay" and that you weren't hurting her. It's amazing when you said she stopped fighting when she started crying. I think it's the most healthful thing she's done—the crying—since she's been in the program.

　　　In the video you could see that she gave you a lot of cues—that this was okay (to cradle her). She would look at you to see the effect on you. I think you were right on with her, and you weren't hurting her. She would quiet down and almost stop crying, and then she would work herself up to crying again, almost as if it felt good to cry. When she quieted down, I thought maybe she's going to stop and maybe when she went to lunch she might stop—but she didn't. It was hard for me, too, part of the time just to allow her to cry because she cried so hard at times. She really felt her body when she cried. She felt alive when she cried.

　　　As the Leader, I felt very good that Aretha cried—a healthy thing for her to do. I felt bad that I wasn't more helpful to Ned. Leaders don't always know the best thing to do; there is no best thing to do sometimes.

Ned: (Softer tone) I feel good about what happened. I think it was very positive. I feel good about that.

Leader: You'll find your relationship with her will be different after this because she will still be with you as her teacher. Her saying during the crying, "I want my Mommy" shows that she connects you to her mother. Calling on her mother gets to you. She needed someone to do exactly what we did—hang out with her and not leave her while she's crying and going through this.

Paul: I want to take back what I said earlier—not being connected to Norm.

Leader: I wondered about that.

Group: (Laughs)

Paul: He was right there today—absolutely right there! He did all kinds of stuff, a lot of it. He wanted to be picked up and carried. He wanted to be held all the time. He still did his break-away stuff, but it was just real different. He spent most of the time in my lap.

Leader: And he did a lot of talking, too.

Paul: Oh, yeah. It was the first time he told me what he wanted. I want my feet done. I want the lotion. I want this; I want that; I don't want that; and he was very verbal.

Leader: When he was doing all this, I thought of what you had said earlier, that you didn't feel connected to him.

Paul: (Laughs) I thought of that. I'm sure you did.

Leader: So you can see the effect on him even when you started late.

Paul: Norm and I started four sessions after everybody else.

Leader: So now do you feel connected to Norm?

Paul: Yes.

Leader: How did that come about?

Paul: Norm did it. He made me feel his presence, and I guess I had something to do with that, too. *I allowed him to reach me.*

Leader: Then there's what he said in Circle Time, in case you have forgotten.

Cora: He was asking for it.

Paul: (Laughing) I was asking for it.

Leader: (To Ned) Are you crying?

Ned: No.

Leader: Say in your own words, "I am moved by what I did today."

Ned: I am moved by what I did today. (Voice trembling)

Cora: I can see that you are moved, Ned. I felt more moved by you than by Aretha, to tell the truth.

Ned: Me, too.

333

Cora: I'm glad you picked her because I wanted to say that to you. (This refers to the time of their choosing their child; at that time, Cora wanted Aretha and because Aretha was absent, Cora started with Celia. From the beginning, Ned wanted no one but Aretha.)

Ned: Me, too. (Crying)

Leader: I would like to hear from the others.

Cora: It took a long time for Celia to settle down. She raced around. She ran over where Paul was and I had to chase her to get her back into our corner. Once we got over there, she slowed down. She asked for the lotion. She wanted the Gingerbread Girl. Then she wanted her feet washed. Then I did the Knock-at-the-Door game. She really liked that because last week she asked for that in Circle Time, and I said we'd do it this week. She really got a kick out of that. I kissed her on her hand, and then she wanted me to kiss her on her mouth. Then as I started to do it, she put her hand over her mouth before I could get there. Then she would laugh. I would say, "I'm going to get you this time," and she'd do the same thing and laugh. She was totally unaware of the camera, or Aretha, or anything else in the room.

Leader: I saw this. Both of you were having such a good time, and both of you were so present, as if no one else was there but you two.

Cora: When we were washing feet she said, "Am I not going to get to go home?" I said, "Why do you say that?" She said, "Because I don't want to go home." Finally, I got the answer.

Leader: She wants to stay with you.

Cora: Yes. That's what she said.

Leader: (To Cora) How do you feel now about what you accomplished with her?

Cora: She's gone a long ways. Takes me back to the first day. I said, "This is not for me (big laugh). I'm not going to make it through these weeks" (laughs). I can remember when I wrote it down the first week. When I traded children that first week, with Ned, and got Celia instead of Aretha, I said to myself that I shouldn't have traded, thinking this is going to be a long time. A lot has been accomplished, and I feel good about it.

Leader: Is there one thing you learned about yourself that stands out?

Cora: To set limits without being too authoritative or too mean, like I want you to sit—to mean it without being mean.

Leader: That's a biggy for you!

Cora: I'm learning that with my daughter, too. *I'm learning to say, "No" and to tell her what I want without being mean.*

Leader: That's pretty important. You feel good about that. Limit setting is an important part of the DP program, but it is limit setting through noticing, touching, and putting out what you want from the child and then responding to their cues as well as through saying "No."

Cora: Once Aretha started crying, Celia sat up and looked. She was concerned. I was talking to her, saying, "You're wondering what's wrong with Aretha."

Leader: The ability to cry is very important. The crying means that the relationship is important. It is a nonverbal communication that says you have a caring self inside. It also says it's okay to allow yourself to receive care from a caring person.

Cora: *You have an inner instinct of what to do, what a child needs.*

Leader: That's what it's all about. There's something inside of you that knows what to do. It comes from inside you. You do it, and you find out from the child's response if it's what the child needs. That's the way you learn.

Clara: (Sighs) I enjoyed myself. I had a good time. Sam wanted to play the Rocking game we played a long time ago. I'd give him a kiss, and he'd rock back and then come up for another. He asked, "Why is this the last day?" He asked me to come back. I said, "I have other things to do." When it was Circle Time he said, "I'm not going to Circle Time. I'm going to stay here all day." In Circle Time he was singing the lullaby. He looks at me when I sing Rock-A-Bye Baby. I sing Rock-A-Bye Sam. Before, he told me to stop doing that. Today, he wanted me to do it. That was nice. (Clara described these events in a quiet, relaxed, somewhat nostalgic tone—different from her usual excited, high energy tone.)

Leader: You sounded really touched by him today. I sensed a very warm feeling between the two of you. I was moved listening to you.

Gill: I didn't have to do anything with Sue today. She chose everything herself. I was really struck by the contrast between the first couple of sessions where she just kind of sat there and waited for me to initiate everything. At one point, she reached over to take one of my shoes. I was going to limit that and then she said, "I'm going to tie them," and so I let her do that. She tied them and I said, "You can do that all by yourself."

The water play fascinated her, and I let her do it all by herself. At the end, she got some soap and said, "Give me your hand." She took my hand. She's confident.

What really bothered me: in the play I said to her, "This is our last time to play together." She went, "Why is that?" I said that we started saying Goodbye two weeks ago and this is the time we have. She went and played some more and then at the end, she came and hugged me, and I said, "Goodbye, Sue." She started to run to the door, and she turned and said, "I'm coming back."

Leader: We gave them the Polaroid pictures to take home as a memory. (In analytical theory, this is called a transitional object.)

Cora: Celia took the one where she was beaming. She told me she wanted to take it home and have mother put it on the wall with the rest of the pictures.

Gill: Sue said, "I want them all" (they had to choose between two pictures). I said, "I know, but you have to choose one." Then she went and touched them to her cheek and said, *"This one is for me, and this one is for you."*

Leader: In Circle Time when I, as the Leader, asked the children what they liked best, Celia gave a most interesting answer. She said, "What I liked best was when we played the Gingerbread Girl and I got burned, she ate me up anyway"—and then she laughed. This is a metaphor that says even if she is damaged, her partner accepts her. This response is also an excellent example of how the abstract and symbolic come out of the concrete and presymbolic. Anything anyone wants to say before we close?

Gill: I just want to say one more thing. Ned, I was thinking of Aretha and what you said was that one of the goals of the program is to really have the children start back at the beginning—like sticking her thumb in her mouth, relaxing, and just lying there is real important. My thought was the crying may have been a last ditch effort. She wanted to feel like a baby but might not feel safe. The crying was just part of that. She is so beautiful. She just comes to life as you play with her.

Leader: You've done a wonderful piece of work with her.

Paul: Do you recognize that?

Ned: Yeah. It's not quite the way I wanted it to end. Nope. Honestly, I thought it was good. I feel like I was the cause. I don't know.

Paul: (Who has recovered from his explosive anger and is more compassionate) You were, but that was healthy. (Said very warmly)

Ned: Sitting there holding her and looking at her face just tore my heart apart, you know. It looked so painful. I guess *I really felt* . . . I don't know. It's not like you knocked a kid down and he cries, and he knows it's your fault, but that's physical, you know, and you feel bad and all, but now, with Aretha, it's not physical. I know it's emotional. It's hard. It's just a totally different feeling, you know, from everything else. I feel like I've hurt her emotionally.

Leader: It's because you love her. You're attached to her. You have a relationship with her. That's different. When you're attached to someone,
you're attached on the emotional and spiritual level, and she gets to
your heart. That's what a relationship means. This is part of your own
growth to be able to experience another's pain and to love them. At the
same time, you discover the loving place inside of you.

COMMENTS

The last session was a very moving and intense one. The ending was connected to the beginning. The ending got its meaning from the beginning. That is,
the trainees saw at the end what they were doing. At the end, they became aware
that they had become attached to their child and that they were in a relationship
with that child. They had experienced what it means to "be-with" a child and to
be in a relationship with a child. Two trainees—Cora and Paul—who didn't like
their child at all in the beginning learned to feel very connected to them—a surprise to both of them at the end!

In learning how to be "with" a child, the trainees learned how to be with
themselves. In learning how to be with Celia, Cora got in touch with her "mean-
ness." Cora got in touch with this hidden part of herself through learning to be in
a relationship with Celia instead of being an army sergeant carrying out a drill. By
learning how to be in a relationship to Norm, Paul got in touch with his inner
core—his loving part and his validating part. Gill learned how to be alive and
present with her child which, in turn, made Sue come alive because she imitated
Gill. Once Gill and her child got attached, Gill learned not to smother her child
with too much attention, attention that distracted Sue from experiencing her
own power. Clara learned what it felt like to have a child love her and how it felt
when a child wants some time to herself. Clara, like Paul, learned that being with
a child is not doing things to a child but rather being with a child. It is being in a
relationship with that child. That means the trainee is part of that relationship.
Clara learned that to be in a relationship with her child doesn't mean she has to
be active, doing something every minute. She can be with a child simply by
quietly observing her. In exploring ways to be with Aretha, Ned (a young man in
his first teaching job) discovered his higher self. In this training group, the trainees witnessed Ned giving birth to his psychological self, and they all were very
moved by him. Ned, the teacher in this agency, was the one trainee who had no
experience as a therapist or as a client.

Finally, the trainees were not the only ones who learned in this training program. As the Leader, or supervisor, I also learned. In writing this book, I saw places
where I could have done it differently, in ways that might have been more helpful

to the trainees. When I made mistakes, it was because I, too, was involved in my own issues and not present. However, I presented what did happen and not what I wished had happened. As you read this book, you may see places where you would have done it differently. I try to emphasize with my trainees that beginners are not supposed to know how to do it and to look at what they do as learning and not mistakes or that they didn't do it "right." Instead of criticizing yourself, look at what you discovered about yourself or your child. Children are wonderful teachers!

POSTPROGRAM SESSION

The trainees said Goodbye to the children in session 13. The goal of this session with the adults only is to provide them with the opportunity to say Goodbye to each other and to the Leader, as well as the opportunity to assess their own growth. Saying Goodbye means sharing their growth experiences with each other. The Goodbye process enables the trainees to review their experiences and to define the meaning and value for them—all shared in the group. They leave, taking these memories with them.

The Leader provided the usual centering, this time ending with inviting the trainees to get an image of their child to whom they had said Goodbye last week. After bringing them back and having them make contact with each other, she passed out paper and pencils and asked them to draw a picture of themselves with their child. Then the Leader handed each one their first drawings done in the beginning (the first Preprogram Session). Each person then shared their before-and-after drawings and pointed out the differences they saw in the two drawings. The first drawings looked static. There was no interaction between child and adult. Although some drawings showed the child on the adult's lap, there was no life or interaction there. In the second drawing—in all of them—the child was active and the two were interacting. The child also had a complete body (the group commented that in one drawing the child looked more like a dog). The adult in the drawing was also more complete. The drawings reflected the changes in the children and in the adults' ability to relate to them. They both came alive in the second drawing.

To help the trainees assess their own growth and to take with them some new sense of who they are, the Leader asked them to write the answers to the following questions. She asked each, in turn, to read them aloud to the group.

The Questions

1. What was the most meaningful experience for you? What did you get in touch with in yourself that you didn't know about before?
2. What was the hardest for you?
3. What moved you the most? What did you like best?
4. What message are you going to take home with you for yourself?

Paul: (Reading) I got in touch with how directive I am with kids when I do therapy with kids—you got to play my way. I used to think I was available and present. I learned much more to follow the kids, follow the kids' direction. I feel like I am much more available—much more.

What I liked best was the very last session when I thought I didn't have a connection, when it was so very obvious we did—Norm and me— there we were. *I really felt that.*

The hardest for me was doing it on my own turf with people I work with being in the program. I didn't disclose as much as I wanted to.

Message I'm going to take home: I get a pretty clear message that I'm pretty competent. I want to correct something. Last time, and the time before, I said I felt like I had been cheated, that I would never do another thing at my shop. I've learned that I don't feel cheated. I learned a lot and enjoyed it, and I'm really glad I did it.

Cora: (Reading) The most meaningful thing I learned was to be present with the child. What I liked was remembering Celia's smile in the Gingerbread Girl game—seeing the joy on her face and she'd say, "Eat me." She really liked it. The hardest to learn was setting limits and following the child without being mean. *The message: to be present.* I learned that it makes a difference by being present, not only physically present, but mentally present when you are with a kid, no matter what kind of mood you're in. I can remember various moods I came in with and realizing during the centering I need to be with her—everything else needs to be put away, It really makes a difference, I've noticed, in playing with my own child—to be with her physically, mentally, and emotionally. It makes a difference! I was more comfortable setting limits without being intrusive with my child and with the children in the Group Home.

Ned: (Reading) What was new for me: The way Aretha responded to me when she asked me if she could take a pee. The moment that gave me the most satisfaction and joy is to see her outside of class. She's a totally different person. She's very outspoken, and she participates more in the activities. The hardest thing was cradling her when she was resisting. The message I'm going to take home: it really had an impact on me.

Leader: What do you see in yourself that's different?

Ned: (Long pause) More sensitive. I can see a difference with the kids when I'm with the kids. (Talks in a very soft, warm voice) I'm more loving. (Self-conscious)

You work hard to make one child happy, and you get it all back. Sam loves me. I really saw it one time. I said, "That's me" when he draws a person. I love him as if he were my own. It gives me tears. It's so weird. Now he's a personal part of me. I almost start crying.

Gill: (Reading) I guess I'm realizing that this approach in its seeming simplicity is very complex. It started out being so simple—just playing with kids. It didn't seem like that was a major deal. I'm constantly aware of how deeply it touched my life and how deeply I feel. The Hellos and Goodbyes—I understand them now. I understand how important they are, how you can generalize this into every aspect of your life.

Leader: Your message?

Gill: I'm not ready to say yet.

Clara: (Reading) One of the big pieces I got—seeing the child in every phase he was at from the beginning to the end. It made me aware that *every place he's at is very important. It made me much more accepting of my own process*—how I can be more accepting of other people which gives me more detachment—which is really nice. I've just been really claiming my richness the last couple weeks. *I got it all experientially!* It's not something somebody told me. (Said emphatically) That's so nice!

Leader: (Closes the session by having the trainees stand in a circle holding hands and making eye contact one more time.) Find your quiet place, or whatever you call it. Feel the hands on each side of you. Now gently let go. Wave Goodbye to someone.

SUMMARY OF CHAPTER 6

This chapter is the story of how six adults (one adult had to leave the program early) and six children came together to learn to be with each other through seeing, touching, and responding. In order to do that and in the act of doing that, they created a community—three communities, in fact: an adult community (when the adults met in the pre- and post-training sessions), a children's community (Circle Time), and a child-adult community (the one-to-one and Circle Time).

Through that community process, the adults were able to provide the children with the conditions they needed to develop their core self; namely, to be touched and seen and responded to so that they could become attached and, in turn, could use this attachment to empower themselves to be independent—to become individuals in their own right.

Through this attachment process, the children in turn provided the adults with the conditions they needed to become aware of parts of themselves—parts of their childhood that had gotten sealed off in their growing up. In other words, learning to be with a child is a reciprocal process. The adult is as much of the process, if not more, as the child is. The children gave as much, if not more, to the adults as the adults gave to the children. Developmental Play therapy is a *relationship process*. You cannot study the child's behavior without studying the adult's behaviors and experiences as she plays with that child.

Lastly, the adult-to-adult community provided the conditions the adults needed to give meaning to their new awareness of themselves. The postsession trainings served to provide a container for the trainees' new awareness of themselves gained from being with their child. That adult meeting gave them time to relive those experiences so that they could remember and integrate them through sharing these experiences with their colleagues. That is the meaning and value of community.

The growth of the individuals in this community—both the adults and the children—demonstrated how verbal language and symbolic thinking evolve out of the experiences of dialoguing through touch. Both the trainees and the children showed this evolution in learning who they really are.

THE EFFECT ON THE TRAINEES

This community of six adults plus a Leader provided the conditions each of the trainees needed to get exactly what they needed. This community provided a safe place in which they could take the risk of being where they are—saying or doing whatever they needed to say or do. In doing that, they became aware of the messages they gave themselves, messages that kept them from being present: You're not doing it right; if you touch the child you might hurt her; if you speak up and say what you want, you are "mean." From that place, they could not be present.

By becoming aware of the messages that kept them from being present, the trainees learned how to focus on their physical bodies and be present in the here and now. As a result of these experiences, the trainees began to be aware that the world looked and felt differently to them. For example, Gill said, *"I'm beginning to let myself see what I'm seeing."* Cora said, *"When I touch my own child, I see more of her.* I feel myself touching her. I am more aware of her." Paul said, *"Norm made me feel his presence,* and I guess I had something to do with that, too. *I allowed him to reach me."* Clara said, "Seeing the child in every phase from the beginning to the end made me aware that every place he's at is very important. *It made me more accepting of my own process.* I've just been claiming my richness the last couple weeks." Ida said, "I liked what I did today." Ned said, "I have so much more respect and caring for others. I feel so much deeper, so much stronger. Today, it was so wonderful I can't talk about it."

What the Leader Provided. As with the children, the Leader started by helping the trainees to experience their physical bodies—the energy and vibration and life within their own bodies. Through simple exercises (meditation), learning to be seen and to see (the Seeing exercise done with a partner), learning to be touched and to touch (the Holding Hands exercise done with a partner), sharing, and some group exercises (Circle Time), the trainees became aware of a new part of themselves, a part that just belonged to them.

A second thing the Leader provided was the experience of being coached. For example, when a pair was practicing saying Hello and the Giver didn't know what to do or was totally lost, the Leader sat near her and guided her. When a trainee didn't know what to do with her child in the one-to-one, sometimes the Leader would guide her.

THE EFFECT ON THE CHILDREN

These six children were seen for one hour weekly for thirteen weeks, each with one specific adult as the therapist or partner. Three of the six adults were staff members (the Director, the teacher, and the social worker).

These children were not like any others with whom I had previously worked. At first, they seemed frozen with fear, especially if invited to do or say anything. One child, who had been a cocaine baby, would open her mouth to say something, and no sounds came out. Yet these children, once they could allow themselves to enjoy being held or cradled, started to assert themselves as early as the sixth week. At the end of the thirteen weeks, the cocaine child looked, talked, and acted like a normal child. The joy on this child's face as she experienced her power was truly a delight for the staff to experience. The staff has already spoken about the change in these children, the way they make themselves more "visible."

The role that touch played in the growth of these children is illustrated in the following examples: Aretha did not know how to use her lips to kiss. Like Jason, she just blew on the therapist's face. She learned to kiss in one or two sessions. Sue made her decision as to which Polaroid picture to select by holding each, in turn, up to her cheek. Then she decided on the basis of how it felt on her cheek. Making use of the Gingerbread Cookie game, Celia created a very complex interactive play with Cora, a drama that showed the evolution of her needs step by step. First she wanted to be overwhelmed with touches (wanting Cora to eat her up); then she just wanted to lie quietly, not doing anything ("I'm not done yet; you forgot to turn the oven on"); then she wanted Cora to be active ("You're supposed to cry now"—when she's not done); and lastly, she competed with Cora and showed her power with much laughter on the part of both. Celia's drama involved concrete (primary thinking) and abstract (symbolic or secondary thinking) behavior.

Three of the children—Sue, Sam, and Celia—used the touching experiences to move them from the attachment stage into the separation stage. Sue not only told her therapist to stay out of her "stuff," defining it as hers (the play in the sink), but she also became very loving and giving. For example, she showed her therapist that she could tie the therapist's shoes and later asked the therapist for her hand so that she could wash it. Thus, she moved from a receiver to a giver. Sam, on the other hand, who wanted to be held a lot, wanted some time just to be by himself and have his therapist only observe. In the last session, Celia had provided a game for her and her therapist—a game in which Celia was the more powerful—the kissing game. They were both so involved that it was as if there was no one else in the world but those two. In the last circle, Celia answered the question, "What did you like best?" with a metaphor: "What I liked best was when we played the Gingerbread Girl game and I got burned, she ate me anyway." Sue defined herself and her therapist as separate when she said, "This one is for me, and this one is for you" as she handed the Polaroid picture to her therapist.

THE EFFECT ON THE PARENT-CHILD RELATIONSHIP

At the end of the thirteen weeks, the preschool social worker (not the one in the program) interviewed the parents, the teacher, and a staff aide.

The Parent (Adult) Interview Questions

1. What differences have you seen in your (this) child the last four months?

2. Does your (this) child talk to you more? What kind of things does the child say to you? Does the child ever mention the play program to you?

3. Do *you* talk to your (this) child more? What kind of things do you say to the child? Are these things new for you to say?

4. Does your (this) child touch you more? Does the child sit on your lap more?

5. Do you hold or rock your (this) child more? Do you like holding this child?

6. If you had to say one thing more than anything else that you like about your (this) child, what would it be?

7. What do you do with your (this) child that is the most fun for you?

Table 1. Reports From Parents, Aide and Teacher On These Six Children

Responses Reported	Parent Report	Aide Report	Teacher Report
Number of children who:			
Talked more to adult (parent)	6	5	2
Mentioned play program	2	3	0
Touched adult more	2	6	2
Sat on adult's lap	3	3	2
Number of adults who:			
Talked more to child	6	5	1
Touched child more	1	2	1
Liked holding child	5	6	4

Comments

The staff social worker who interviewed the parents said, "I was interested to see that these parents were able to see the things we asked them. It's hard for our clients. We don't get much from them a lot of the time. I was pretty impressed that the parents could notice the changes."

According to the interview reports, all six parents reported that the children talked more to them and that they talked more to their children. There was also a trend toward more touching and holding by the parents. Some parents said they did not touch their children more, but they held them more. The parents also expressed their love and empathy toward their children. Three parents said, in almost the same words, "I love her (him)." Two parents said, "She's a warm, loving child." One parent (a stepfather) said, "I like watching him enjoy himself."

THE EFFECT ON THE AGENCY

The Interview Report (Table 1) made this agency aware of the role of their staff (aides) in providing the support and relationships these very deprived children needed. It made the agency aware of how much some of their aides do for

344

these children. For example, the report showed that two of the children who expressed very little to the parent, the teacher, or their DP partner, did share with one particular aide their sadness, disappointments, and even their tears. This information should be shared with the whole staff, especially with this particular aide.

Aides receive little, if any, feedback on how their work affects the children (except when things go wrong). It is important that good things be made public, too. When the staff feels seen and feels good about themselves because they belong to a group that interacts with them, the energy in the agency changes. It would be very therapeutic to offer DP training to the agency staff—both for the children and the staff.

APPLICATIONS

The focus of Chapter 6 is training. The training approach in Developmental Play is unique: first, the training begins with the adults—not with what to do with the children. The training is organized around helping the adults be present with themselves and with each other, first through touch and seeing. Second, the trainees practice with each other the seeing and touching they will be doing with the children. Being present is a basic need for all humans. Therefore, this training has applications to others outside of the Developmental Play group program (Brody, 1976, 1978). Below is a list of groups who have received and benefited from this type of training.

College Students, especially in classes in child therapy, play therapy, child development, and early childhood education. The Developmental Play training (illustrated and demonstrated in Chapter 6) furnishes an experiential foundation needed to understand the theoretical concepts. When concepts are expressed experientially, the concepts then have meaning. For example, when the students in my Play Therapy class read about attachment and separation as stages of development, they will also be experiencing these concepts in their bodies, their emotions, and their relationships right in class. One college student told me that as a result of being in my class, she found out that she had an "inner self."

In addition, this book includes verbatim case studies illustrating how a DP therapist works with three very different children. College students need to know what it would be like to carry out a therapeutic approach as well as to know the theory. This book does that.

Teacher and Parent Groups. Teachers and parents of handicapped children need something for themselves and some new ideas on what to do with the children. Children can make dramatic changes from being in individual therapy, but many need support at school and at home to maintain that gain. That was

345

true of Kenny (Chapter 4) when I worked with his mother. Teachers and parents who have participated in the DP training report that it is very effective (Brody, 1976, 1978).

Adolescent Boys. DP therapists have used these exercises with a group of adolescent boys and found them very effective.

Therapists Who Lead Groups. Therapists could use these exercises to build a sense of community. These DP training exercises would be excellent to do with any care-taking population: nurses, teachers in preschools, therapeutic schools, staffs of day care centers, Head Start (where I first started doing DP therapy), and with those who make decisions about children: HRS administrators, attorneys, and judges.

Brief Review of the Training Exercises in Chapter 6

» Meditation and centering exercises
» Circle Time activities (Hello song, Follow-the-Leader, I See You song)
» Seeing and Being Seen exercise (partners, sharing, sharing in big group)
» Touching and Being Touched exercise (handholding with partners, sharing, etc.)
» Saying Hello exercise (partners)
» The Goodbye song

Chapter 6 describes how one group of adults experienced these exercises and how it changed their sense of who they are. Participants in this group expressed surprise that these simple exercises could move them so quickly into deep places.

As said before, there is no magic in these exercises by themselves. It is the quality of the energy of the Leader and her intent and ability to be present that makes them effective.

EXAMPLES OF DEVELOPMENTAL PLAY INTERACTIONS

The following snapshots of the Children's Hour were taken during session 12. Unfortunately, pictures taken in the beginning are not available. However, these snapshots do show the quality and form of the adult-child interactions that take place in a Developmental Play program when the goals are met: relationships that express joy, fun, comfort, closeness, action, nurturing, and security.

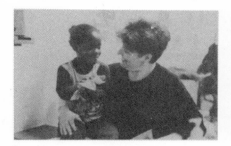
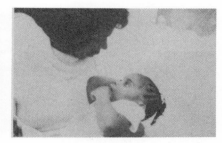

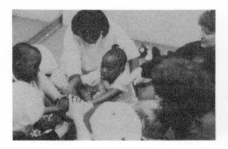
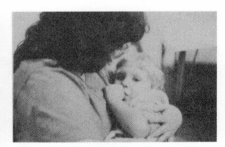

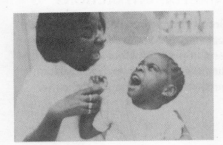
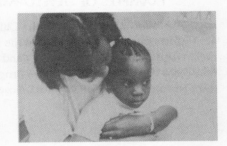

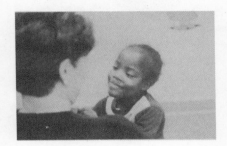
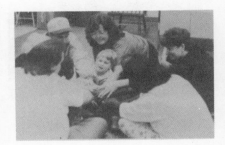

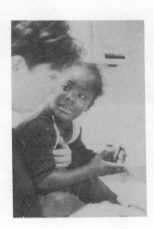

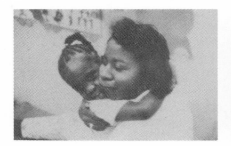

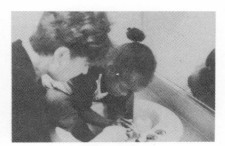

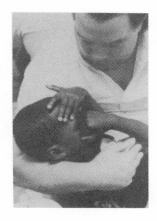

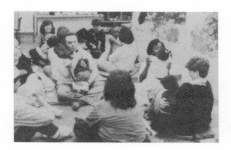

REVIEW

Chapters 5 and 6 described the Developmental Play approach through verbatim material that gave you an idea of what it would be like for a child to be in this program, what it would be like to be an adult partner to a child, what it would be like to receive training to become an adult partner, and what it would be like to be the Leader or Supervisor. The Developmental Play group program provides individual and group therapy for children, training for adults, and experience being the Leader.

Developmental Play is a highly compact, structured developmentally-based therapy program. Its goal is to provide the conditions the child needs to develop her inner self, her core self, her inner guide. The conditions that the DP therapist provides is a relationship initiated through touch—the first relationship between a parent and a child.

The purpose of the touch is not to regress the child (although that may happen) but to enable her to experience her physical body, to experience her energy and her aliveness, and to experience the pleasure of discovering this new sense of self—*her living body self.* The purpose of the touch is to enable the child to experience the physical presence of the therapist: there is someone there for her—to see her, to touch her, to support her and, more importantly, someone with whom she can relate.

The Developmental Play Relationship. The relationship is the vessel within which the interaction between child and therapist takes place. Everything that happens between child and therapist has to be seen as a working out of and a product of that relationship. It makes no sense at all to look at different things a therapist does without first defining the framework or relationship within which those actions take place.

Developmental Play is an "I-Thou" relationship (Buber, 1958). This means that the therapist is *in* the relationship *with* the child. *Both* the child and the therapist are participants, or co-creators, in this relationship (Landreth, 1991, pp. 5-6). When I set limits, these limits are also mine (Moustakas, 1992, pp. 7-11). Every therapy session is created anew by both the child and the therapist. Therefore, nothing is preplanned ahead of time, at least nothing specific— how could it be if the child is to be free to be where she needs to be as she moves from one stage to the next? For example, as Mira's therapist (Chapter 5), I never quite knew what she would do or where she would be. The best thing I could do was to get myself present so I would be available to her in whatever way she was.

Being *in* the relationship as opposed to just being an observer who interprets behavior, as happens in some play therapy and child analysis, I learn about myself. For example, I learned about myself when I had to deal with the intensity of Mira's resistant behavior in session 3 (Chapter 5). Working with these children also made me aware of some things that I do that I was not aware of— behavior that I never learned about from the many years of therapy. In other words, my DP relationship with these children was a two-way street. In Buber's terms, I was a "You" for Mira so that she could experience her "I." She, in turn, was a "You" for me so that I could experience my "I" more fully.

This "I-Thou relationship, illustrated many times in this book, is reflected in the quality of the interaction between child and therapist. What stands out is the focused quality of the energy and the interaction between child and DP therapist as if the two were the only ones in the world. Clearly, the two have a relationship. For example, the things that Mira did or brought up had to do with where she was in building our relationship. What I did in responding to her had to do also with where we were in our relationship. In other words, what she or I did had nothing to do with people in the outside world. Whatever was going on between Mira and me—whether it be her time of resistance in the beginning, or her time of anger in the middle, or time of her creations (poems and games) at the end—there was always a focused, quiet energy between us and a quality of intimacy. Those are qualities that describe an "I-Thou" relationship. Both people are working for and with each other, each from her respective place—one as the adult and one as the child.

For Future Research: I would like to see a group of therapists conduct a study on the effect of different therapy approaches on the development of the child's core self. Studies have been done on the effect on IQ, and some have been done on behavior—but behavior and IQ are only part of the story. Studies on IQ and behavior do not give us any insight into the child's inner experience.

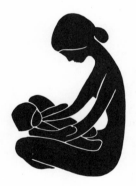

REFERENCES

Adler, Janet (1981). *Who is the Witness?* Unpublished paper.

Buber, Martin (1958). *I and Thou*. New York: Charles Scribner.

Barnum, K.E., & Brazelton, T.B. (1990). *Touch: The Foundation of Experience*. Connecticut: Universities Press.

Brody, V.A. (1963). Treatment of a Prepubertal Twin Girl with Psychogenic Megacolon. In *The American Journal of Orthopsychiatry*, Volume XXXIII, No. 3.

Brody, V.A. (1978). Developmental Play: A Relationship-Focused Program for Children. In *Child Welfare*, Volume LVII, No. 9, November.

Brody, V.A., Fenderson, C., Stephenson, S. (1976). *Sourcebook for Developmental Play*.

Cline, F. (1988). Jeremy: An Abbreviated Case History. In K. Magid & C. McKelvey, *High Risk Children Without a Conscience*. New York: Bantam Books.

Des Lauriers, A. (1962). *The Experience of Reality in Childhood Schizophrenia*. Connecticut: International Universities Press.

Erikson, E.H. (1940). Studies in the Interpretation of Play: Clinical Observation of Play Disruption in Young Children. *Genet. Psychol. Monograph* 22, pp. 557-671.

Erikson, E.H. (1965). *Childhood and Society*. London: Hogarth.

Jernberg, A. (1979). *Theraplay*. San Francisco: Jossey-Bass.

Landreth, G.L. (1991). *Play Therapy: The Art of the Relationship*. Muncie, Indiana: Accelerated Development, Inc., Publishers.

Levin, D.M. (1987). *The Body's Recollection of Being*. London: Routledge & Kegan Paul.

Levin, D.M. (1988). *The Opening of Vision*. London: Routledge & Kegan Paul.

Levin, D.M. (1989). *The Listening Self*. London: Routledge & Kegan Paul.

Lovaas, I. (1971). Infantile Autism. In *Considerations in the Development of a Behavioral Treatment Program for Psychotic Children*, edited by D. Churchill, G. Alpern, & M. DeMeyer. Springfield, Illinois: Charles C. Thomas.

Lovaas, I. (1977). *The Autistic Child: Language Development Through Behavior Modification*. New York: Irvington Press.

Magid, K., & McKelvey, C. (1988). *High Risk Children Without a Conscience*. New York: Bantam Books.

Moustakas, C.E. (1953, 1992). *Psychotherapy with Children*. Greeley, Colorado: Carron Publishers, pp. 7-11.

Stern, N. (1985). *The Interpersonal World of the Infant*. New York: Basic Books.

Welch, M.G. (1988). *Holding Time*. New York: Simon and Schuster.

Winnicott, D. W. (1953). Transitional Objects and Transitional Phenomena. In *International Journal of Psycho-Analysis* 34, pp. 89-97.

Zaslow, R., & Menta, M. (1975). *The Psychology of the Z-Process*. San Jose, California: San Jose State University.

APPENDIX: DEVELOPMENTAL PLAY GAMES

These Developmental Play games were created by me in my work with autistic and psychotic children. These games, or contact activities, were immensely successful in enabling these children to bond with me because almost immediately they set up a dialogue of touch. They are games for adults (parents, teachers, therapists) to use with children who have difficulty relating. However, these games are not to be used indiscriminately. The adult needs to understand the child and fit these games to her needs. You need to be present when you do them. However, if done sensitively and creatively, they can be extremely effective and work where other methods fail. Even "normal" children love these games. They have the universal quality of the "Peek-A-Boo" and "This Little Pig Goes to Market" games.

There is no single way to play these games. Each child-adult pair has a unique way of playing them. One way to play these games and the effect of these games on the child has already been illustrated in this book with Jason, Kenny, Mira, and the children in Chapter 6 (see Chapters 3, 4, 5, 6).

THE SLIPPERY HAND GAME

This game is especially good with children who do not relate at all, such as autistic children. You need a bottle of hand lotion. First, you put a little lotion on your own hand and rub it around to warm it. Then you hold your hand out, inviting the child to put her hand in yours. Then you rub lotion on her hand and arm. You encircle the child's arm with your hands, going across the muscles and moving up the arm to the shoulder. Then you tell the child to pull, and her arm will slide through your hands from her shoulder down to her hands and fingertips. You will be moving down the muscles lengthwise. In case the child doesn't understand the word "pull," you slide your hands down as you say, "Pull," until the child gets the idea and pulls her arm through herself (see Chapter 3, page 46).

THE SLIPPERY FOOT GAME

This game is the same as the Slippery Hand except that you do it on the feet. Some children like the foot version even better, and many ask for both. You do it slowly and firmly so as not to tickle the child. Tickling is verboten in Developmental Play (see Chapter 3).

HILLS AND VALLEYS GAME

Taking the child's hand in yours, say, "Did you know that your hand has hills and valleys in it?" Starting on the outside of the child's thumb, you move your finger up over it and down on the other side between the thumb and first finger. Then move your finger over the child's pointer finger and repeat this with each finger, saying, "You go up a little hill and down the hill, and up a big hill and down the hill" until you've done all five fingers. You do it slowly and firmly, putting a little more pressure at the base of the fingers so as not to tickle the child. (Tickling is a definite No-No in Developmental Play.)

THE GINGERBREAD COOKIE GAME

This game is one of the all-time favorites. Of all the games, it is the one most effective and most enjoyed by most children, especially young children. This game enables the child to experience her body being touched by the adult, her body boundaries as separate from the adult's, and the pleasure of just being held and touched while she images this wonderful cookie being created. In reality, this game is a birthing fantasy, the oven being the womb.

As with all the games, there are many ways to do it. I do the Gingerbread Cookie game as follows: I tell the child that I think I'll make her into a wonderful Gingerbread Cookie, or maybe I'll make a "Nancy" (her name) Cookie. I take her on my lap, hold her tight and say, "I'm putting you in the mixing bowl to mix you up" as I turn on the mixing bowl. I shake her around, making the sound of the mixing bowl. Then I take her out and lay her in front of me. I take my pretend rolling pin and flatten her out. I do all this very slowly and gently. Then I take my cookie cutter to shape the cookie. In doing this, I go all around the child's body—her head, neck, shoulders, limbs, hands, feet, and every finger and toe. I make her face. Finally, I put her in the oven by picking her up and laying her across my lap. I put down the cover to the oven and say that now she is cooking. I move my hands slowly over her, making a little "Shh" sound of her cooking in the oven. (The idea of this is to help her just relax and be.) Then I raise the lid and ask her if she is done yet. Some children say "Yes" right away; others say "No" several times (these children enjoy just lying still there).

Eventually, I take her out of the oven and say, "Do you know what comes next?" I say, "You smell so good I'm going to eat you up," as I proceed to kiss her. I do this in small amounts, waiting for cues from the child as to how much she wants. Some children will hold up a hand or a foot for me to kiss. Cora's child, Celia, kept asking Cora to eat her up.

The child will guide you. You need to pay attention to the child's cues. For example, Celia's responses to this game (see Chapter 6, page 301) went through a series of developments. At first she wanted the loud, active touching in the act of eating her up all over. She wanted to be kissed all over (eaten up). Later, she would say, "I'm not done yet" (which she did for several sessions). She wanted to lie relaxed in Cora's arms (the oven). Then she and Cora created a little play. Cora would add her part, saying she wanted Celia to be done and would pretend to cry, saying she was hungry. Celia would say, "Cry," and both of them would laugh. Then Celia would say she is a burnt cookie (because she stayed in the oven too long), but Cora would eat her anyway. Thus, this game may start out very simply, but it develops into a two-character play. It was a metaphor that said you are accepted no matter how you are or what color you are.

KNOCK AT THE DOOR GAME
A Traditional Kindergarten Action Song

This game is another favorite. The area focused on is the face. The child gets to experience her face and the part of her that makes contact with others through eye contact in addition to touch. Vision is added to touch. This game also starts out very simply, usually the child's response being, "Do it again." As the game is played over time, it gets more complicated and symbolic from the contributions of both the child and the adult. See Chapter 5 for the way Mira and Vi played this game. In Mira's last session, she asked to play that game one more time. "That game is so much fun. I love that game."

Knock at the Door

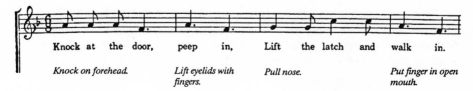

Knock at the door,   peep   in,   Lift   the latch   and   walk   in.

Knock on forehead.   *Lift eyelids with fingers.*   *Pull nose.*   *Put finger in open mouth.*

359

When an adult initiates this game with a child, the child can respond by following the script or by creating her own script. For example, instead of opening her mouth to let the other "walk in," she may choose to keep her mouth shut. Then both the child and the adult have to deal with a closed door.

THE PORTRAIT GAME

This game also focuses the child to experience her face. Again, the effectiveness and beauty of this game depends upon the presence and creativity of the adult painting this portrait of the child. The adult begins by saying that the child looks so wonderful today you think you would like to paint a picture of her. Would that be all right with her? I take her left hand and pretend that holds the paint. I use her right hand as the palette, where I mix the paints to get them just the right color. I use my finger and hand as the paint brush. First, I paint (touch) the whole face, putting on the basic color. Then I proceed to paint each part— her eyebrows, her eyes, eyelashes, nose, etc., touching each one rather lightly. At the end, I take the child's hand, saying, "Pretend this is a mirror and look at yourself now. What do you see?" Some children can say how they see themselves. Others can only say they see a hand. Hence, their response tells you if they are still presymbolic (primary thinking) or whether they have moved to the symbolic level (abstract or secondary thinking).

THE MAGIC BUTTON

This game requires greater participation and concentration from the child. You begin by saying, "I wonder if I can find the magic button that makes your pointer finger move." Then you start touching the child gently in different places—her head, shoulder, the back of her hand, etc., saying, "Is this it?" The child responds either "Yes" or "No." Sometimes you never find it. In that case, you say, "I guess I'm not going to find it today." And you let it be. Sometimes the child will show you. Then you choose another place, if the child seems interested, such as, "I wonder if I can find the magic button that makes you say Hello."

THE OWL GAME

Very young children love the Owl Game. The child doesn't have to do anything but respond or experience it. The adult takes the child's head in her two hands—placing a hand on each side of the child's head—and moves her face toward the child, touching noses and saying, "Close your eyes. Now open them. Boo!" The child usually giggles and wants to play it again.

THE BUTTERFLY KISS

The adult gives the child a butterfly kiss by putting her cheek close to the child's cheek in a position where her eyelashes will touch the child's cheek. The adult blinks her eyes, and her eyelashes brush against the child's cheek. It is a very soft, brushing touch. Often the child responds by saying, "Let me do it to you."

THE ROW, ROW, ROW YOUR BOAT GAME

The adult sits on the floor with the child's back to her front and with her arms around the child, holding her fairly tightly. The adult rocks back and forth as she sings, Row, row, row your boat, gently down the stream. Merrily, merrily, merrily, life is but a dream." At that point the adult says, "There's a storm coming up. I have to hold you tight so that you won't fall out of the boat," and the adult begins to roll around from side to side as if she were a boat in stormy waters, holding the child closer and closer. Children who cannot tolerate touch love this game, saying, "Do it again." Because there is movement, they don't resist the touch. They are distracted by the activity, and they like being held tightly.

THE CRADLING

Of all the touching activities, the cradling is the most therapeutic and growth stimulating. You may have to offer other kinds of touching that are briefer and have a focus to them before the child can allow herself just to be held without having to do anything. In the cradling, the adult is not doing anything but creating a space and a container for the child to experience her inner self. As said before, the child is not regressing in the cradling. She is getting in touch with her own body and her core self, and she doesn't need anyone to tell her what to do. She finds this special place inside her. Some children do this by lying in a trance and sucking their thumbs. This is excellent.

At other times, and later on, children like to do things while being cradled: for example, holding up a foot and saying, "This foot needs ten kisses." One child said to me while being cradled, "Guess which part wants to be touched."

What If? What if the child asks you to touch her in the genital area? One boy, age four, asked me to touch his penis. I said immediately, "That is something I am not going to do. That part of your body belongs to you. No one should touch it but you." Depending upon the response of the child, I continue what we were doing, or I might just hold him quietly if that felt right to him and to me.

Provided you do these games sensitively and appropriately, you will notice something: the child will move out of this concrete, presymbolic level of behavior into a more symbolic and verbal form of communication. The child will begin to empower herself and show the joy of being able to do something on her own. That's the reward if you do it well and *if you are totally present and attuned to your own quiet energy*. What makes these "games" effective is the experience of the quiet flow of energy between child and therapist.

In the beginning, these were not "games." They were ways of touching a disturbed child so that she felt my presence. In the beginning, each "game" was created to fit the needs of one specific child. However, other children liked them so much that in order to identify them, I gave them names. At present, I seldom play these "games" with a client. I just do whatever seeing or touching seems appropriate for that child.

Therefore, I recommend that you also create your own ways of seeing and touching a child because you will then be more apt to be in tune with that child. However, if you don't know how to start, you could start with one of these "ready-made" games.

INDEX TO SESSIONS

Jason begins the process of attachment.
Once I stopped his running by grabbing his
hand, he returned to have contact repeated.
He made a beginning by wanting at some
level to be touched.
Since Jason has no speech and little eye contact, the avenue for contact is through his
body by touch. He initiates taking his shoes
off to get a foot message. There's a small
core self emerging.
Jason has bonded with me, the therapist, and
with his mother.

      Trainees shared how moved they were by
      their child from seeing the tape last week.
      The trainees were moved by realizing the
      shift in themselves—that they are now more
      available to themselves. Their denials were
      changing to owning their own value.
      All the trainees and the Leader had to deal
      with their reactions and response to Aretha's
      crying in the last Circle Time. Then they
      could focus on looking at their own work and
      growth of their child.
      The trainees assess their own growth by writ-
      ing the answers to a set of questions and then
      reading them out loud to the group.

ABOUT THE AUTHOR

Viola A. Brody is the originator of the Developmental Play Therapy approach.

Former chief psychologist of the Child Guidance Clinic in St. Petersburg, Florida, she has been an adjunct professor at the University of South Florida and at Eckerd College in St. Petersburg. Under a grant from the U.S. Office of Education to offer the Developmental Play group program within the school system, she saw over a thousand early elementary-age children and adults-in-training over a ten-year period. She has presented workshops in Developmental Play throughout the U.S. and in Canada, Ireland, and London.

In 1995 Dr. Brody initiated a program to provide training for the pre-K division of the Orlando, FL public schools, and was the keynote speaker for the 1996 Association for Play Therapy International Conference. Her current interest is in the study of how touch and the child's use of his body provides the foundation for everything he does.

This book represents a culmination of Dr. Brody's work begun more than forty years ago at the University of Chicago, the University of Illinois College of Medicine, the Chicago Institute for Psychoanalysis, and Michael Reese Psychiatric and Psychosomatic Institute. She is now writing a second book, *The Magic of Touch*.